D1595999

Forensic Pathology Reviews, Volume 5

FORENSIC PATHOLOGY REVIEWS, VOLUME 5

Michael Tsokos, MD, SERIES EDITOR

Volume 1 *(2004)* ● Hardcover: ISBN 1-58829-414-5
Full Text Download: E-ISBN 1-59259-786-6

Volume 2 *(2005)* ● Hardcover: ISBN 1-58829-414-3
Full Text Download: E-ISBN 1-59259-872-2

Volume 3 *(2005)* ● Hardcover: ISBN 1-58829-416-1
Full Text Download: E-ISBN 1-59259-910-9

Volume 4 *(2006)* ● Hardcover: ISBN 1-58829-601-6
Full Text Download: E-ISBN 1-59259-921-4

Volume 5 *(2008)* ● Hardcover: ISBN 978-1-58829-832-4
Full Text Download: E-ISBN 978-1-59745-110-9

Forensic Pathology Reviews

Volume 5

by

Michael Tsokos

Institute of Legal Medicine and Forensic Sciences,
Charité-Universitätsmedizin Berlin, Berlin, Germany

Editor
Prof. Michael Tsokos
Institute of Legal Medicine
and Forensic Sciences
Turmstr. 21 (Hausl)
10559 Berlin
Germany

ISSN: 1556-5661
ISBN: 978-1-58829-832-4   e-ISBN: 978-1-59745-110-9
DOI: 10.1007/978-1-59745-110-9

Printed on acid-free paper

9 8 7 6 5 4 3 2 1

springer.com

To my son Julius

Preface

The *Forensic Pathology Reviews* series has gained considerable attention worldwide over the last years and thus I am very pleased to present another, now the fifth, volume of this series.

As with previous volumes, it is an attempt to focus on both practical and scientific aspects of the different areas of expertise within the broad field of forensics. Advances in forensic sciences and a profound knowledge of the results will strengthen and enhance the role of forensic medicine and pathology in the courtroom and will thereby help to solve crimes and bring justice.

The future of forensic sciences depends, more than ever, on attracting outstanding individuals to research and it is hoped that this book not only imparts the state-of-the-art of special topics of forensic medicine and pathology to those working in the field of forensics but also helps to encourage and inspire young forensic scientists for future research projects.

I gratefully acknowledge the help and support of the authors who contributed to this book.

Michael Tsokos, MD

Contents

Contributors

Michael J. P. Biggs, MB, ChB, MRCS
Dept. of Histopathology, Leicester Royal Infirmary, Leicester,
United Kingdom

Andreas Büttner, MD
Institute of Legal Medicine, University of Munich, Munich, Germany

Roger W. Byard, MBBS, MD
Depts. of paediatrics and Pathology, University of Adelaide, Adelaide,
South Australia, Australia

Glenda E. Cains
Forensic Science South Australia, Adelaide, South Australia, Australia

Tracey S. Corey, MD
University of Louisville, School of Medicine and Office of the Kentucky
Medical Examiner, Louisville, KY

Gunther Geserick, MD
Institute of Legal Medicine and Forensic Sciences, Charité – University
Medicine Berlin, Berlin, Germany

James R. Gill, MD
Office of Chief Medical Examiner, New York, NY

Mark A. Hilts, BA
Behavioral Science Unit, Federal Bureau of Investigation, Quantico, VA

Lai Siang Hui, MBBS, MRCPath, DMJ(Path)
Centre for Forensic Medicine, Health Sciences Authority, Singapore

Ionut Ichim, BDS, MDS
Dept. of Oral Rehabilitation, University of Otago, New Zealand

Bernd Karger, MD
Institute of Legal Medicine, University of Münster, Münster, Germany

Jules Kieser, BSc, BDS, PhD, DSc, FLS, FDSRCS Ed, FFSSoc
Dept. of Oral Sciences, University of Otago, New Zealand

Holger Lach, MD
Institute of Legal Medicine, University of Hamburg, Hamburg, Germany

Gilbert Lau, MBBS, FRCPath, DMJ(Path), FAMS
Centre for Forensic Medicine, Health Sciences Authority, Singapore

Burkhard Madea, MD
Institute of Forensic Medicine, Rheinische Friedrich-Wilhelms-University
Bonn, Bonn, Germany

Helen Nicholson, BSc(Hons), MB ChB, MD
Dept. of Anatomy and Structural Biology, University of Otago, New Zealand

Andreas Olze, DDS
Institute of Legal Medicine and Forensic Sciences, Charité – University
Medicine Berlin, Berlin, Germany

Klaus Püschel, MD
Institute of Legal Medicine, University of Hamburg, Hamburg, Germany

Johanna Preuß, MD
Institute of Forensic Medicine, Rheinische Friedrich-Wilhelms-University
Bonn, Bonn Germany

Walter Reisinger, MD
Institute of Radiology, Charité – University Medicine Berlin, Berlin, Germany

David T. Resch, MA
Behavioral Science Unit, Federal Bureau of Investigation, Quantico, VA

Andreas Schmeling, MD
Institute of Legal Medicine, University of Münster, Münster, Germany

Friedrich Schulz, MD
Institute of Legal Medicine, University of Hamburg, Hamburg, Germany

Mary N. Sheppard, MD FRCPath
Dept. of Pathology, Royal Brompton Hospital, London, United Kingdom

Ellie K. Simpson, PhD
Forensic Science South Australia, Adelaide, South Australia, Australia

Michael Swain, BSc, PhD
Dept. of Oral Rehabilitation, University of Otago, New Zealand

Benjamin Swift, MB, ChB, MD, MRCPath(Forensic), MFFLM
Forensic Pathology Services, Culham Science Centre, Oxfordshire,
United Kingdom

Michael Taylor, BSc(Hons), PhD
Institute for Environmental Science and Research, Christchurch, New Zealand

Michael Tsokos, MD
Institute of Legal Medicine and Forensic Sciences, Charité – University
Medicine Berlin, Berlin, Germany

Elisabeth E. Türk, MD
Institute of Legal Medicine, University of Hamburg, Hamburg, Germany

J Neil Waddell, MDipTech, HDE, PGDipCDTech
Dept. of Oral Rehabilitation, University of Otago, New Zealand

Serge Weis, MD
Laboratory of Neuropathology and Brain Research, The Stanley Medical
Research Institute and Depts. Psychiatry and Pathology, Uniformed Services
University of the Health Sciences, Bethesda, MD

Kelly Whittle, BSc
Dept. of Anatomy and Structural Biology, University of Otago, New Zealand

Regula Wick, MD
Forensic Science South Australia and Department of Histopathology,
Women's and Children's Hospital, Adelaide, South Australia, Australia

Brittany Wong, BSc, PGDip Sci
Dept. of Anatomy and Structural Biology, University of Otago, New Zealand

About the Editor

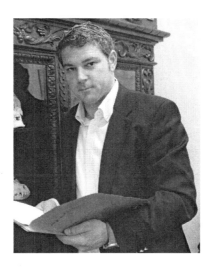

Professor Michael Tsokos is the Director of the Institute of Forensic Sciences and Legal Medicine, Charité – Universitätsmedizin Berlin, in Berlin, Germany. He is also the Director of the Governmental Institute of Forensic and Social Medicine in Berlin, Germany. He is the primary or senior author of more than 200 scientific publications in international peer-reviewed journals and the author as well as editor of a number of books dealing with topics of forensic pathology.

In 1998 and 1999, Professor Tsokos worked for a time with the exhumation and identification of mass grave victims in Bosnia-Herzegovina and Kosovo under the mandate of the UN International Criminal Tribunal. In 2001, he was honored with the national scientific award of the German Society of Forensic and Legal Medicine for his research on micromorphological and molecularbio-locical correlates of sepsis-iinduced lung injury in human autopsy specimens. In December 2004 and January 2005, Prof. Tsokos worked with other experts from national and international disaster victim identification teams in the region of Khao Lak/Thailand for the identification of the victims of the tsunami that struck South East Asia on December 26, 2004.

He is a member of the International Academy of Legal Medicine, the German Identification Unit of the Federal Criminal Agency of Germany, the German Society of Forensic and Legal Medicine, the National Professional Association of Forensic Pathologists, and the American Academy of Forensic Sciences. Professor Tsokos is one of the Editors of *Rechtsmedizin*, the official publication of the German Society of Forensic and Legal Medicine, member of the Advisory Board of *the International Journal of Legal Medicine*, member of the Editorial Board of *Legal Medicine and Current Immunology Reviews* and the *European Editor of Forensic Science, Medicine, and Pathology.*

Part I
Death from Environmental Conditions

Chapter 1
Death Due to Hypothermia

Morphological Findings, Their Pathogenesis and Diagnostic Value

Burkhard Madea, Michael Tsokos and Johanna Preuß

Contents

Abstract Morphological findings in fatalities due to hypothermia are variable and unspecific. If body cooling is rapid and the duration of the cooling process until death is short, autopsy findings can be scarce or even completely missing. Typical morphological findings in hypothermia are frost erythema, hemorrhagic gastric erosions, lipid accumulation in epithelial cells of renal proximal tubules and other organs. Although being unspecific as exclusive findings, they are of high diagnostic value regarding the circumstances of the case. The main pathogenetic mechanisms of morphological alterations due to hypothermia are disturbances of microcirculation, changes of rheology, cold stress, and hypoxidosis. Typical morphological findings can be found in two thirds of all cases.

Keywords Hypothermia · Wischnewsky spots · Frost erythema · Morphological findings · Pathogenesis

B. Madea
Institute of Forensic Medicine, Rheinische Friedrich-Wilhelms-University Bonn,
Bonn, Germany
e-mail: b.madea@uni-bonn.de

M. Tsokos (ed.), *Forensic Pathology Reviews, Volume 5,*
doi: 10.1007/978-1-59745-110-9_1, © Humana Press, Totowa, NJ 2008

1.1 Introduction

Cold is a common but underestimated danger to man [1, 2, 3, 4]. Hypothermia may develop not only at temperatures around 0°C or below but also at temperatures above 10°C. Hypothermia is defined as a body core temperature of below 35°C. In homeothermic organisms, the normal body temperature is maintained at a much greater range of ambient temperature than the so-called "indifferent temperature" [5] (Fig. 1.1). The term "indifferent temperature" refers to the ambient temperature at which the basic metabolic rate is sufficient to maintain the normal body temperature. When body temperature decreases, heat transfer is lowered by vasoconstriction and piloerection as first counter-regulation mechanisms. Simultaneously, heat production is increased by shivering and chemical thermogenesis [5].

If these counterregulation mechanisms become insufficient, the body temperature will decrease. How long the normal body temperature can be maintained or when the counterregulations become insufficient mainly depends on the quotient between heat transfer and heat production. The heat transfer to the surrounding medium is directly proportional to the difference between body temperature and ambient temperature: the higher the difference, the more rapid

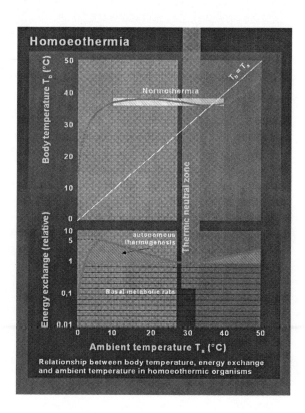

Fig. 1.1 Relation between body temperature, energy exchange and ambient temperature in homeothermic organisms. The normal body temperature may be maintained over a much wider range than the indifferent temperature due to counterregulation mechanisms as vasoconstrictions, pilaerections, and chemical thermogenesis (modified according to [73])

the decrease of body temperature; however, the drop of body temperature slows down when it approaches the ambient temperature.

The velocity of the drop of body temperature depends on the extent of the surface of the medium and the "stored heat". The greater the surface, the more rapid the cooling of a body. Since the surface/volume-ratio is increasing with increasing body height, small children are cooling more rapidly than adults.

Furthermore, the velocity of cooling depends upon whether there is a convective or a conductive heat transport, for instance in water. In immersion hypothermia, the body heat loss is about three times faster than in exposure to the same temperature in dry cold air [3, 4].

Understanding the aforementioned pathophysiology of hypothermia is also of importance for the understanding of the morphological findings seen in hypothermia deaths. If the body cooling is very rapid and the duration of the cooling process until death is short, autopsy findings due to hypothermia can be scarce or even completely absent, especially in cases of immersion hypothermia [2, 3, 4, 6, 7, 8, 9, 10, 11, 12, 13, 14, 15, 16, 17, 18]. However, data on the duration of exposure to cold before death, which is of course positively correlated to the surrounding temperature, can only rarely be found in the literature. In immersion hypothermia with a water temperature of about 5°C, death occurs after about 1 h [4, 15, 19].

For dry ambient temperature, Hirvonen [20] has published his experiences regarding the duration of exposure. The estimated duration of exposure ranged from approximately 1.5 h at –30°C to 12 h at +5°C; in the majority of his cases estimated duration of exposure was between 3 and 6 h at –10°C. Normally, death occurs at body core temperatures of about 25°C [4, 15, 19]. However, lower temperatures may be survived, especially when body cooling is rapid [15]. The final cause of death is either ventricular fibrillation or asystolia [5, 19]. Internal asphyxiation or hypoxia due to a left shifting of the oxygen-hemoglobin-dissociation-curve, failing of enzymes, and electrolyte dysregulations may contribute to the final cause of death. According to animal experiments, ventricular fibrillation seems to be more predominant compared to asystolia.

For didactical purposes, several phases of hypothermia are differentiated, beginning with the excitatory phase and followed by an adynamic phase, a paralytic phase, and the phase of apparent death (Table 1.1). Although body core temperatures are given for these different phases, it has to be kept in mind that the clinical picture at a given body temperature may vary widely [3, 4, 21]. The clinical phases are mainly characterized by functional alterations, e.g., within the musculature from shivering over a drop of muscular tonus to a rise of muscular rigidity, within the cardiovascular system from tachycardia over sinus bradycardia to bradyarrhythmia, and within the pulmonary system from hyperventilation over depression of ventilation to bradypnoe.

Hemodynamic and rheological alterations in hypothermia are of importance for the development of morphological changes, which is especially true for the rise of resistance due to vasoconstriction and increase of blood viscosity [22, 23, 24].

Table 1.1 Clinical phases of hypothermia

	Phase 1 36–33°C	Phase 2 33–30°C	Phase 3 30–27°C	Phase 4 Below 27°C
Muscular system	Shivering	Drop of muscular tonus	Rise of muscular rigidity	Either further decrease of vital functions or cardiocirculatory arrest due to *ventricular fibrillation* or *asystolia*
Heart	Tachycardia	Sinus bradycardia	Bradyarrhythmia	
Circulatory system	Reduced perfusion of Body-surface	Rise of resistance due to vasoconstriction	Rise of resistance due to increased viscosity of the blood	
Ventilation	Stimulation of Respiration, Hyperventilation	Central Depression of Ventilation	Bradypnoe, apnoic pause; Decrease of compliance	Cessation of breathing, apnoea
Nervous system	Raised vigilance, confusion; Painful acra	Disorientation, apathy; Passing off pain	Unconsciousness, loss of reflex	
	"Excitation"	"Exhaustion"	"Paralysis"	"Vita reducta" – apparent death

These functional changes are already of great medicolegal importance since the rise of muscular rigidity must not be mistaken for rigor mortis [25, 26]. However, the differential diagnosis can in any case easily be made since, in muscular rigidity due to hypothermia, postmortem lividity is missing whereas in cases with rigor mortis, postmortem lividity is present. There are several case reports in the literature of living persons being pronounced dead due to great muscular rigidity mistaken for rigor mortis [25, 26].

1.2 Epidemiology and Death Scene Findings

As outlined above, deaths due to hypothermia are not only restricted to the winter season but can also be encountered in spring or autumn in colder periods. Furthermore, hypothermia deaths not only occur outside buildings but also indoors, especially in the elderly. In various earlier autopsy series, death due to hypothermia was mainly seen in people over 60 years of age [18, 20, 27, 28, 29, 30, 31, 32, 33, 34, 35]; beside senile mental deterioration and immobility, lack of fuel for heating and open windows for fresh air were identified as special risk factors. Other groups of persons most liable to suffer from accidental hypothermia are the following:

- Intoxicated persons (mainly by alcohol but also by other drugs as well as tranquilizers or opiates)
- Newborns
- Persons engaged in hazardous outdoor activities such as climbing, mountaineering, sailing, or fishing [7, 13, 15, 31, 36]

In outdoor as well as indoor deaths due to hypothermia, persons may be found partly or completely unclothed with scratches and hematomas on knees, elbows, and feet or situated in a hidden position under a bed or behind a wardrobe [2, 9, 20, 37, 38]. This paradoxical undressing and hide-and-die syndrome may be observed in up to 20% of cases. The hide-and-die syndrome seems to be a terminal primitive reaction pattern while paradoxical undressing may be caused by a paradoxical feeling of warmth of the affected individual [38]. However, up to now the pathophysiology of both phenomena is not clearly understood.

1.3 Morphological Findings in Fatalities Due to Hypothermia

The diagnosis of hypothermia is based on circumstantial evidence, the exclusion of concurrent causes of death, and temperature measurements (e.g., if body temperature is much lower than it has to be expected for the given postmortem interval) [39, 40]. However, by the end of the nineteenth century, the morphologic changes with the highest diagnostic validity for death due to hypothermia

Table 1.2 Classification of morphological and biochemical findings in fatal cases of hypothermia (concerning regulation of body temperature, pathogenesis)

Examination of organs which contribute to body temperature
- Thyroid
- Adrenals

Biochemical changes due to counterregulation mechanisms in hypothermia
- Loss of glycogene in various organs
- Release of catecholamines and excretion in urine
- Fatty changes of organs

Examination of organs which are responsible for death
- Myocardial damage

Examination of freezing tissues and tissues at the surface-core-border
- Frost erythema
- Muscle bleeding in core muscles

Other organ damages (cold stress)
- Hemorrhagic gastric erosions
- Pancreatic changes
- Hemorrhagic infarcts
- Microinfarction

had been described: frost erythema reported by Keferstein in 1893 [22] and in 1895 hemorrhagic spots of the gastric mucosa named after Wischnewsky [41, 42, 43, 44, 45, 46, 47, 48]. Morphologic alterations due to hypothermia can be classified as follows (see also Table 1.2) concerning regulation of body temperature, counterregulation and pathogenesis. In Table 1.3, all morphological changes due to hypothermia as reported in the literature are arranged according to their main pathogenetic pathway and diagnostic significance.

1.3.1 Bright Red Colour of Blood and Lividity

Of course, in victims of hypothermia a bright red colour of blood as well as of postmortem lividity may be found, but it was already shown in the nineteenth century that this is not a specific finding of death due to hypothermia since this may be seen as well in other causes of death taking place at low ambient temperatures. The mechanism leading to the bright red colour of blood and lividity is the left-shifting of the oxygen-hemoglobin-dissociation curve.

In hypothermia, the blood within the left ventricle is often found to be of brighter red when compared to that of the right ventricle [49]. The explanation is that the blood later appearing within the left ventricle was cooled down when it passed the lungs and thereby turned to bright red. However, this finding is not constant and a pink red colour may also be seen in postmortem freezing.

Table 1.3 Morphological changes in hypothermia

Left shifting of oxygen-hemoglobin-dissociation curve	Diagnostic significance
▪ Bright-red colour of blood and lividity	−
▪ Blood of the left ventricle bright red compared to that of the right ventricle	−
Postmortem artefacts	
▪ Cutis anserina	−
▪ Skull fractures due to freezing of the brain	−
Hemorrhages and erythemas	
▪ Frost erythema	+
▪ Hemorrhagic gastric erosions	+
▪ Hemorrhagic pancreatitis	−
▪ Hemorrhages into muscles of the core	(+)
▪ Hemorrhages of the synovia, bleeding into synovial fluid	?
Fatty changes	
▪ Liver	−
▪ Kidney	+
▪ Heart	(+)
Unspecific changes	
▪ Brain edema	−
▪ Subendocardial hemorrhages	−
▪ Pneumonia	−
▪ Contraction of spleen	(?)
Counterregulation mechanisms	
▪ Vacuolisation of liver-, pancreas-, renal (proximal tubules), adrenal cells, loss of glycogen	(+)
▪ Colloid depletion and activation of thyroid	(+)

1.3.2 Skin Changes

Skin changes in general hypothermia are different from those seen in local hypothermia. In local hypothermia three grades of frostbites are seen [50, 51, 52]:

1. Violaecous discoloration, mainly on tips of fingers, toes, or nose (*dermatitis congelationis erythematosa*)
2. Blisters filled with clear or bloody fluid (*dermatitis congelationis bullosa*)
3. Bluish discoloration with blister formation and tissue necrosis (*dermatitis congelationis gangrenosa*)

The main mechanisms leading to frostbites are freezing of the tissues and obstruction of blood supply to the tissues [12, 23, 52]. Microscopically, there might be a damage of endothelial cells, a leakage of serum into the tissues and sludging of red blood cells [3, 24].

In general hypothermia, frostbite-like injuries may be seen as swelling of ears, nose, and hands but more striking findings are red or purple skin and

(A)   (B)

(C)

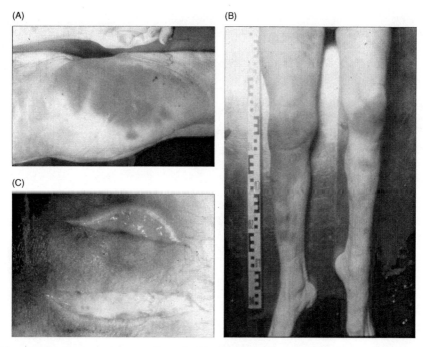

Fig. 1.2A–C Frost erythema. **A** Over the hip joint. **B** Over the knee. **C** No subcutaneous bleeding but a hemolytic reddish appearance of subcutaneous tissue

violet patches on knees or elbows or at the outside of the hip joint [2, 9, 20] (Fig. 1.2). Frost erythemas must not be mistaken for hematomas since they are macroscopically and histologically free of extravasation of erythrocytes. The pathogenesis is still unclear. However, they may develop due to capillary damage and plasma leaking into the tissue [4, 22]. Obviously, plasma hemoglobin due to frost damage of erythrocytes is leaking into the tissue (Fig. 1.3) as could be shown by an immunhistochemical visualisation of hemoglobin in frost erythema [53]. By 1893 Keferstein [22] had assumed that the blood flow in

(A)   (B)

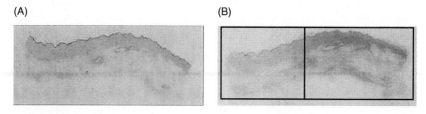

Fig. 1.3A,B Diffuse positive reaction of intra- and extracellular structures in hemoglobin immunostaining of frost erythema

Table 1.4 Frequency of violet patches (frost erythema)

	n	%
Mant [34]	19/43	44%
Gillner and Waltz [7]	18/25	72%
Hirvonen [20]	12/22	54%
Thrun [73]	10/23	43%
Own material (Bonn and Greifswald)	82/145	56.6%

exposed skin areas first ceases and after rewarming, a diffusion of hemoglobin into the extravascular tissue takes place. By an immunohistochemical study, the proposal of hemoglobin diffusion, especially in exposed skin areas, could be supported although the rewarming – as suggested by Keferstein over 100 years ago – does not occur [53]. Why this diffusion takes places or how exposure to cold triggers it will, however, still remain a matter of speculation and will have to be examined by further investigations in the future.

Development of swollen ears and nose in cold ambient temperatures is due to edema formation. Skin changes can be found in about 50% of cases in hypothermia (Table 1.4).

1.3.3 Hemorrhagic Spots of the Gastric Mucosa

Wischnewsky [41] was the first to describe multiple hemorrhagic gastric lesions as a sign indicative of hypothermia (Fig. 1.4). The lesions vary in diameter from 1 mm to about 2 cm and in quantity from only a few up to more than 100 scattered throughout the mucosa of the stomach. The lesions must not be mistaken for bleedings (true hemorrhagic erosions) of the gastric mucosa [3, 45, 54, 55, 56, 57]. Histologically, these so-called Wischnewsky spots are characterized by a necrosis of the mucosa with hematin formation [6].

(A)   (B)

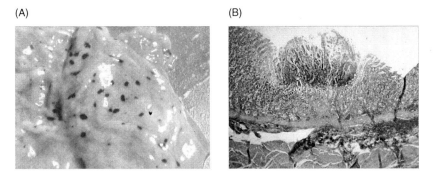

Fig. 1.4A,B Wischnewsky spots. **A** Gross appearance. **B** Histology

Wischnewsky spots are an unspecific finding concerning the underlying etiology: similar changes of the gastric mucosa are found as a consequence of drug or alcohol abuse and in stress or shock. Disturbances of microcirculation (hemoconcentration) and tissue amines histamine and serotonine seem to be involved in their pathogenesis [10]. Local hypothermia or freezing of the gastric mucosa can be ruled out as pathogenetic factor since local hypothermia of the stomach was used as therapy in upper gastrointestinal bleedings and a local gastric temperature of 2–6°C for 24 h has been estimated to be harmless [4, 58, 59]. A most recent immunohistochemical study on the pathogenesis of Wischnewsky spots using a specific antibody against hemoglobin revealed immunopositivity against hemoglobin [60, 61]. Perhaps cooling of the body in the sequel of cold ambient temperature primarily leads to circumscribed hemorrhages of the gastric glands in vivo or during the agonal period, respectively. Subsequently, due to autolysis, erythrocytes are destroyed and hemoglobin is released. After exposure to gastric acid, hemoglobin is then hematinized which leads to the typical blackish-brownish appearance of Wischnewsky spots seen at gross examination [60]. The incidence of gastric erosions is variable (Table 1.5). They seem to be more frequent in elderly people exposed to cold stress for a long period but they may also be found in newborns [4].

1.3.4 Other Gastrointestinal Lesions

Hemorrhagic erosions can be found not only in the gastric mucosa but also in the duodenum and jejunum but much less frequently [32, 33, 34, 59, 62, 63, 64]. When these lesions were observed in other gastrointestinal localizations, they

Table 1.5 Frequency of hemorrhagic gastric erosions ("Wischnewsky spots")

	N	%
Wischnewsky [41]	40/44	90.9%
Krjukoff [45]	44/61	72%
Dyrenfurth [56]	–	–
Altmann/Schubothe (animals), Müller/Rotter (humans)	very frequent	
Mant [34]	37/43	86%
Gillner and Waltz [7]	22/25	88%
Hirvonen [20]	10/22	45%
Thrun [73]	21/23	91.3%
Birchmeyer and Mitchell [54]	15	60%
Takada et al. [57]	17	88%
Dreßler and Hauck [55]	29	86%
Kinzinger et al. [37]	30	40%
Mizukami et al. [76]	23	44%
Own material (Bonn and Greifswald)	117/145	80.7%

(A)   (B)

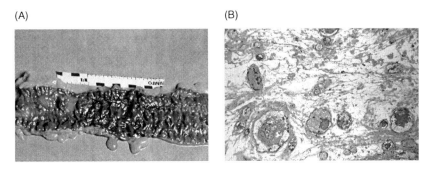

Fig. 1.5A,B Hemorrhagic infarction of the colon in a fatality due to hypothermia. **A** Gross appearance. **B** Histology: hemorrhages into the colonic wall with thrombosis of the veins of the submucosa and an acute inflammatory infiltrate

had always been present in the stomach, too. Besides ulcerations of the colon and ileum, hemorrhagic infarctions of the colon have been described as well (Fig. 1.5). These infarctions are due to rheologic and hemodynamic alterations during hypothermia with sludge formation of red blood cells and subsequent thrombosis of the veins of the submucosa (Table 1.6). They are very rare findings; these authors have seen such infarctions of the large bowel in association with fatal hypothermia in two cases; they were associated with an episode of hemorrhagic shock prior to death [62].

1.3.5 Pancreas Changes

A variety of pancreas changes has been described in association with hypothermia: focal or diffuse pancreatitis, hemorrhagic pancreatitis, patches of fat necrosis over the organs surface, increased levels of serum amylase, hemorrhages, and focal or diffuse interstitial infiltration of leukocytes [20, 29, 30, 32, 33, 35, 65, 66, 67] (Table 1.7). At autopsy, hemorrhages into the pancreas parenchyma as well as under the mucosa of the pancreatic duct may be seen. In animal experiments, Fisher et al. [66] were able to reproduce these pancreatic changes; they found a nonhemorrhagic pancreatitis with fat necrosis in 10% of their cases. A recent retrospective analysis of 143 cases of death due to hypothermia revealed that pancreatic bleedings are of no diagnostic significance in deaths due to

Table 1.6 Hemodynamic and rheological response in phase III (paralysis) of hypothermia

Hemodynamic response		Rheological response	
Heart rate	↓	Hematocrit	↑
Blood pressure	↓	Plasma volume	↓
Blood pressure amplitude	↓	Viscosity	↑
Venous pressure	↓	Red blood cells sludge-formation	↑
Resistance	↑		

Table 1.7 Pancreatic changes in hypothermia according to different authors

Pancreatic changes in Hypothermia	Author
Focal or diffuse pancreatitis in 10% of patients (n = 50) who were treated with hypothermia	Sano and Smith [67]
Among 13 cases of hypothermia 2 cases of hemorrhagic pancreatitis, 3 cases of pancreatitis with fat necrosis over its surface (38%)	Duguid et al. [28]
Focal pancreatitis or hemorrhagic pancreatitis in 29 of 43 cases (67%)	Mant [34]
Hemorrhage into the gland in 4 of 22 cases (18%)	Hirvonen [20]
Raised serum amylase in 11 of 15 cases (73%)	Duguid et al. [28]
Focal, non-hemorrhagic pancreatitis with patches of fat necrosis in 10% of animals in experimental hypothermia	Fisher et al. [66]
Empty vacuoles in adenoid cells of the pancreas	Preuß et al. [68]

hypothermia [68] – they are observed only very rarely and are seen in other causes of death with the same frequency.

The high incidence of pancreatic changes described by Mant [32, 33, 34] might be caused by the composition of his case material – mostly older people; in such a biased autopsy population the delimitation of preexisting diseases may be difficult.

Preuß et al. [68] found in 24 out of 62 cases of fatal hypothermia (38.7%) in microscopic investigations seemingly empty vacuoles in the adenoid cells of pancreas (Fig. 1.6). These vacuoles were not observed in a control group without hypothermia prior to death and in a control group of chronic alcoholics. Although these vacuoles seem to be diagnostically significant, their pathogenesis still remains unclear.

1.3.6 Hemorrhages into Core Muscles

Hemorrhages into muscles belonging to the core of the body, for instance the iliopsoas muscle, as a diagnostic criterion of death due to hypothermia were first described by Dirnhofer and Sigrist [69]. This morphological alteration

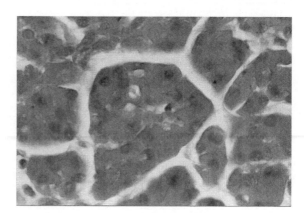

Fig. 1.6 Vacuoles in pancreatic adenoid cells

seems to be known only in the German literature [70, 71]. Muscular hemorrhages in cases of hypothermia have, however, already been described in the textbook of von Hofmann and Haberda [42], but it remained unclear whether these hemorrhages developed during life as a response to hypothermia or postmortem as a resuscitation or transportation artefact. The observation of hemorrhages into core muscles especially in the iliopsoas muscle has been confirmed by other authors but seems to be a rare finding. Histologically, a vacuolated degeneration of subendothelial layers of the vascular walls with a lifting of epithelial cells is seen. These changes were thought to represent a hypoxic damage and the hemorrhages as due to diapedesis. The hypoxic damage of vessels of core muscles is interpreted as a result of insufficient circulation due to hypothermia induced vasoconstriction. However, compared to the muscles of the surface, the oxygen requirement of the core muscles is not reduced. The misbalance of reduced perfusion and normal oxygen requirement is thought to be the cause of hypoxic damage of epithelial cells with resultant raised permeability [69].

1.3.7 Lipid Accumulation

Fatty changes in heart, liver, and kidneys have been described repeatedly in fatalities due to hypothermia [46] but data on their diagnostic value and the sensitivity of this finding are still missing. As fatty changes of the liver may have many causes and are frequently found, they are of no diagnostic significance for the diagnosis of death due to hypothermia.

Recent investigations show that lipid accumulation in epithelial cells of proximal renal tubules seem to be of high diagnostic significance, pointing towards hypothermia of the affected individual prior to death [72, 73] (Fig. 1.7). This lipid accumulation is always seen at the base of the epithelial cells; there are no concomitant changes of cell nucleus or plasma. The fatty changes may be either a result of energy depletion after shock-induced hypoxia or caused by tubular resorption after raised mobilisation of triglycerides [72, 73]. There is a strong positive correlation between the grade of fatty change with the occurrence of macroscopic signs of hypothermia (frost erythema and Wischnewsky spots) [72]. In control cases, only slight fatty changes can be found. The degree of fatty degeneration of renal tubules can therefore be used as a very helpful marker for the diagnosis of death due to hypothermia and has an equal value of diagnostic sensitivity compared to that of Wischnewsky spots [72]. Also for the cardiac muscle, a fatty degeneration of myocytes may be observed in cases of fatal hypothermia (Fig. 1.8) [74]. However, this fatty degeneration is only of diagnostic significance if a lipofuscin staining is also carried out and a marked difference between lipid staining and lipofuscin staining is obvious in the case in question (Fig. 1.9). There is also a correlation between fatty degeneration of cardiac myocytes and Wischnewsky spots. However, fatty degeneration of the cardiac muscle does not have the diagnostic sensitivity of fatty degeneration of proximal renal tubules [72, 74].

(A)

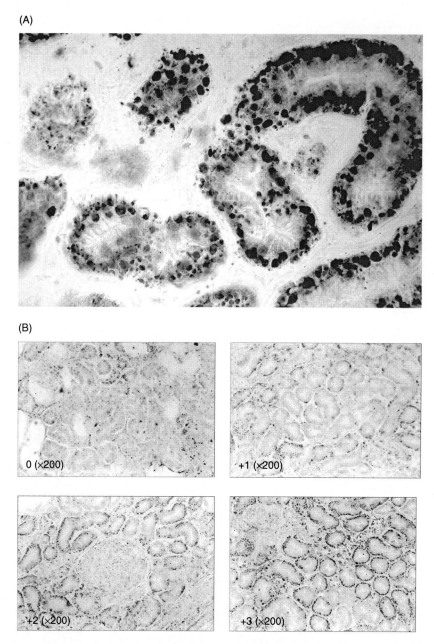

(B)

Fig. 1.7A,B Lipid accumulation in renal proximal tubules. A The lipid stains are always located the base of the cells. B Fatty changes in cells of in renal proximal tubules

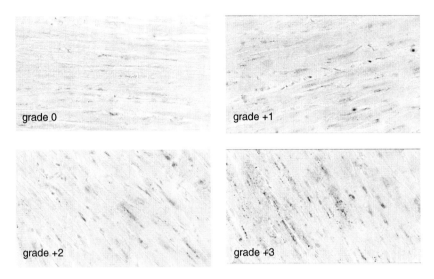

Fig. 1.8 Fatty changes of cardiac myocytes in hypothermia

1.3.8 Endocrine Glands

Since endocrine glands are responsible for the maintenance of normal body temperature, a decrease of body temperature activates the function of most of the endocrine glands, especially the thyroid and adrenals [6, 10, 11, 75].

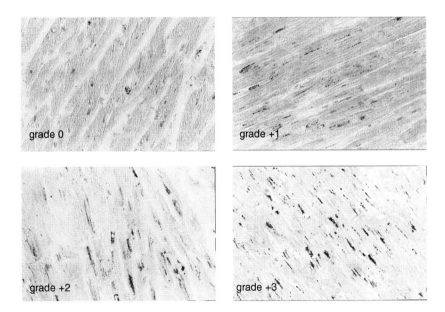

Fig. 1.9 Lipofuscin staining of cardiomyocytes

However, morphological findings can be expected only in long-lasting hypothermia, not after the usual exposition to cold ambient temperatures for only a few hours [6]. In animal experiments, no morphologic changes have been detected after exposure to cold temperatures for 49 h, but an activation of the thyroid has been observed after long lasting exposure (5–9 days with temperature drops from 37.5 to 36°C; morphologic changes: depletion of colloid, raise of epithelial cells). Only after long lasting hypothermia has a lipid depletion of adrenal cortex been found in animal experiments (10 days with core temperatures of 33°C) not after short exposures of 4–7 h [6].

1.4 Conclusions

Vital morphological alterations due to exposure to cold may be scarce in hypothermia fatalities. Most of the findings are unspecific and clinically of no relevance. However, external and internal findings are of diagnostic significance, not only as the sole finding of frost erythema but especially when they are found in combination like the presence of both frost erythema and Wischnewsky spots. Although unspecific as an exclusive finding, frost erythema and Wischnewsky spots are specific for hypothermia in combination. This is also true for fatty changes of proximal renal tubules which have a strong correlation with the aforementioned macroscopic signs of hypothermia. The pathogenesis of morphologic alterations caused by hypothermia differs widely (hypoxic changes, stress, disturbances of microcirculation with vasoconstriction and increased hematocrit) due to the different organs and tissues affected.

References

1. Blatteis CM (1998) Physiology and pathophysiology of temperature regulation. World Scientific Publishing, Singapore
2. Hirvonen J (2004) Kälte. In: Brinkmann B, Madea B (eds.) Handbuch Gerichtliche Medizin, Bd. 1. Springer, Berlin Heidelberg New York, pp 875–889
3. Madea B, Preuß J, Lignitz E (2003) Unterkühlung: Umstände, morphologische Befunde und ihre Pathogenese. Rechtsmedizin 14: 41–49
4. Madea B, Preuß J, Henn V, Lignitz E (2004) Morphological findings in fatal hypothermia and their pathogenesis. In: Oehmichen M (ed) Hypothermia. Clinical, pathomorphological and forensic features. Schmidt-Römhild, Lübeck, pp 181–204
5. Singer D (1991) Pathophysiologie der akzidentellen Hypothermie – eine Betrachtung aus vergleichend-physiologischer Sicht. In: Siegenthaler W, Haas R (ed) Publikationen der Jung Stiftung für Wissenschaft und Forschung, Bd. 3, Thieme, Stuttgart
6. Büchner F (1943) Die Pathologie der Unterkühlung. Klin Wschr 22: 89–92
7. Gillner E, Waltz H (1971) Zur Symptomatik des Erfrierens. Kriminal Forens Wiss 5: 179–185
8. Gordon J, Shapiro HA, Berson SD (1988) Forensic medicine. A guide to principles, 3rd edn. Churchill Livingstone, Edinburgh London Melbourne New York

9. Hirvonen J (1977) Local and systemic effects of accidental hypothermia. In: Tedeshi CG, Eckert WG, Tedeshi LG (eds) Forensic medicine, vol 1. WB Saunders Co, Philadelphia London Toronto, pp 758–774
10. Hirvonen J, Elfving R (1974) Histamine and serotonin in the gastric erosions of rats dead from exposure to cold: a histochemical and quantitative study. Z Rechtsmed 74: 273–281
11. Hirvonen J, Huttunen P, Lapinlampi T (1987) The markers of hypothermia deaths. Abstract J Canad Soc Forens Sci 20: 226
12. Killian H (1981) Cold and frost injuries. Springer, Berlin Heidelberg New York
13. Klöss Th (1983) Pathophysiologie, Diagnose und Behandlung akzidentieller Unterkühlungen. I Anästh Intensivmed 24, 6-11. II Anästh Intensivmed 24: 43–50
14. Knight B (1987) Legal aspects of medical practice, 4th edn. Churchill Livingstone, Edinburgh London Melbourne New York
15. Oehmichen M (2004) Hypothermia. Clinical, pathomorphological and forensic features. Schmidt-Römhild, Lübeck
16. Polson L, Gee D, Knight B (1985) The essentials of forensic medicine. Pergamon Press, Oxford New York Sydney Paris Frankfurt
17. Simpson K, Knight B (1985) Forensic medicine, 9th edn. Edward Arnold, London
18. Unterdorfer H (1977) Statistik und Morphologie des Unterkühlungstodes. Ärztl Praxis 29: 459–460
19. Hegenauer AH (1959) Lethal hypothermic temperatures for dog and man. Ann N Y Acad Sci 315–319
20. Hirvonen J (1976) Necropsy findings in fatal hypothermia cases. Forensic Sci 8: 155–164
21. Kahle W, Burchard E (1984) Überleben in der Kälte: Entstehung allgemeiner Kälteschäden und therapeutische Maßnahmen. Dtsch Ärztebl 81: 3743–3748
22. Keferstein (1893) Leichenbefund beim Erfrierungstod. Z Medizinalbeamte 6: 201–208
23. Killian H (1966) Der Kälteunfall. Allgemeine Unterkühlung. Dustri Verlag, München
24. Staemmler M (1944) Die Erfrierung. Thieme, Leipzig
25. Madea B (2006) Die Ärztliche Leichenschau. Rechtsgrundlagen – Praktische Durchführung – Problemlösungen, 2 nd edn. Springer, Berlin Heidelberg New York
26. Rautenberg E (1919) Ein bemerkenswerter Fall von Scheintod. Dtsch Med Wochenschrift 45: 750–751
27. Coe JI (1984) Hypothermia: autopsy findings and vitreous glucose. J Forensic Sci 29: 289–395
28. Duguid H, Simpson G, Stowers J (1961) Accidental hypothermia. Lancet 2: 1213–1219
29. Emslie-Smith D (1958) Accidental hypothermia. Lancet 2: 492–495
30. Fruehan AE (1960) Accidental hypothermia. Arch Int Med 106: 218–229
31. Gee G (1984) Deaths from physical and chemical injury, starvation and neglect. In: Mant AK (ed) Taylor's principles and practice of medical jurisprudence. Churchill Livingstone, Edinburgh London Melbourne New York
32. Mant AK (1964) Some post-mortem observations in accidental hypothermia. Med Sci Law 4: 44–46
33. Mant AK (1967) The pathology of hypothermia. In: Simpson K (ed.) Modern trends in forensic medicine, vol 2. Butterworths, London, pp 224–232
34. Mant AK (1969) Autopsy diagnosis of accidental hypothermia. J Forensic Med 16: 126–129
35. Read AE, Emslie-Smith D, Gough KR, Holmes R (1961) Pancreatitis and accidental hypothermia. Lancet 2: 1219–1221
36. Coniam WS (1979) Accidental hypothermia. Anaesth 34: 250–256
37. Kinzinger R, Risse M, Püschel K (1995) "Kälteidiotie": Paradoxes Entkleiden bei Unterkühlung. Arch Kriminol 187: 47–56
38. Rothschild MA, Mülling C, Luzar (2004) Lethal hypothermia: the phenomena of paradoxical undressing and hide and die syndrome. In: Oehmichen M (ed.) Hypothermia. Clinical, pathomorphological and forensic features. Schmidt-Römhild, Lübeck, pp 167–173

39. Madea B, Henßge C (1990) Electrical excitability of skeletal muscle postmortem in casework. Forensic Sci Int 47: 207–227
40. Püschel K, Türk EE (2004) Determination of the rectal temperature as an important tool for establishing the diagnosis of vital hypothermia. In: Oehmichen M (ed) Hypothermia. Clinical, pathomorphological and forensic features. Schmidt-Römhild, Lübeck, pp 175–180
41. Wischnewsky S (1895) Ein neues Kennzeichen des Todes durch Erfrieren. Bote f gerichtl Med 3: 12
42. Hofmann E v, Haberda A (1927) Lehrbuch der gerichtlichen Medizin, 11th edn. Urban und Schwarzenberg, Wien
43. Ignatowsky (1901) Über die Ursachen der Blutungen in der Schleimhaut des Magens beim Tode des Erfrierens. Bote d gerichtl Med 10: 1649
44. Kratter J (1921) Lehrbuch der gerichtlichen Medizin. Enke, Stuttgart
45. Krjukoff A (1914) Beitrag zur Frage der Kennzeichen des Todes durch Erfrieren. Vjschr gerichtl Med 47(3F); 79–101
46. Meixner K (1932) Ein Fall von Tod durch Erfrieren. Dtsch Z gerichtl Med 18: 270–284
47. Reuter F (1933) Lehrbuch der gerichtlichen Medizin. Urban und Schwarzenberg, Berlin Wien
48. Strassmann F (1895) Lehrbuch der gerichtlichen Medizin. Enke, Stuttgart
49. Richter M (1905) Gerichtsärztliche Diagnostik und Technik. Hirzel, Leipzig
50. Bourne MH, Piepkorn MW, Clayton F, Leonard LG (1986) Analysis of microvascular changes in frostbite injury. J Surg Res 40: 26–35
51. Kreyberg L (1946) Tissue damage due to cold. Lancet 338–340
52. Wilkerson JA, Bangs CC, Hayward J (1986) Hypothermia, frostbite and other cold injuries. The Mountaineers, Seattle
53. Türk EE, Sperhake JP, Madea B, Preuß J, Tsokos M (2006) Immunohistochemical detection of haemoglobin in frost erythema. Forensic Sci Int 158: 131–134
54. Birchmeyer MS, Mitchel EK (1989) Wischnewski revisited: the diagnostic value of gastric mucosa ulcers in hypothermic deaths. Am J Forensic Med Pathol 10: 28–30
55. Dreßler J, Hauck JG (1996) Zum Beweiswert kälteassoziierter histologischer Befunde beim Verdacht auf "Kältetod". Kriminol Forens Wiss 85:39–44
56. Dyrenfurth F (1916) Über den Wert zweier neuer Kennzeichen des Todes durch Kälteeinwirkung. Vjschr gerichtl Med 51: 234–241
57. Takada M, Kusano I, Yamamoto H, Shiraishi T, Yatani R, Haba K (1991) Wischnevsky's gastric lesions in accidental hypothermia. Am J Forensic Med Pathol 12: 300–305
58. Cali JR, Glaubitz JP, Crampton RS (1965) Gastric necrosis due to prolonged local gastric hypothermia. JAMA 191: 154–155
59. Tidow R (1943) Kälteschäden des Magendarmkanals unter besonderer Berücksichtigung der Abkühlung. Münch Med Wschr 90: 597–600
60. Tsokos M, Rothschild MA, Madea B, Risse M, Sperhake JP (2006) Histological and immunhistochemical study of Wischnewsky spots in fatal hypothermia. Am J Forensic Med Pathol 27: 70–74
61. Sperhake JP, Rothschild MA, Risse M, Tsokos M (2004) Histomorphology of Wischnewsky spots: contribution to the forensic histopathology of fatal hypothermia. In: Oehmichen M (ed) Hypothermia. Clinical, pathomorphological and forensic features. Schmidt-Römhild, Lübeck, pp 211–220
62. Madea B, Oehmichen M (1989) Ungewöhnliche Befunde in einem Fall von Unterkühlung. Z Rechtsmedizin 102: 59–67
63. Otto HF, Wanke M, Zeitlhofer J (1976) Darm und Peritoneum. In: Doerr W, Seifert G, Uehlinger E (eds) Spezielle pathologische Anatomie, Bd 2, Teil 2. Springer, Berlin Heidelberg New York
64. Stoddard JC (1962) Mesenteric infarction during hypothermia. Brit J Anaesth 34: 825–830
65. Becker V (1973) Bauchspeicheldrüse. In: Doerr W, Seiffert G, Uehlinger E (eds) Spezielle pathologische Anatomie, Bd. 6, Springer, Berlin Heidelberg New York
66. Fisher ER, Fedor EJ, Fischer B (1957) Pathology and histochemical observations in experimental hypothermia. Arch Surg 75: 817–827

67. Sano ME, Smith CW (1940) Fifty post-mortem patients with cancer subjected to local or generalized refrigeration. J Lab Clin 26: 443
68. Preuß J, Dettmeyer R, Lignitz E, Madea B (2007) Pancreatic changes in cases of death due to hypothermia. Forensic Sci Int 166: 194–198
69. Dirnhofer R, Sigrist T (1979) Muskelblutungen im Körperkern – ein Zeichen vitaler Reaktion bei Tod durch Unterkühlung? Beitr Gerichtl Med 37: 159–166
70. Schneider V, Klug E (1980) Tod durch Unterkühlung. Z Rechtsmed 86: 59–69
71. Schneider V, Wessel J (1987) Zum gehäuften Auftreten von Todesfällen an Unterkühlung bei überraschenden Kälteeinbrüchen. Lebensvers Med 39: 58–61
72. Preuß J, Dettmeyer R, Lignitz E, Madea B (2004) Fatty degeneration in renal tubule epithelium in accidental hypothermia victims. Forensic Sci Int 141: 131–135
73. Thrun C (1992) Verfettung der Tubulusepithelien der Niere – ein Hinweis für Hypothermie? Rechtsmedizin 2: 55–58
74. Preuß J, Dettmeyer R, Lignitz E, Madea B (2006) Fatty degeneration of myocardial cells as a sign of death due to hypothermia versus degenerative deposition of lipofuscin. Forensic Sci Int 159: 1–5
75. Simon A, Müller E (1971) Einige Aspekte zur Physiologie und Morphologie des Kältetodes unter besonderer Berücksichtigung der sogenannten Kälteschilddrüse. Kriminal Forens Wiss 6: 131–138
76. Mizukami H, Shimizu K, Shiono H, Uezono T, Sasaki M (1999) Forensic diagnosis of death from cold. Legal Med 1: 204–209

Part II
Trauma

Chapter 2
Fatal Falls from Height

Elisabeth E. Türk

Contents

Abstract Especially in urban settings, falls from height are a phenomenon that significantly contributes to population morbidity and mortality. The injuries sustained vary depending on the falling height, the composition of the impact surface, the position of the body when landing and individual factors such as age, body weight and preexisting disease. Cases of fatal falls from height can carry a high forensic relevance, because at the time the body is found, the manner of death is often unclear. Injuries sustained prior to the actual fall that might have been inflicted by another person might well be masked by the impact injuries. It is thus especially important in these cases to take into account not only the autopsy findings but also toxicology results, findings at the death scene, and the medical, psychiatric, and social history of the victim. The aim of this review is to summarize the most important findings in cases of fatal falls from height and to discuss the possibilities and limits in interpreting these findings with special regard to the manner of death.

Keywords Fall from height · Blunt trauma · Injury pattern · Forensic pathology

E.E. Türk
Institute of Legal Medicine, University of Hamburg, Hamburg, Germany

M. Tsokos (ed.), *Forensic Pathology Reviews, Volume 5,*
doi: 10.1007/978-1-59745-110-9_2, © Humana Press, Totowa, NJ 2008

2.1 Introduction

Most cases of fatal falls from height are suicidal. Although compared to other suicide methods, falls from height are relatively rare, they have been observed to be a preferred method in elderly suicides [1, 2]. Accidents occur at work, for example on construction sites or amongst roofers and window cleaners, as well as in domestic settings and during recreational sports activity like climbing or mountaineering. Cases of homicide are relatively rare. In homicides, additional injuries may be present that cannot be explained by the fall alone, like defence or offence injuries. But they can also be absent if the victim was taken by surprise, if the perpetrator was physically significantly stronger than the victim, or if the victim was defenceless, for example due to intoxication. Furthermore, those injuries will in most cases be very difficult to differentiate from injuries attributable to the fall itself. Thus, a forensic pathologist dealing with such cases will depend on every additional piece of information he can get and effective interdisciplinary work between all involved parties, namely forensic pathologists, police officers, physicians and sometimes relatives is essential.

2.2 Death Scene Findings

First of all, the location of the death scene can already carry some valuable information regarding the classification of the fatality. Falls or jumps from places where people normally do not go, like house roofs, cliffs or bridges where no pedestrians are allowed, are highly suspicious of suicide [3, 4]. Furthermore, descents from heights that happen from windows of psychiatric wards are likely to be suicidal in nature. Suicides also often occur at peoples' homes, as do homicides, while accidental falls from a height have been shown to happen rarely at the victims' homes and more often at their work-places [3, 5]. Especially at dangerous work-places like building sites, most falls from height will be accidental, although, of course, a suicidal or even a homicidal fall can never be excluded at first sight. It has been demonstrated that higher buildings are preferred if someone jumps from a height with suicidal intention, whereas in accidents the heights are more randomly distributed [3, 4]. This observation is in line with the finding that the victims are usually dead when found if the manner of death is suicide, whereas more victims survive at first in accidental falls [5]. Several studies indicate that falls from less than four stories can be survived, whereas falls from over seven stories are almost exclusively fatal [6, 7, 8, 9].

Expectedly, working accidents have been demonstrated to occur exclusively at working hours, whereas suicides often happen in the evening or at nighttime [3].

Suicide notes are always clearly indicative of a suicidal fall, but they are certainly not found in all suicidal falls from height. Frequencies range from under 10% to approximately 25% and are thus less frequently found in suicidal falls than in suicides by other causes [3, 5, 11].

Signs of a fight at the death scene always suggest homicide. In accidental falls, scene findings might suggest that the person had been working in a dangerous position prior to the fall, for example cleaning windows. Signs of substance use prior to the fall, like empty bottles, syringes and the like, might suggest an accidental fall due to a substance-related lack of coordination or over-estimation of the person's physical abilities (for example under the influence of cocaine or psychedelic drugs). The barrier preventing an accidental fall, like windows, railings, fences etc., should always be thoroughly documented. An accident is unlikely if this barrier is higher than the person's center of gravity [4]. In suicides, chairs or ladders might be present as means to get over the barrier. Likewise, the security measures preventing falls at building sites should be thoroughly investigated. Although falls through closed windows would in most cases suggest an accidental fall, they can also be suicidal as observed in a previous study [5].

Some authors suggest that the distance of the body from the jumping site can be used as an additional tool to determine the manner of death. Studies have demonstrated that in intentional jumps the distance to the jumping site is likely to be higher than in accidental falls [11, 12].

Although the distance from a building can be valuable in determining the manner of death, caution should be used in the interpretation of these findings for a variety of reasons. Suicidals do not necessarily jump actively but can also just let themselves fall down. Furthermore, distances can overlap between intentional jumps and passive falls [12]. Moreover, an active jump does not necessarily indicate suicidal intention. Some users of psychedelic drugs, for example, might jump down a building under the impression that they can fly [3, 5]. Psychotic patients might try to escape their "pursuers", or perfectly healthy people might jump out of the window/down a building to escape real dangers like fires [3, 5]. The distance from the jumping site will also vary depending on the part of the body to hit the ground first [14]. In addition, in many cases the exact distance or position of the body in relation to the jumping site cannot be determined as it might have been changed prior to death scene investigation, for example by rescue teams.

In summary, a thorough death scene investigation is always the first important piece of the puzzle when it comes to the assessment of a fatal fall from a height.

2.3 Psychiatric History

A history of psychiatric illness is most frequently found in suicidal falls from height. Psychiatric illnesses most often include depressions, schizophrenia and/or substance abuse, but also personality disorders [3, 5, 13, 14, 15]. In accidental falls, substance abuse is the most frequent psychiatric disease, whereas a history of depression is suggestive of a suicidal fall. In many of these cases, previous suicide attempts can be elucidated. The denial of suicidal ideation by the victim's medical care giver cannot be taken as absolute in these cases, as there is often a potential conflict of interest involved and the care giver might be accused of wrong assessment of the patient's mental situation [5]. Schizophrenia is found in suicides, but also in unclarified cases (like in escapes from "pursuers"). In many cases, a combination of psychiatric illnesses can be found, especially substance abuse in combination with others [3, 5, 13].

2.4 Injury Patterns

The injury pattern in falls from height is, of course, dependent on the part of the body that hits the ground first, as well as on the falling height, the age and body weight of the victim, the clothing and the ground composition.

2.4.1 External Examination

The examination of the clothing can already provide some clues about the nature of a fall from a height. In feet-first impacts, longitudinal tears in the loin region of trousers due to inguinal stretching may be present [3, 5, 10, 16]. In falls from great heights, clothing might not be regularly situated after the impact. Soiling and tissue defects due to direct ground surface contact can hint towards the site of the impact.

In general, injuries seen at external examination tend to be relatively mild compared to the severe injuries that are frequently revealed at autopsy (Fig. 2.1A,B). This is especially true for falls into water but has also been observed in descents onto solid ground [3, 4, 17].

Postmortem lividity may be sparse due to major external or internal blood loss [3]. In accordance with the clothing, in feet-first impacts, longitudinal tears of the inguinal regions can be seen occasionally. In addition, plantar injuries with open fractures of the ankle joint or calcaneus are characteristic in these cases [3, 5, 10, 16]. Bruising in the perineal region as a sequel of relative movement of that region against clothing also occurs in feet-first impacts and may be misinterpreted as a sign of sexual abuse prior to the fall, thus wrongly leading to the assumption of a homicidal fall [13].

In a recent study it was observed that palmar skin tears and open comminuted fractures of the wrists and knees are also common injuries in fatal free falls and might be a sign of the victim's attempt to cushion the impact [3]. Blunt injuries such as abrasions and hematoma at the site of primary impact, termed planar impacts, are a frequent finding [3, 5]. Depending on the structure of the impact surface, the ground texture might be reflected in patterned injuries [13]. If the victim strikes protruding intermediate objects on the way down, for example balconies, additional, non-planar injuries may be present. Depending

(A)   (B)

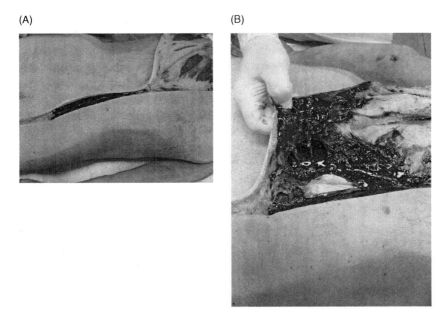

Fig. 2.1 **A** No visible external injury on the back of a free-fall victim. **B** Extensive soft tissue hematoma in the same region as revealed by dissection during autopsy

on the impact surface(s) and ground composition, the body or parts of it can be severely dismembered [3, 13].

Some injuries are not typically caused directly by falls from a height and may therefore be revealing regarding the circumstances surrounding a fall. Palmar injuries such as abrasions ("rope burns"), resulting from the attempt of the victim to hold on to objects preventing a fall, suggest a homicidal or an accidental fall. In contrast, old or fresh wrist incisions ("hesitation marks") are indicative of a suicidal intention [5]. As a caveat, however, it has to be noted that especially old hesitation marks can of course be present in accidents and homicides independent of the present fall [3]. Signs of complex suicide, for example additional shot or stab wounds, may be present in suicides but can, of course, also be found in homicides. Hematoma of the inner surface of the upper arms, in keeping with grab marks, are usually not found in accidental or suicidal falls from a height and are therefore strongly suggestive of infliction by another person [3].

2.4.2 Internal Examination

Severe injuries of the internal organs and/or the musculoskeletal system can be found in all fatal falls from height. It is generally accepted that the falling height is a major determinant of the severity of injuries sustained in a fall, and multiple injuries are more frequent in greater falling heights. Mathematical models have been developed to correlate the severity of injuries with the falling height, and it has been found that the falling height and the age of the victim are the major factors determining injury severity. Accordingly, it has been proposed to use the injury severity score, age and type of organ injuries to calculate an estimated falling height band [18]. It has, however, also been demonstrated that the injury severity score alone does not allow an exact estimation of the falling height due to a wide variation of injuries and dependence on too many additional factors [3, 13, 19, 20, 21, 22, 23, 24].

In feet-first impacts, the vertical deceleration trauma causes characteristic injuries like aortic lacerations and ring fractures of the skull base. Aortic lacerations have also been shown to be frequent in falls with other landing positions [3, 5, 7, 10, 13, 16, 25]. Depending on the site of first impact, a large variety of injury patterns can be observed.

2.4.2.1 Head Injuries

Head injuries are frequently seen in falls from heights and include subarachnoid, subdural and epidural hemorrhage, intracerebral hemorrhage and brain contusion as well as severe disruption and the complete or partial loss of brain structures. Severe head trauma with intracranial bleeding and/or disruption of brain structures has been shown to be mostly associated with skull fractures and are rarely seen in falls onto water surface [3, 4, 13]. Open comminuted skull fractures with additional facial bone fractures and splattering of the brain over wide areas is mostly seen in head-first impacts. In theses cases, the head seems to cushion most of the impact as severe injuries of other internal organs have been observed to be rare in falls from heights below 25 m resulting in severe head trauma [3]. Brainstem injuries such as lacerations, contusion or transection are frequently found in feet-first impacts with ring fracture of the skull base [13]. Traumatic subarachnoid hemorrhage can be seen in cases where no evidence of direct head trauma is present, suggesting that shearing and rotational forces also play a role in head injury caused by falls from a height. This has been corroborated by the occasional observation of corpus callosum lacerations. However, diffuse axonal injury is rarely seen at histological examination, in keeping with the mostly short survival times of free fall victims [13]. Interestingly, although some authors have described an increasing number and severity of head injuries with an increasing falling height [5], others have shown that severe head trauma predominantly occurs in falls from smaller (below 10 m) and very great (over 25 m) heights, while it is less frequent in falls from intermediate heights [3, 13].

2.4.2.2 Neck Injuries

When neck injuries are present, the forensic pathologist always has to consider strangulation prior to the fall, and the possibility of a homicidal infliction of the injuries must always be taken into account, especially if additional conjunctival petechial hemorrhages are present [26, 27]. In falls from height, however, blunt force neck injuries directly attributable to the fall are frequently found and may be misleading regarding the manner of death in the first place. Such injuries include mild to moderate hemorrhage in subcutaneous and muscular layers as well as thyroid hematoma, but severe injuries like hyoid bone and thyroid cartilage fractures can also be present in nonhomicidal free falls [3, 13, 28]. Altogether, blunt neck injuries have been observed with a frequency of up to 33% in falls from heights [3].

2.4.2.3 Thoracic Injuries

Thoracic Cage

Thoracic cage injuries like abrasions and bruises of the chest wall and rib fractures are found in nearly all fatal falls from height. Rib fractures can be solitary, but are most commonly bilateral. In falls from heights above 25 m, multiple fractures of the whole thoracic cage, including the sternum and thoracic spine, are often found [3, 4, 5, 7, 13]. In falls into water, the prevalence of rib fractures is a little lower than in falls onto solid ground, but rib fractures a still a common finding even in these cases [3, 4, 25]. Penetrating rib fractures can cause secondary injuries to the thoracic organs or may result in pneumothorax and/or hemothorax. Significant intrathoracic bleeding has, however, been reported to be relatively rare given the high prevalence of severe organ and major blood vessel injuries. This has been attributed to the immediate occurrence of death in many such cases [13].

Heart

Cardiac injuries are frequently seen in fatal falls from height. In a recent autopsy-based study, blunt injuries to the heart were seen in 54% of all cases, 79% of which were multiple [29], a percentage which is well in line with previous observations [13]. These injuries contribute significantly to mortality in descents from height. The frequency and severity of cardiac trauma increases with increasing height of the fall [13, 29].

Pericardial tears are found in the majority of cases, most of which show additional cardiac injuries. Pericardial tears are most likely to occur in the right posterior part of the pericardium and tend to be of longitudinal orientation, although irregular tears are also common. Epicardial tears that can be attributed to stretching of the epicardium as well as epicardial hemorrhage can frequently be detected and appear to occur preferably in falls from heights below 15 m [29]. The area most vulnerable to epicardial injuries is the vicinity of the entry of the inferior vena cava into the right atrium. In contrast to pericardial tears, endocardial tears are more likely to be found in falls from greater heights.

Complete or incomplete transmural tears of the heart (Fig. 2.2A,B) affect the right heart more often than the left heart and may affect both the atria and

(A)   (B)

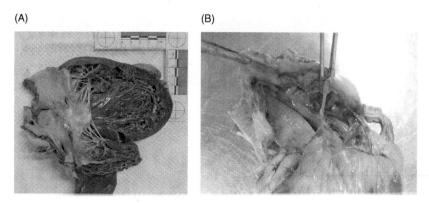

Fig. 2.2 **A** Incomplete tear of the left ventricle. **B** Full-thickness rupture of the right atrium

ventricles [13, 29, 30]. Tears of the interatrial septum are more common than interventricular septal tears. In the atria, the areas of vascular attachment are most frequently affected. Frequency and severity of full-thickness cardiac ruptures correlate positively with the falling height. Although these injuries are survivable [30, 31, 32], transmural rupture especially of the left ventricle or more than one heart chamber will in most cases be the cause of death or contribute significantly to fatal outcome.

Papillary muscle ruptures are less commonly seen and can involve the valves.

Myocardial hematoma is not rarely observed in fatal descents from height and can be extensive, thus contributing to fatal outcome, or might even be the only cause of death. The left heart is more frequently involved than the right heart, and the hemorrhage is confined to the left ventricular myocardium in the majority of cases [29].

Especially in falls from greater heights, the cardiac valves of the heart might rupture. Again, the right heart is more frequently affected than the left heart, and overall, the atrioventricular valves rupture more easily than the aortic and pulmonary valve [13, 29]. Complete coronary artery ruptures are rare and almost exclusively limited to great falling heights.

In falls from very great heights, the heart can be completely or subtotally torn off from the great vessels, which is frequently associated with further cardiac injuries such as multiple full-thickness atrial and/or ventricular tears that usually result in death immediately.

In a clinical trial, it has been suggested that cardiac injuries are more likely to occur when sternal fracture is present [33], an observation well in line with the correlation of the two injury types seen at autopsy [29]. However, there seems to be no significant correlation between sternal fractures and the type of cardiac injury.

Minor injuries, especially cardiac contusion/concussion, can be present in blunt chest trauma and may contribute to fatal outcome but are, due to minor morphological changes, difficult to detect at autopsy without histological investigations. Their relevance and the mechanism of death is still relatively poorly understood. In surviving victims of blunt chest trauma, it is important to diagnose cardiac contusion/concussion. The use of troponin as a marker has been suggested in these cases [34, 35].

Thoracic Blood Vessels

Ruptures of the thoracic aorta (Fig. 2.3) are a common finding in free fall victims and are mostly located in the isthmus area [3, 5, 13]. Complete or incomplete circumferential involvement is frequently found. The rupture margins are smooth in the majority of cases, giving the injury an appearance of sharp transection. Full thickness but not circumferential rupture can be present and can be survived in case of early diagnosis and operative intervention [36]. The frequency of aortic rupture increases with greater falling heights [3, 13, 24]. Mediastinal hemorrhage occurs as a sequel of aortic rupture, but hemothorax of the left thoracic cavity may also be present. Aortic rupture can be multiple and is not rarely accompanied by cardiac injuries [3, 13]. Pulmonary artery and venous ruptures are seen less frequently. The frequency of other major artery ruptures, for example of the axillary arteries, is not known as they might escape detection at autopsy due to the prominence of other major injuries and the necessity of a very diligent search in order to find such ruptures [13].

Lungs

Minor or major contusions of the lungs can be found in almost all fatal falls from height, with prevalence and severity increasing with greater falling distance. Especially in greater falling heights, pulmonary ruptures or complete hilus ruptures can be found. In the majority of cases, pulmonary injury is accompanied by (multiple) rib fractures. Penetrating rib fractures with associated pulmonary injury are also common [3, 13]. Blood aspiration, either as a secondary phenomenon in pulmonary injuries or as a sequel of head injuries, is frequently found and does not appear to show a preference for greater falling heights [3].

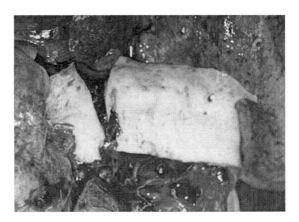

Fig. 2.3 Complete transverse rupture of the descending aorta

Diaphragm

Diaphragmatic rupture can result not only in respiratory failure but can also be associated with further severe injuries such as displacement of abdominal organs into the thorax. Diaphragm ruptures are relatively rare in falls from height.

2.4.2.4 Abdominal Injuries

Liver

Liver ruptures are more frequent in falls from height than in other mechanisms of blunt abdominal trauma [37]. They have been observed with a frequency between 52% and 68% of all cases [3, 5, 13]. The right lobe of the liver is involved more often than the left lobe [24]. Tears are often irregular in nature but have been shown to be almost parallel in many cases (Fig. 2.4) [13]. Depending on the falling height, severe disruption of the whole liver as well as vascular avulsion and hilar rupture are also common findings [13]. It has been observed that even if extensive ruptures of the liver are present, associated abdominal bleeding is often minimal [3, 13].

Spleen

Spleen ruptures are common in falls from height and are often multiple [13]. Like liver ruptures, they rarely result in extensive intraabdominal hemorrhage.

Gastrointestinum

Ruptures or bruises of the intestinal root are a common finding in greater falling heights [3, 13], but traumatic ruptures of the esophagus, stomach and

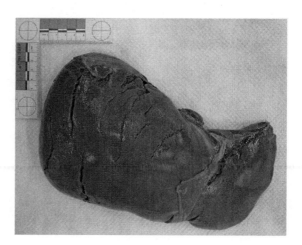

Fig. 2.4 Liver ruptures in a free-fall victim. Note the parallel nature of the tears

bowel are relatively rare. This has been attributed to their compliance and relative mobility within the thoracic/abdominal cavity [13].

Retroperitoneal Organs

Rupture of the abdominal aorta is, in contrast to thoracic aortic rupture, relatively rare [3, 13]. Retroperitoneal hemorrhage has been observed. Whereas some authors state that retroperitoneal hemorrhage is often extensive and can lead to fatal outcome [7], others report that it is rarely extensive in nature [13, 38]. Psoas muscle bleeding can be a result of inguinal stretching especially in feet-first impacts. Adrenal ruptures are an occasional finding in fatal falls from height. Renal injuries have been reported to occur rarely in falls from height [7, 39, 40] but may be overlooked – especially if only minor injuries are present – and have thus been suggested to be under-represented in many studies [38]. Renal injuries can be severe and thus contribute to fatal outcome. Most frequently, renal fat capsule bleeding without actual renal injury is found. Parenchymal ruptures of the kidneys are rare events. The most common injuries occur at the sites of fixed and mobile organ portions, namely the ureter and the vascular entrance sites. Frequency and severity of renal injuries seem to be independent of the falling height. Instead, the site of impact is crucial for the extent of renal injuries, with victims landing on their sides being most likely to suffer renal injury [38].

2.5 Cause of Death, Survival Times

The majority of victims of fatal falls from height die at the scene instantly or within minutes. Of the survivors, most victims die in emergency departments shortly after admission, and only a minority of victims survives longer than a few hours [3, 13]. In instantaneous deaths, the most frequent cause of death is polytrauma, followed by head trauma and (mostly internal) blood loss. Head trauma has been shown to be the most common cause of death in free-fall victims who survive for hours to days [3]. In victims who survive a few days, other possible causes of death include septic multiple organ failure and pulmonary embolism. In jumps or falls into water, drowning may be the cause of death or contribute to fatal outcome [4, 5, 41].

2.6 Toxicology

Ethanol has been reported with a frequency of 15–20% up to 35% in free-fall fatalities and seems to be equally distributed between accidents and suicides [3, 13, 42]. The range of blood alcohol concentration generally seems to be wider in suicides than in accidents. In accidents, blood alcohol levels tend to be generally higher. Illicit drugs appear to be more frequent in suicidal descents from height than in other manners of death [3]. Psychiatric medications are much more frequent in suicides than in accidents or homicides [3, 5]. Benzo-diazepines and antidepressants are most common [5, 13]. In many cases a history of psychiatric illness is present. In almost all cases alcohol and/or drug levels are not found in lethal concentrations, and thus do not significantly contribute to fatal outcome [13, 41].

2.7 Conclusions

The main questions of medicolegal relevance in fatal falls from height concern the manner of death and the toxicology of the fatality in question. The determination of the manner of death is often quite difficult in falls from height, as many findings that are usually suggestive of homicide, like neck injuries or defence-type injuries of the extremities, can be present as a mere sequel of the fall. Thus, it is essential in these cases to base one's assessment of such a fatality not only on the autopsy examination of the body but also on as much additional information as possible. A thorough death scene investigation should always be performed, the social and medical history should be evaluated, and toxicology results should always be taken into account. In some cases, however, all these investigations will not provide good enough clues to clarify the case, and the manner of death will remain unclear.

References

1. Bennett AT, Collins KA (2001) Elderly suicide: a 10-year retrospective study. Am J Forensic Med Pathol 22:169–172
2. Abrams RC, Marzuk PM, Tardiff K, Leon AC (2005) Preference for fall from height as a method of suicide by elderly residents of New York City. Am J Public Health 95:1000–1002
3. Türk EE, Tsokos M (2004) Pathologic features of fatal falls from height. Am J Forensic Med Pathol 25:194–199
4. Cetin G, Günay Y, Fincanci SK, Özdemir Kolusayin R (2001) Suicides by jumping from Bosporus Bridge in Istanbul. Forensic Sci Int 116:157–162
5. Gill JR (2001) Fatal descent from height in New York City. J Forensic Sci 46:1132–1137
6. Lewis WS, Lee AB Jr, Grantham SA (1965) "Jumper's syndrome". The trauma of high free falls as seen at Harlem Hospital. J Trauma 5:812–818
7. Scalea T, Goldstein A, Philips T, Sclafani SJ, Panetta T, McAuley J, Shaftan G (1986) An analysis of 161 falls from a height: the "jumper syndrome". J Trauma 26:706–712
8. Roshkow JE, Haller JO, Hotson GC, Sclafani SJ, Mezzacappa PM, Rachlin S (1990) Imaging evaluation of children after falls from a height: review of 45 cases. Radiology 175:359–363
9. Risser D, Bonsch A, Schneider B, Bauer G (1996) Risk of dying after a free fall from height. Forensic Sci Int 78:187–191
10. Li L, Smialek JE (1994) The investigation of falls and jumps from height in Maryland (1987–1992). Am J Forensic Med Pathol 15:295–299

11. Shaw KP, Hsu SY (1998) Horizontal distance and height determining falling pattern. J Forensic Sci 43:765–771
12. Wischhusen F, Patra S, Braumann M, Türk EE, Püschel K (2006) Analysis of jumping/falling distance from a height. Forensic Sci Int 156:150–153
13. Chao TC, Lau G, Teo CES (2000) Falls from a height: the pathology of trauma from vertical deceleration. In: Mason JK, Purdue BN (eds) The pathology of trauma, 3rd edn. Arnold, London
14. Lecomte D, Fornes P (1998) Suicide among youth and young adults, 15 through 24 years of age. A report of 392 cases from Paris, 1989–1996. J Forensic Sci 43:964–968
15. Chute D, Grove C, Rajasekhara B, Smialek JE (1999) Schizophrenia and sudden death: a medical examiner case study. Am J Forensic Med Pathol 20:131–135
16. Gupta SM, Chandra J, Dogra TD (1982) Blunt force lesions related to the height of a fall. Am J Forensic Med Pathol 3:35–43
17. Harvey PM, Solomons BJ (1983) Survival after free falls of 59 m into water from the Sydney Harbour Bridge 1930-1982. Med J Aust 1:504–511
18. Lau G, Ooi PL, Phoon B (1998) Fatal falls from height: the use of mathematical models to estimate the height of fall from the injuries sustained. Forensic Sci Int 93:33–44
19. Goodacre S, Than M, Goyder EC, Joseph AP (1999) Can the distance fallen predict serious injury after a fall from a height? J Trauma 46:1055–1058
20. Steedman DJ (1989) Severity of free-fall injury. Injury 20:259–261
21. Isbister ES, Roberts JA (1992) Autokabalesis: a study of intentional vertical deceleration injuries. Injury 23:119–122
22. Katz K, Gonen N, Goldberg I, Mizrahi J, Radwan M, Yosipovitch Z (1988) Injuries in attempted suicide by jumping from a height. Injury 19:371–374
23. Mathis RD, Levine SH, Phifer S (1993) An analysis of accidental free falls from a height: the "spring break" syndrome. J Trauma 34:137–143
24. Atanasijevic TC, Savic SN, Nikolic SD, Djokic VM (2005) Frequency and severity of injuries in correlation with the height of fall. J Forensic Sci 50:608–612
25. Lucas GM, Hutton JE Jr, Lim RC, Mathewson C Jr (1981) Injuries sustained from high velocity impact with water: an experience from the Golden Gate Bridge. J Trauma 21:612–618
26. Bockholdt B, Maxeiner H (2000) Cervical findings and petechial hemorrhages in falls from high positions [Article in German]. Arch Kriminol 205:53–58
27. Plattner T, Kopp A, Bolliger S, Zollinger U (2004) External injuries to the neck after free fall from great height. Am J Forensic Med Pathol 25:285–287
28. De la Grandmaison GL, Krimi S, Durigon M (2006) Frequency of laryngeal and hyoid bone trauma in nonhomicidal cases who died after a fall from a height. Am J Forensic Med Pathol 27:85–86
29. Türk EE, Tsokos M (2004) Blunt cardiac trauma caused by fatal falls from height: an autopsy-based assessment of the injury pattern. J Trauma 57:301–304
30. Perchinsky MJ, Long WB, Hill JG (1995) Blunt cardiac rupture. Arch Surg 130:852–856
31. Fang BR, Kuo LT, Li CT, Chang JP (2000) Isolated right atrial tear following blunt chest trauma: report of three cases. Jpn Heart J 41:535–540
32. Duda AM, Ilada PB, Molnar RG, Bachulis BL (1999) Successful repair of blunt cardiac rupture involving both ventricles. Cardiovasc Surg 7:263–265
33. De Waele JJ, Calle PAA, Blondeel L, Vermassen FEG (2002) Blunt cardiac injury in patients with isolated sternal fractures: the importance of fracture grading. Eur J Trauma 3:178–182
34. Moulin A (2002) Cardiac contusion diagnosed by cardiac troponin. Am J Emergency Med 20:382–383
35. Salim A, Velhamos GC, Jindal A, Chan L, Vassiliu P, Belzberg H, Asensio J, Demetriades D (2001) Clinically significant blunt cardiac trauma: role of serum troponin level combined with electrocardiographic findings. J Trauma 50:237–243

36. Santaniello JM, Miller PR, Croce MA, Bruce L, Bee TK, Malhotra AK, Fabian TC (2002) Blunt aortic injury with concomitant intra-abdominal solid organ injury: treatment priorities revisited. J Trauma 53:442–445
37. Matthes G, Stengel D, Bauwens K, Seifert J, Rademacher G, Mutze S, Ekkernkamp A (2005) Predictive factors of liver injury in blunt multiple trauma. Langenbeck's Arch Surg Nov 1:1–5
38. Brandes SB, McAninch JW (1999) Urban free falls and patterns of renal injury: a 20-year experience with 396 cases. J Trauma 47:643–650
39. Velmahos GC, Demetriades D, Theodoru D, Cornwell EE III, Belzberg H, Asensio J, Murray J, Berne TV (1997) Patterns of injury in victims of urban free-fall. World J Surg 21:816–820
40. Lowenstein SR, Yaron M, Carrero R, Devereux D, Jacobs LM (1989) Vertical trauma: injuries to patients who fall and land on their feet. Ann Emerg Med 18:161–165
41. Coman M, Meyer AD, Cameron PA (2000) Jumping from the Westgate Bridge, Melbourne. Med J Aust 172:67–69
42. Perret G, Flomenbaum M, La Harpe R (2003) Suicides by fall from height in Geneva, Switzerland, from 1991 to 2000. J Forensic Sci 48:821–826

Chapter 3
Understanding Craniofacial Blunt Force Injury: A Biomechanical Perspective

Jules Kieser, Kelly Whittle, Brittany Wong, J Neil Waddell,
Ionut Ichim, Michael Swain, Michael Taylor and Helen Nicholson

Contents

Abstract One of the most important tasks in forensic investigation of blunt force trauma is to determine accurately the nature and magnitude of the forces applied to the skin. The primary emphasis of research into blunt force trauma has focused on analysing the demographics rather than the mechanobiology of such injuries. Nevertheless, a large body of literature has accumulated on the biomechanics of skin. Here we review this evidence, together with the complex role of intrinsic factors such as age, sex and ethnicity on the wounding suscept-ibility of skin. We also review how the skin responds to blunt trauma, and try to relate this to the estimation of the force of impact. Finally, we review the current biomechanical models of blunt force trauma, and introduce our own model and its preliminary findings. Contrary to the impression gained from the literature, wounding can be modelled in a basic simulation of the contact events during blunt force impact, and the results be evaluated quantitatively. We conclude that subject-specific parameters could be calculated from a more sophisticated model in order to provide a more robust set of values that can be used to predict forces used in generating skin wounds.

Keywords Blunt force · Mechanical trauma · Biomechanics · Biomechanical properties of skin · Elastic behaviour of skin · Lacerations · Langer's lines

J. Kieser
University of Otago, Dunedin, New Zealand
e-mail: jules.kieser@stonebow.otago.ac.nz

3.1 Introduction

Forensic scientists and pathologists have long recognised the importance of understanding the mechanics of blunt force wounding in the craniofacial region, and also the factors influencing the different clinical or postmortem presentation of such wounds [1, 2, 3, 4]. Blunt force trauma typically results in laceration, defined as full-thickness separation of the skin caused by tearing, splitting, or crushing [5]. While the incidence, clinical presentation, assessment and treatment of such injuries have been described extensively, the biomechanics of lacerations that occur as a result of blunt trauma has received little attention [6]. Moreover, the lack of quantitative data on the force needed for a given blunt object to lacerate human skin makes it highly difficult to reconstruct blunt force trauma mathematically with any degree of confidence. This clearly presents a problem to the forensic expert, since it is impossible to infer whether a specific laceration was necessarily the result of a deliberate blow. Ankers et al. [7] have stressed the importance of an ability to quantify the force used in a particular traumatic incident. Not only will this enable the pathologist to determine the effort and speed involved in single or repetitive blows, but knowledge of the biomechanics of the production of lacerations relative to location on the body will enable clinicians to make appropriate assessments of the severity of blunt force injuries.

The forensic investigator is also interested in the following (in approximate order of importance):

1. Is the wound part of a significant injury and/or related to the cause of death?
2. What type of instrument caused the wound? Could it be the one the police has as an exhibit?
3. How much force was used, and was it intentional and/or excessive?
4. Is there likely to have been bleeding associated with the wound, and if so what sort (spurt, drip, spray, pooled, etc.) and how much? This of course relates to the added issues of DNA identification and bloodstain pattern analysis.

Considerable experimental and epidemiological research has focused on sharp force and ballistic injuries, with the primary emphasis of blunt force trauma focusing on analysing the demographics of such injuries [8]. However, over the past 20 years or so a strong research theme has emerged in medicine and dentistry that exploits the relationship between the structure and material properties of biological tissues and which seeks to understand more about aspects of structure-property correlations during normal function, pathology and treatment. This review traces some of the questions that have been raised and attempts to show how some of these questions have in turn raised new questions to be answered. The first obvious question is, what are the biomechanical properties of the human skin? This is followed by questions about the intrinsic and extrinsic determinants of blunt force injury, and finally, about how blunt force trauma can be modelled. However, to set the scene, we first have to briefly review what is known about craniofacial blunt force trauma.

3.2 Craniofacial Blunt Force Trauma

Blunt force trauma is injury caused by the impact of an object whose surface is blunt or rounded (in other words, not sharp) with the skin, and can result from direct or indirect contact [9]. The agents of direct blunt trauma range from assault (e.g., feet, fists or rounded objects) to accidental injury (e.g., motor vehicle accidents, sport). Indirect injury results from the body making forceful contact with a stationary object (e.g., stairs, concrete paving) [10]. The literature on this is extensive, and suggests that assaults and falls contribute to most of the injuries sustained in blunt force events, with victims being predominantly males between the age of 21 and 40 years. It appears that most victims of blunt force attacks are acquaintances, that these attacks usually involve a single weapon and that they mostly occur within the victim's own domicile. In contrast to sharp force injuries, blunt force trauma mostly involves blows to the left side of the craniofacial region [8, 10, 11, 12, 13, 14, 15, 16].

Forces are constantly being applied to the skin, which are usually absorbed. When these exceed the threshold that the skin in that area can sustain, its integrity is breached and wounding results [5]. The degree of injury is determined by a number of factors, including the amount of force applied to the target area, the contact area of both object and target, the tissue structure at the target and the shape of the weapon used [17]. Soft tissue trauma resultant from blunt force injury may be classified into abrasions, contusions and lacerations. Abrasions result from either the skin being pulled along a rough surface (scrape abrasion), or from perpendicular impact of a rough object with the skin (pattern abrasion), and is limited to the epidermal layer [5, 17]. Contusions occur when a blunt force ruptures small vessels, which bleed subcutaneously without the skin being breached. In contrast, lacerations occur when the compressive force of a blunt impact stretches the skin and subcutaneous tissues against bone, with the resultant pressure causing the skin to breach in the form of a laceration. A laceration is characterised by a deep wound with uneven margins that often have a crushed appearance. Often, bruising and abrasions surround the wound site. The resilience of some cutaneous and subcutaneous structures may result in bridging of connective tissue which span the laceration, and assists the pathologist in differentiating between sharp and blunt force injury [18].

The role of the shape and direction of the assaulting weapon in the determination of the appearance of a laceration is complex and not well understood. Lacerations are often classified into linear, stellate and Y-shaped wounds [19], and are thought to vary according to the direction of the force and the underlying structure of the contact area [18]. While perpendicular impacts with hammers have been shown to result in stellate wound patterns, tangential impacts are thought to result in separation of dermal tissue from the underlying bone at the edge of the wound, in the direction of the blow [18]. The important question that emerges now is whether it is possible to make estimates of the shape and severity of blunt force trauma from our knowledge of the biomechanical properties of human skin.

3.3 Biomechanics of Skin

Despite being the largest organ of the body (about 15% of the total body weight) and also the most visible, skin has received surprisingly little attention from biomechanical scientists until recently [20]. Human skin behaves as a non-homogenous, anisotropic, non-linear viscoelastic material subject to prestress. Because one of its primary functions is to protect the internal organs from mechanical trauma, skin is viscoelastic. These properties are related to the structure of collagen and elastin fibres and to proteoglycans found in the dermis [21, 22]. The skin's response to mechanical loading involves firstly, a viscous component associated with the dissipation of energy and secondly, an elastic response associated with energy storage. Energy applied to the skin is initially dissipated through viscous sliding of dermal collagen fibres during alignment in the direction of the force. The changes in collagen assembly during deformation are critical to the maintenance of the large extensibility of the skin [21]. In contrast, the elastic behaviour of skin is important in the recovery of shape after deformation [23]. The viscoelastic properties of skin also dictate that the rate of impact will determine the effective contact pressure generated, as dissipation and damping of such forces are dependent upon the fluidic content of skin.

At a gross anatomical level, however, it is important to remember that skin is a large continuous organ. This means that while the stress required to rupture a small area of skin is the same as that needed to break a large one, the large area will require a greater force to achieve the same stress. This may involve a greater volume of skin stretching further than the small one before it breaks and hence will require more energy to break it. In other words, a large area of skin cushions a sudden blow by stretching elastically under the load, until the transient stresses that result from the blow are dissipated [24]. This quality to store strain energy and deflect elastically under load without breaking is an important property of skin, referred to as its resilience.

The literature on the biomechanical behaviour of skin, both in vivo and in vitro, is extensive and has been reviewed elsewhere [20, 25]. Although the collagen and elastin are considered to be linearly elastic, the stress-strain

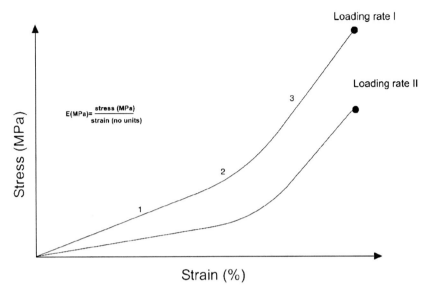

Fig. 3.1 Generic stress-strain diagram for skin. The curve for skin may be divided into three phases; elastin is responsible for the skin stretching, resulting in a linear, elastic phase (1); gradual straightening of collagen results in an increase in stiffness hence a viscoelastic phase (2); and when all collagen fibres are aligned another, elastic phase results (3). Viscoelastic behaviour of skin is rate dependent; loading rate I is fast loading, loading rate II slower

curve for skin under unidirectional tension is non-linear because of the non-uniformity of its structure (Fig. 3.1). The stress-strain curve is divided into three phases. In the first stage, collagen offers little resistance to deformation and the behaviour is dominated by elastic fibres, resulting in a linear relation, with a Young's modulus of approximately 5 kPa [26]. In the second phase, a gradual recruitment of collagen results in increased stiffness, followed by a third phase where all collagen fibres are aligned and the stress-strain relation becomes linear again. Beyond this phase, yield and eventual rupture of the skin takes place. However, in the case of impact, a considerable volume of skin experiences complex compressive and shear stresses directly below the contact area, about which little information is available in the literature.

Skin has evolved to fill needs posed by the ways in which animals function. One of these is the resistance to fracture when exposed to static and dynamic loads. The mechanical efficiency of skin as opposed to other biological structures may be quantified and compared by a performance chart [27] that shows toughness plotted against Young's modulus (Fig. 3.2). This clearly shows skin stores significant energy per unit volume and hence has unique flexural properties.

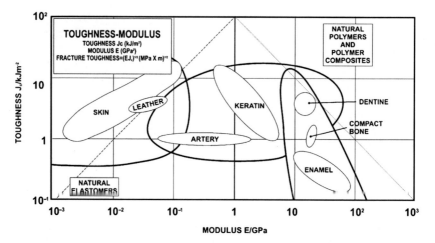

Fig. 3.2 Material property chart for a number of natural materials, with toughness plotted against Young's modulus, showing the unique toughness and flexural properties of skin (according to [27])

3.4 Intrinsic Factors

The role of intrinsic factors such as age, sex, and ethnicity on the wounding susceptibility of skin is complex. Silver et al. [28] have studied the viscoelastic mechanical properties of the human dermis in young (23-years-old) and old (87-years-old) donors, and found a significant decrease in the viscosity of skin with age (Fig. 3.3). This, they postulated, was attributable to a decrease in

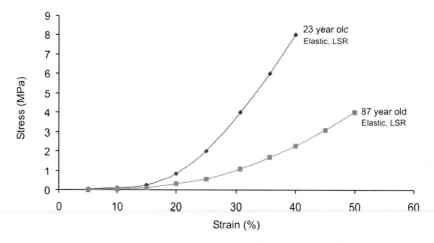

Fig. 3.3 Stress-strain curves for the dermis of a 23-year-old male donor and an 87-year-old male donor, showing loss of elasticity (low strain rate LSR) in the older individual (adopted from [28])

collagen fibril viscosity. With ageing, skin transforms itself in terms of composition, structural organisation and hence its properties. However, in spite of numerous studies, it has not been possible to obtain an accurate picture of the changes induced either by the passage of time (true ageing) or by repeated exposure to sunlight or smoking (actinic ageing). In general, skin becomes intrinsically less extensible as a result of an increase in the modulus of elasticity, and there is a notable decrease in the skin's ability to return to its original shape after being subjected to deformation [29]. This raises the question of the forensic significance of the parameters measured. While we know anecdotally that older skin is more fragile than younger skin, the notions of fragility, firmness, tone or elasticity cannot be reduced to simple physical measurements. Hence it remains difficult for forensic experts to take advantage of the published literature in reconstructing traumatic events in the elderly.

Site- and sex-dependent variations in skin thickness and mechanical properties were examined in vivo by Diridollou et al. [30]. They showed that skin is thicker, stiffer and less tense and elastic on the forehead than on the ventral forearm. They also showed that the skin on the forehead of men was significantly greater than women by about 13%, and that *Young's modulus* for forehead skin was not significantly higher for women than for men.

Ethnic differences in the biomechanical properties of skin have been minimally explored. Much of what is known about human skin is derived from studies of caucasoid skin, yet most of the population of the earth are darkly pigmented. However, marked differences between ethnic groups in skin extensibility, recovery and elastic modulus have been documented [31, 32]. Moreover, more darkly pigmented subjects have been shown to retain younger skin properties compared with the more lightly pigmented groups [33]. Although differences in intercellular cohesion are apparent between different ethnic groups, these findings are of doubtful use in the current interpretation of blunt force trauma.

One intrinsic property of skin that has a huge bearing upon the forensic interpretation of lacerations is the existence of skin tension lines (Langer's lines). In a series of papers Langer described the results of his method of systematically stabbing what he referred to as 'relatively fresh' cadavers [34, 35]. He found that stab wounds caused by a circular object would, in most cases, have an oval shape. This suggested that skin was under different amounts of natural tension in different directions. From these he derived a map of the lines of least cross-sectional tension of the human body – lines that are now referred to as Langer's lines. Since then Lee et al. [6] have shown that in response to blunt trauma to the face, skin breaks along these lines of least resistance, and hence the patterns of laceration generated are determined by inherent structural and biomechanical properties of the skin, rather than of subcutaneous attachments. Byard et al. [36] have recently called attention to the way in which Langer's lines may complicate the assessment of wounds at autopsy. Skin tension lines may transform round skin wounds into slit-like defects resembling sharp force stab wounds. Hence these lines need to be taken into consideration when craniofacial blunt force trauma is assessed at autopsy.

3.5 Extrinsic Factors

An obvious question that arises from what we know about the skin and its response to blunt trauma relates to the estimation of the force of the impact. For a given location and a given area of skin, does the force of impact determine the shape of the resultant laceration? In other words, can an observer infer the force of an attack from the shape of the blunt force injuries? As we have seen, a number of intrinsic factors affect wound morphology. The question now is, how do we quantify the blunt force needed to penetrate human skin?

The problem, of course, is that skin is so highly deformable. It has been said that skin is stressed at levels far below those of engineering materials, but may be strained at orders of magnitude more. Hence, the strain energy stored in the cheek skin during yawning is similar to that in mild steel at normal engineering stress [37]. As a result, measuring the resistance to fracture is difficult. Doran et al. [37] have, however, calculated the resistance of human skin samples to be $2.32 \pm 0.40\,\mathrm{kJm}^{-2}$.

Simplified, skin is a thin, multilayer membrane overlying muscle, fat and bone. The thickness of this arrangement is location dependent. Modelling of contact events is very important for a wide range of materials and engineering structures and has resulted in the development of a strong basic mechanics of this problem. Impact events play an important role in the tribology as well impact damage to structures especially at a localised impact site. For instance, the onset of cracking induced behaviour in brittle materials is very important to ensure their reliability. Deliberate contact events are the basis of simple methods to determine the mechanical properties such as hardness and elastic modulus of materials. This approach has become ever more popular with the development of thin coatings on most materials especially in the optical and micro-electronics industries. The pioneering studies of contact mechanics were initiated more than 100 years ago with the classic studies of Bousinesq and Hertz who investigated the stresses generated by a point contact and spherical or blunt contact [38]. An initial response may be had by considering simple elastic contact between the objects of relevance, namely say for instance a baseball bat of 60 mm diameter in contact with the skull which may be considered a sphere of 150 mm diameter. Knowing the elastic properties of both materials one may determine the contact dimensions and shape generated by a specific force. In the case of skin overlying bone the problem is more complex in that the thickness and properties of the skin and underlying bone need to be included. This is a major issue for the contact loading of multilayer materials. Again, as a first approximation, the contact may be considered elastic as this will enable the stresses in the skin tissue to be quantified and assist with identifying the locations of maximum tensile stress and the directions cracking is most likely to extend.

Shergold and Fleck [39] have sought to understand the fracture mechanics of human skin and a simulant (silicone rubber) by developing a micromechanical

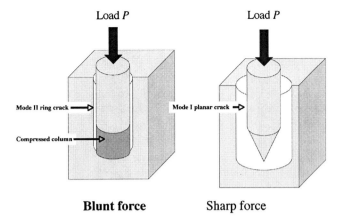

Fig. 3.4 Shergold and Fleck's model for the penetration of skin by a blunt punch (*left*) and a sharp punch (*right*) (according to [38])

model for deep penetration of a blunt and sharp-tipped cylindrical punch. Their model shows that the mechanism of penetration depends upon the geometry of the punch tip. While a blunt tip penetrates by the growth of a ring (mode II or tearing) crack, a sharp tip wedges open a planar (mode I – opening) crack. The blunt punch penetrates by an unstable crack advance and results in a compressed column of material at the bottom of the cylindrical cavity thus created (Fig. 3.4). In contrast, the sharp punch tunnels into the tissue at a penetration pressure several times lower than that of a blunt punch. This implies that blunt force injury requires more energy than sharp force injury, and that the former will result in larger, more irregular wounding.

3.6 Biomechanical Modelling

Blunt force trauma plays a central role in the forensic reconstruction of injuries. As we have seen, there is considerable empirical, experimental, and theoretical evidence that such interpretations are highly complex and multifactorial. What is needed is a simple model of blunt force trauma that can be used to reveal the basic biomechanical mechanisms that control for given wounding patterns under variable loads and from various impact surfaces. One such model is that of Thali et al. [40] which employed a drop tube with a weighted body impacting at an angle onto a skin-skull-brain model. Although they did not analyse their results, they did document close resemblance with real blunt force injuries, such as tissue bridges of the artificial skin.

Our own drop-tube model consisted of a medium density open-celled polyurethane foam to which is bonded a silicone skin simulant. The foam is allowed

Fig. 3.5 *Top*: typical
postmortem view of linear
laceration (courtesy of Prof
Michael Tsokos, Berlin,
Germany). *Bottom*:
characteristic linear wound
shape generated from a
perpendicular blunt impact
onto fluid-filled sponge

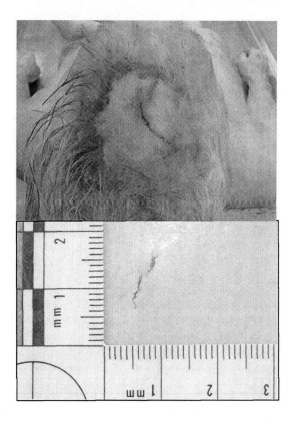

to absorb water, whereupon it is placed beneath the droptube and subjected to
various levels of impact energy. As stated earlier, skin exhibits rate-dependent
elastic properties (Fig. 3.1), which are highly fluid dependent. In other words,
skin has a threshold of energy absorption per unit time; hence, fast impact will

(A)   (B)

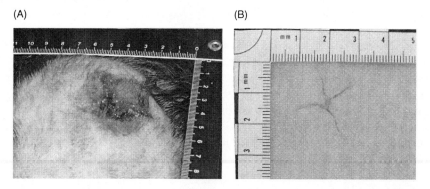

Fig. 3.6 *Top*: typical postmortem view of stellate laceration (courtesy of Prof Michael Tsokos,
Berlin, Germany). *Bottom*: characteristic stellate wound shape generated from a perpendicular blunt impact onto fluid-filled sponge

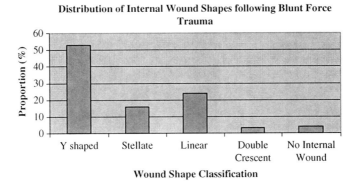

Fig. 3.7 The distribution of internal wound shapes generated by a skin simulant model subjected to perpendicular blunt force trauma

be met with more rigidity than slower impact. To mimic this, we allowed the sponge to absorb water before the wounding experiment.

Initial, unpublished results indicate that there were four discrete wound shapes created by perpendicular 5 kg blunt impact on our skin simulant models. These were classified as stellate, linear, double crescent or Y-shaped and corresponded to blunt force lacerations seen at autopsy (Figs. 3.5 and 3.6). The percentage distribution of internal wound types generated by our skin simulant model (subjected to 49 N and 24.5 J) is given in Fig. 3.7, and suggests that Y-shaped lacerations are the most common result of perpendicular blunt force trauma, followed by linear and stellate forms.

Regardless of whether an external laceration was created following perpendicular impact, an internal "wound" was created. Intriguingly, this suggests that in life, blunt force trauma may result in subcutaneous cavitation, even when the skin is not actually breached. This might result in haematoma formation, and may have implications for bloodstain pattern analysis, as such blood-filled cavitation may become a reservoir of blood to be spattered by subsequent blows.

References

1. Messerer O (1884) Experimentelle Untersuchungen über Schädelbrüche. Rieger, München
2. Walcher K (1929) Ueber traumatische Spalt- und Höhlenbildungen innerhalb der weichen Schädelbedeckungen und deren praktische diagnostische Bedeutung. Dtsch Z Gerichtl Med 28:128–134
3. Tornheim P, Liwnicz B, Hirch C, Brown D, McLaurin R (1983) Acute responses to blunt head trauma. J Neurosurg 59:431–438
4. Zugibe F, Costello J (1986) Identification of the murder weapon by intricate patterned injury measurements. J Forensic Sci 31:773–777
5. Saukko P, Knight B (2004) Knight's forensic pathology, 3rd edn. Arnold, London

6. Lee RH, Gamble WB, Mayer MH, Manson PN (1997) Patterns of facial laceration from blunt trauma. Plast Reconstr Surg 99:1544–1554
7. Ankers J, Birkbeck AE, Thomson RD, Vanezis P (1999) Puncture resistance and tensile strength of skin simulants. Proc Inst Mech Eng (H) 213:493–501
8. Ambade V, Godbole H (2006) Comparison of wound patterns in homicide by sharp and blunt force. Forensic Sci Int 156:166–170
9. Murphy G (1991) Beaten to death: an autopsy series of homicidal blunt force injuries. Am J Forensic Med Pathol 12:98–101
10. Strauch H, Wirth I, Taymoorian U, Geserick G (2001) Kicking to death – forensic and criminological aspects. Forensic Sci Int 123:165–171
11. Ong T, Dudley M (1999) Craniofacial trauma presenting at an adult accident and emergency department with an emphasis on soft tissue injuries. Injury 30:357–363
12. Stron C, Nordenram A, Johanson G (1991) Injuries due to violent crimes: a study of police reported assaults during 1979, 1982 and 1985 in a police district of Stockholm, Sweden. Med Sci Law 31:251–258
13. Avis SP (1996) Homicide in Newfoundland: a nine-year review. J Forensic Sci 41:101–105
14. Rogde S, Hougen HP, Poulsen K (2003) Homicide by blunt force in two Scandinavian capitals. Am J Forensic Med Pathol 24:288–291
15. Henderson JP, Morgan SE, Patel F, Tiplady ME (2005) Patterns of non-firearm homicide. J Clin Forensic Med 12:128–132
16. Lo S, Aslam N (2005) Mechanisms and pattern of facial lacerations in the accident department. Int J Clin Pract 59:333–335
17. DiMaio V, DiMaio D (1993) Forensic pathology. CRC Press, Boca Raton
18. Henry T (2003) Blunt force injuries. In: Froede R (ed) Handbook of forensic pathology, 2nd edn. College of American Pathologists, Illinois
19. Pollak S, Saukko P (2000) Blunt injury. In: Siegel J, Saukko P, Knupfer G (eds) Encyclopaedia of forensic sciences. Academic Press, San Diego
20. Payne P (1991) Measurement of properties and function of skin. Clin Res Physiol Meas 12:105–129
21. Dunn MG, Silver FH (1983) Viscoelastic behaviour of human connective tissues: relative contribution of viscous and elastic components. Connect Tiss Res 12:59–70
22. Silver FH, Kato YP, Ohno M, Wasserman AJ (1992) Analysis of mammalian connective tissue: relationship between hierarchical structures and mechanical properties. J Long-term Effect Med Implants 2:165–198
23. Silver FH, Freeman JW, DeVore D (2001) Viscoelastic properties of human skin and processed dermis. Skin Res Tech 7:18–23
24. Gordon JE (1978) Structures. Plenum, New York
25. Bischoff JE, Arruda EM, Grosh K (2000) Finite element modeling of human skin using an isotropic, nonlinear elstic constitutive model. J Biomech 33:645–652
26. Daly CH (1982) Biomechanical properties of dermis. J Invest Dermatol 79(Suppl 1): 17s–20s
27. Ashby MF, Gibson LJ, Wegst U, Olive R (1995) The mechanical properties of natural materials. 1 Material property charts. Proc Math Phys Sciences 450:123–140
28. Silver FH, Seehra GP, Freeman JW, DeVore D (2002) Viscoelastic properties of young and old human dermis: a proposed molecular mechanism for elastic energy storage in collagen and elastin. J Appl Polym Sci 86:1978–1985
29. Batisse D, Bazin R, Baldeweck T, Querleux B, Leveque JL (2002) Influence of age on the wrinkling capacities of skin. Skin Res Tech 8:148–154
30. Diridollou S, Black D, Lagarde JM, Gall Y, Berson M et al. (2000) Sex and site dependent variations in the thickness and mechanical properties of human skin in vivo. Int J Cosmet Sci 22:421–435
31. Berardesca E, DeRigal J, Leveque JL, Maibach HI (1991) In vivo biophysiological characterisation of skin physiological differences in races. Dermatologica 182:89–93

32. Wesley NO, Maibach HI (2003) Racial (ethnic) differences in skin properties. Am J Clin Dermatol 4:843–860
33. Rawlins AV (2006) Ethnic skin types: are there differences in skin structure and function? Int J Cosmet Sci 28:79–93
34. Langer K (1978) On the anatomy and physiology of the skin I. Cleavability of the cutis. Brit J Plastic Surg 31:3–8
35. Langer K (1978) On the anatomy and physiology of the skin II. Elasticity of the cutis. Brit J Plastic Surg 31:185–199
36. Byard RW, Gehl A, Tsokos M (2005) Skin tension and cleavage lines (Langer's lines) causing distortion of ante- and postmortem wound morphology. Int J Legal Med 119:226–230
37. Doran CF, McCormack BAO, Macey A (2004) A simplified model to determine the contribution of strain energy in the failure process of thin biological membranes during cutting. Strain 40:173–179
38. Lawn BR, Wilshaw TR (1973) Indentation fracture: principles and applications. J Mater Sci 10:1049–1073
39. Shergold OA, Fleck NA (2004) Mechanisms of deep penetration of soft solids, with application to the injection and wounding of skin. Proc Roy Soc A Math Phys Eng Sci 460:3037–3058
40. Thali MJ, Kneubuehl BP, Dirnhofer R (2002) A skin-skull-brain model for the biomechanical reconstruction of blunt forces to the human head. Forensic Sci Int 125:195–200

Chapter 4
Electrocution and the Autopsy

Regula Wick and Roger W. Byard

Contents

Abstract Deaths due to the passage of electric current through the body are most often accidental, although suicides and homicides may occasionally occur. Electrical energy represents electron flow, or current, between two points with

R.W. Byard
University of Adelaide, Adelaide, South Australia, Australia
e-mail: byard.roger@saugov.sa.gov.au

M. Tsokos (ed.), *Forensic Pathology Reviews, Volume 5*,
doi: 10.1007/978-1-59745-110-9_4, © Humana Press, Totowa, NJ 2008

different potentials, measured in voltage. The amount of current is determined by the resistance of the conducting material. Electrocutions involving humans may be due to low voltages (<1000 V), high voltage (>1000 V), or to lightning. Deaths are caused by a direct effect of current on the heart, resulting in ventricular fibrillation, on respiratory muscles resulting in respiratory paralysis or on the brainstem respiratory centers. Deaths may also be caused by thermal effects of current, or by trauma or drowning associated with exposure to an electrical current, or to multiorgan failure complicating initial injuries. The autopsy assessment of possible electrocution is complicated by the non-specificity and subtlety of lesions. Victims may have classical targetoid electrical burns of the skin with central charring, surrounding pallor and hyperemic rims. There may also be adjacent nodules of burnt keratin due to arcing of current. Victims of lightning strikes may demonstrate the typical ferning pattern of Lichtenberg figures. Conversely, other cases, e.g., electrocutions occurring in water, may have no pathological indicators of electrical injury. For this reason, the investigation of possible electrocution requires careful evaluation of the death scene and assessment of the electrical safety of the building and any electrical equipment that had been used. Meticulous examination of all body surfaces for subtle electrical burns with histological sampling is also required.

Keywords Electrocution · Lightning · Electrical burn · Entry mark · Metallization · Forensic pathology

4.1 Introduction

Electrocution refers to death caused by the passage of an electric current through the body. While not all cases are lethal, the potential effects of contact with electricity are well recognized, with the word "electrocution" deriving from a combination of the words "electricity" and "execution". Such deaths are unusual and are usually due to accidents caused by faulty devices, or by carelessness or misuse of electrical equipment. Suicides and homicides associated with electricity are even less common. Judicial execution by electricity occurs in countries such as the United States [1, 2].

Electricity may have a variety of effects on the body, ranging from only minor shocks not associated with any injuries, to lethal cardiac arrhythmias. The morphological findings following fatal exposure to an electric current may also vary considerably, with some cases having no demonstrable pathological features, others showing characteristic electrical burns that may be patterned reflecting the nature of the surface contacted, and yet others demonstrating extensive and deep burning. This wide range of findings sometimes makes the diagnosis of electrocution at postmortem difficult and emphasizes the need for a careful death scene investigation in all cases [1, 2].

4.2 Electricity

Electricity is a form of energy resulting from the flow of electrons between two points with a potential difference. The flow of electrons, or current, is measured in amperes (A), and the potential difference in volts (V). The rate-limiting step in current flow is often the resistance to electron flow of the material between the points of different potential. This is measured in ohms. The relationship of amperes, volts and ohms is expressed in Ohm's law as amperes = volts/ohms (A = V/R). This means that the amount of the current flow (amperes) is proportional to the voltage of the source and inversely proportional to the resistance of the material conducting the current [1].

For an electrical current to pass through the body a circuit has to be completed [2]. The amount of tissue damage and physiological effects of exposure to an electrical current then depend on the type of current (AC = alternating current or DC = direct current), the amount of current, the voltage, the resistance encountered, the duration of the event, and the route of the current [3].

4.2.1 Type of Current

Alternating current is more dangerous than direct current as it causes fatalities at lower amperage, is more likely to generate cardiac arrhythmias, and may prevent a victim from releasing his/her grasp of a conductor due to tetanic spasm of muscles. It has been deemed four to six times more likely to cause death [4, 5].

4.2.2 Current

The amperage is the most important factor in electrocution, but is obviously related to both voltage and resistance through Ohm's Law. It has been estimated that an individual exposed to a current of 40 mA will lose consciousness and that death is likely after several seconds of exposure to current over 50–80 mA [5]. The effects of increasing current are summarized in Table 4.1.

Table 4.1 The effects of increasing current flow (according to [1]); mA = milliamperes, A = amperes

1 mA	Barely perceptile tingle
16 mA	Current that can be grasped and released
16–20 mA	Muscular paralysis
20–50 mA	Respiratory paralysis
50–100 mA	Ventricular fibrillation
>2000 mA	Ventricular standstill

4.2.3 Voltage

Deaths caused by electrocution are attributed to low-voltages (<1000 V), high-voltages (>1000 V) or lightning [3, 6], with most deaths occurring at voltages of 110–380 V, which is the voltage range of homes and industrial works [7]. Electrocutions at very low voltages (<80 V) are rare, although this may occur if humidity reduces resistance or there is prolonged contact [8, 9]. High-voltage electrocutions may occur without direct contact between the victim and a conductor due to arcing through air. Arcs can generate extremely high temperatures (up to 5000°C) and so deaths may be due to the flow of current itself, or to severe burns [1]. Significant injuries may also result from falls if the victim is flung away from the conductor due to muscle contractions; for example a worker who falls from a high voltage power line.

4.2.4 Resistance

Body tissues have very variable resistance to electric currents with the highest levels found in bones, fat and tendons, and the lowest in nerves, blood, mucous membranes, and muscles. Thus, exposure of different parts of the body to the same voltage will generate different current (amperage). Internal resistance is estimated to be between 500 and 1000 ohms. Skin has an intermediate resistance depending on the thickness and also on the dampness. For example, dry skin may have a resistance of 100,000 ohms, whereas for water- or sweat-soaked skin the resistance often drops to 1000 ohms [1,6,10]. The very low resistance of moist and thin mucous membranes increases the danger of severe orofacial injuries in young children who may put electrical leads in their mouths [11, 12]. Thickened and callused hands have the greatest resistance.

4.2.5 Duration of Contact

The possibility of a lethal event often increases with the time of contact with a conductor. For this reason, deaths have been reported with voltages as low as 24 V when contact has been maintained for several hours. This also explains the paradox of survival with high voltage electrocution, when muscle spasms result in the victim being thrown back away from the conductor, thus dramatically decreasing the duration of current exposure. Conversely, muscle spasm causing a victim to grip a conductor may have the opposite effect by prolonging contact.

4.2.6 Route of the Current

The path of current through the body is another important factor determining outcome, and passage of current through the heart or through the brain increases the risk of a fatal outcome [2, 13]. Current generally passes from the contact point to the nearest earthed point. This is often from hand to foot or from hand to hand.

4.3 Lightning

Lightning is caused by atmospheric electricity and can produce temperatures of up to 30,000°C with currents of 20,000 A and potentials of up to 100,000,000 V [14]. Deaths due to lightning are rare events and result from the effects of high voltage direct current with a variety of mechanisms [15]. Lightning may directly strike a victim or may be conducted through another object. Examples of these two situations include a golfer being directly struck while standing on a course, or being indirectly struck through an upraised metal club. A side flash strike refers to the situation where an object adjacent to the victim suffers a direct strike that is followed by a secondary discharge from the object; e.g., a golfer sheltering beneath a tree may be hit secondarily. With step potentials, lightning hits the ground and then enters a victim's body through one foot and exits from the other. Finally, a victim may be so highly charged during a strike that they discharge an upward "streamer" [14]. Lightning may be quite capricious in its effects with cases occurring where only one person in a group exposed to the same conditions suffered lethal injury [16].

The flash-over phenomenon refers to the passage of electrical current from lightning over the surface of the body, often causing vaporization of surface water with a blast effect to clothing and shoes [1]. Torn clothing and shoes may suggest to investigators that the victim has been subject to blunt force trauma such as a motor vehicle accident rather than a lightning strike. Very rarely deaths have occurred indoors when a victim was using a telephone and the line was struck by lightning. One death per year has been attributed to telephone-related lightning injuries in the United States, with survivors manifesting deafness from ruptured tympanic membranes, transient vertigo, ataxia, neurological deficits and convulsions [17, 18]. In addition to the pathological findings of lightning strike detailed below, victims may have singed hair and retinal detachments [14].

4.4 Mechanism of Death

In deaths from electrocution the lethal event may be directly due to the electrical energy itself, or to the secondary effects of burns or blunt injuries due to falls precipitated by the electric shock [10]. The immediate mechanism of death due to the passage of current through the body usually involves one or more of the following [2, 19]. Delayed deaths may be due to multisystem complications following the initial event [20].

4.4.1 Ventricular Fibrillation

This is considered to be the commonest cause of death and follows the passage of electrical current through the heart. The precise effect of electrical current on the myocardium is ill understood; however it is most likely involves a direct action on cardiac myocytes, nodal tissue and conduction tracts.

4.4.2 Respiratory Paralysis

This is much less common than cardiac arrhythmias and involves passage of current through the chest with respiratory paralysis due to severe contraction of respiratory muscles, such as the diaphragm and intercostal muscles, with resultant asphyxia and cardiac arrest. It is more often seen in high voltage deaths.

4.4.3 Paralysis of the Respiratory Centre

This may rarely occur if current passes through the respiratory centre in the brainstem causing disruption of neural function due to the direct effect of electrical current or secondarily to hyperthermia.

4.4.4 Blunt Trauma

Contact with electrical current may cause an individual to be thrown back with considerable force resulting in potentially lethal traumatic injuries.

4.4.5 Drowning

Cases have been reported where individuals in swimming pools have drowned following electrical shocks [21].

4.5 Environmental Factors

The amount of electric current passing through a victim is often heavily influenced by environmental conditions and this is another reason why a full evaluation of the death scene should be undertaken by personnel experienced in the assessment of electrical deaths. For example, an individual wearing rubber boots and standing on dry insulating material may sustain only a minimal shock from the same faulty circuitry that might kill a second person standing with bare feet on a wet metal surface.

4.6 Autopsy Findings

4.6.1 General Remarks

Electrical injuries can be separated into three main groups: direct tissue damage caused by the electric current itself, thermal damage from the conversion of electrical to thermal energy, and traumatic injuries from muscle contractions causing bone fractures or injuries from falls [1, 13, 22]. Particular injury patterns may occur in different parts and tissues of the body.

4.6.2 Skin

Characteristic skin lesions due to an electrical current generally appear in low-voltage injuries as burns at the entry and the exit sites of current. They are not always present, however, being found in only 57–83% of cases, as the occurrence and severity of burns depends on several factors, such as the amount of current flow per unit time, the voltage and the length of time of exposure. For example, if there is a low current passing for a short time, no burns will necessarily be produced and no marks may be detected on the skin [1, 2, 6, 15, 23]. Electrical burns of the fingers may also be difficult to visualise if finger flexion is maintained by rigor mortis.

The initial effect that an electrical current has on skin when there is good contact is to cause heating and vaporization of fluid resulting in blister formation. After the current stops, the blister collapses, sometimes with splitting of the epidermis. The usual appearance is of a small, circumscribed, crater-like, indurated lesion that has a grey or black centre (if there is charring) surrounded by a zone of pallor caused by arteriolar spasm and coagulative necrosis. Sometimes there is a

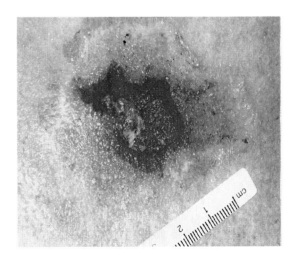

Fig. 4.1 A typical electrical burn of the skin demonstrating charring of the center with surrounding blanching and a hyperemic rim

Fig. 4.2 A series of "spark" lesions caused by arcing of high voltage current resulting in nodular coalescence of melted keratin

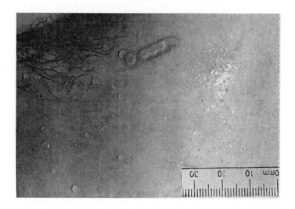

surrounding zone of hyperemia (Fig. 4.1) with small vesicles. Spark burns occur when the contact is less firm and the voltage is high resulting in arcing of current with melting of keratin into small nodules (Fig. 4.2). Electrical burns often show an admixture of these two kinds of lesions. It is also possible for such lesions to be produced after death and so antemortem and postmortem lesions are not able to be separated histopathologically if death occurs rapidly before a tissue inflammatory response has occurred.

The entry mark generally shows the shape and the size of the conductor [2]; for example a linear burn from a live wire (Fig. 4.3), or three evenly spaced burns from an electric plug. The pattern of electrical burns may give an indication of torture or homicide. No marks on the skin may be seen if the contact point was broad, for example with electrocution in a bath, where much of the body surface is exposed to the conductor and resistance is considerably reduced due to the water, that also cools the skin, thus preventing burns [21]. In these circumstances there may be linear marking of the skin at the level of the water, although this is not specific to electrical deaths [24].

Occasionally the phenomenon of "metallization" may be observed, providing evidence that a burn was due to an electrical current. Metallization occurs when

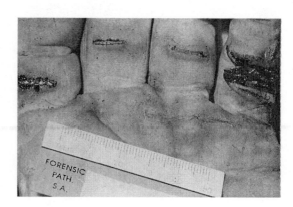

Fig. 4.3 Linear burns of the fingers caused by grasping a live electrical wire

Fig. 4.4 Deep charring of the side of the foot in a case of high voltage electrocution

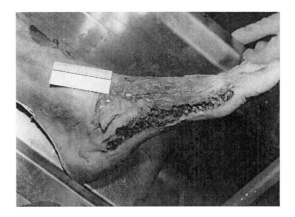

tissue anions combine with the metal of an electrode to form metallic salts that may be seen on the surface of the skin. If an electrical arc forms, the skin may be coated with a thin layer of vaporized metal. A bright green colour may be seen with brass or copper electrodes. Metal residue can also be demonstrated by chemical testing or visualised by scanning electron microscopy [5].

High voltage electrocution may cause severe burning of multiple areas of the body with deep charring (Fig. 4.4). There may also be multiple current arcs so that numerous spark burns occur (Fig. 4.5) producing a "crocodile skin" effect. High voltages due to lightning may also cause so-called arbors, ferns, Lichtenberg figures or keraunographic markings. These are multiple brick-red to brown linear macules in a ferning pattern on the skin possibly caused by heat denaturation of red blood cells resulting in a distinctive pattern of hemolysis [6]. Histological examination of Lichtenberg figures shows no specific features other than dermal and subcutaneous vascular congestion [16]. This pattern will disappear within 24 h if the victim survives [18]. More common than Lichtenberg figures are linear burns that follow skin creases (Fig. 4.6).

Fig. 4.5 Multiple punctate burns of the arm from contact with a high voltage power line. The victim was moving a boat when the metal mast came in contact with overhead power lines. The lesions were caused by arcing of current

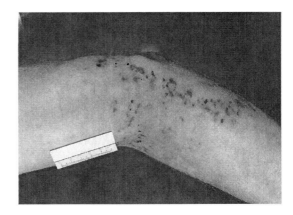

Fig. 4.6 Irregular linear
burns of the flank in a case
of lighting strike are more
common than the classical
arborising pattern of
fine branching, so-called
Lichtenberg figures

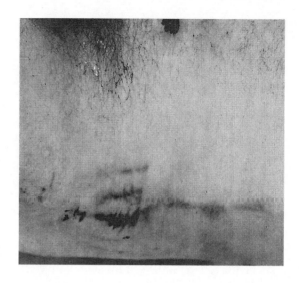

While conjunctival and internal petechiae have been reported in up to three
quarters of cases of electrocution in some series, this is not the general experience
[15, 23].

Histological findings in electrical injuries are essentially due to thermal
effects with no pathognomonic lesions, despite earlier literature that suggested
this. There is often an abrupt transition from normal to abnormal skin, with
separation of the cells of the lower epidermis with microvesicle formation
(Fig. 4.7), coagulative necrosis extending into the dermis [2]. Cell nuclei show
pyknosis and elongation with alignment. Although this "nuclear streaming"
was thought to be due to the passage of electrical current, it is not a specific
finding and may be found in other types of burns and in hypothermia [24].

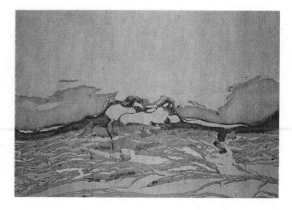

Fig. 4.7 Histologic section
of an electrical burn with
focal coagulative necrosis
and blistering of the
epidermis

4.6.3 Other Organs

The heart may show scattered foci of myocardial necrosis with subendocardial hemorrhages and contraction bands; however these are essentially non-specific findings. Vascular injuries may result in damage to vessel intima and media that may lead to subsequent thrombosis, rupture or aneurysm formation if there is survival [10, 13].

Soft tissue and visceral injuries may result from falls due to electricity causing muscle contractions. Long bone fractures, vertebral crush fractures and joint dislocations may be directly caused by muscle contractions, in addition to impact from falls [1, 22]. Intramuscular hemorrhages are a rare finding caused by tetanic current-induced muscle contractions [25]. Contraction bands in skeletal muscle are a regular but non-specific finding [26]. High voltage electrocution may result in marked heating of bones with so-called "osseous pearls" found on the cortices of the burnt bones [2].

Prolonged exposure to an electric current may also cause internal markings. For example, Anders et al. reported a suicide by electrocution where the victim was connected to current for several days. At autopsy, a blackish linear mark with histological changes attributed to an electrical current was found in the parietal pleura of the left thoracic cavity between external skin markings [24].

Central nervous system effects are similarly non-specific with reports of cerebral edema, petechial hemorrhages, demyelinization and cellular vacuolisation [10, 13]. Rupture of the tympanic membrane of the ear has been described following lightning strike [16, 27, 28].

4.7 Manner of Death

4.7.1 Accidents

Accident is the most common manner of death in electrocution and is the fifth leading cause of occupation-related death in the United States. Typically, the victim is a young male and the accident occurs in the summer months [7, 15, 29, 30], most likely related to increased outdoor activities during this time of the year, and possibly sweating decreasing skin resistance [7]. Accidental electrocutions may be even more common in countries where housing standards are suboptimal and electrical safety requirements are not strictly enforced [2].

Low-voltage accidents usually occur with household and work activities. High-voltage accidents occur with certain outdoor or work-related activities. Lightning strikes are invariably outdoor occurrences. Autoerotic fatalities, where the victim has been using an electrical device for sexual stimulation, form a distinct and uncommon subgroup of accidental electrical deaths [31, 32].

4.7.2 Suicide

Suicidal electrocution is uncommon and may be separated into two groups. One group consists of individuals who have some knowledge of electricity such as electricians or electrical engineers. They often use complicated systems with time switches, sometimes in combination with drugs. The other group consists of those who opportunistically use electricity to terminate their lives, such as individuals who sit in a bath and drop a device such as a hairdryer or lamp into the water [4, 9, 15, 24, 33, 34, 35].

4.7.3 Homicide

Very few cases of homicidal electrocution have been reported; Karger et al. found two homicides in 37 cases, Wright and Davis found only one homicide out of 220 cases of electrical fatalities, and other studies have reported no homicides [3, 6, 15, 23].

4.8 The Investigation of Electrical Deaths

The investigation of deaths possibly due to electrocution requires a team approach with a clear description of the death scene, including photographic documentation of the body, scene and any nearby electrical devices or conductors. An analysis of the electrical circuitry within, and sometimes connecting to, the building where the victim was found is required in addition to examination of any equipment that was near the body by individuals fully qualified in electrical assessment [6]. A complete autopsy with careful examination of clothing and body surfaces for subtle electrical burns is then required. Clothes may show burns corresponding to contact with metallic conductors and torn clothing with burned shoes may implicate lightning [13, 28]. Examination of the body for evidence of underlying natural diseases such as cardiovascular conditions is also important, as these may have predisposed the victim to coming in contact with live circuitry, or may have reduced the victim's capacity to survive an electric shock.

The most difficult cases are often those where a body is presented to autopsy with a history of "collapse" or being "found dead", with no indication that electrocution is a possibility. It may be necessary to ask police to return to a scene and check for electrical devices if electrocution is suspected. A history of screaming, swearing, or shouting followed by collapse may indicate electrocution. Early or partial development of rigor mortis may also indicate electrocution as tetany from electrical current may accelerate the development of rigor [6]. Careful examination of all body surfaces, including the flexor surfaces of the fingers, with photography and histological sampling of possible electrical burns is required.

A not insignificant part of identifying electrocution as a cause of death lies in need to protect others who may be exposed to the same dangerous environment or unsafe piece of equipment unless an accurate assessment of the factors leading up to the fatal episode is made.

References

1. Koumbourlis AC (2002) Electrical injuries. Crit Care Med 30:S424–430
2. Al-Alousi LM (1990) Homicide by electrocution. Med Sci Law 30:239–246
3. Mellen PF, Weedn VW, Kao G (1992) Electrocution: a review of 155 cases with emphasis on human factors. J Forensic Sci 37:1016–1022
4. Budnick LD (1984) Bathtub-related electrocutions in the United States, 1979–1982. JAMA 252:918–920
5. Saukko P, Knight B (2004) Knight's forensic pathology, 3rd edn. Arnold, London, pp 326–338
6. Wright RK, Davis JH (1980) The investigation of electrical deaths: a report of 220 fatalities. J Forensic Sci 25:514–521
7. Fatovich DM (1992) Electrocution in Western Australia, 1976–1990. Med J Aust 157:762–764
8. Peng Z, Shikui C (1995) Study on electrocution death by low-voltage. Forensic Sci Int 76:115–119
9. Marc B, Baudry F, Douceron H, Ghaith A, Wepierre J-L, Garnier M (2000) Suicide by electrocution with low-voltage current. J Forensic Sci 45:216–222
10. Leibovici D, Shemer J, Shapira SC (1995) Electrical injuries: current concepts. Injury 26:623–627
11. Thompson JC, Ashwal S (1983) Electrical injuries in children. Am J Dis Child 137:231–235
12. Yamazaki M, Bai H, Tun Z, Ogura Y, Wakasugi C (1997) An electrocution death of an infant who had received an electrical shock from an uncovered oval shaped lamp switch in his mouth while in a hospital. J Forensic Sci 42:151–154
13. Anders S, Tsokos M, Püschel K (2002) Nachweis der Stromwirkung und des Stromweges im Körper. Rechtsmedizin 12:1–9
14. Blumenthal R (2005) Lightning fatalities on the South African highveld. A retrospective descriptive study for the period 1997–2000. Am J Forensic Med Pathol 26:66–69
15. Hyldgaard L, Søndergaard E, Leth P (2004) Autopsies of fatal electrocutions in Jutland. Scand J Forensic Sci 1:8–12
16. Resnik BI, Wetli CV (1996) Lichtenberg figures. Am J Forensic Med Pathol 17:99–102
17. Andrews CJ (1992) Telephone-related lightning injury. Med J Aust 157:823–826
18. Qureshi NH (1995) Indirect lightning strike via telephone wire. Injury 26:629–630
19. Lee WR (1965) The mechanisms of death from electric shock. Med Sci Law 18:23–28
20. Bailey B, Forget S, Gaudreault P (2001) Prevalence of potential risk factors in victims of electrocution. Forensic Sci Int 123:58–62
21. Goodson ME (1993) Electrically induced deaths involving water immersion. Am J Forensic Med Pathol 14:330–333
22. Martinez JA, Nguyen T (2000) Electrical injuries. South Med J 93:1165–1168
23. Karger B, Süggeler O, Brinkmann B (2002) Electrocution – autopsy study with emphasis on "electrical petechiae". Forensic Sci Int 126:210–213
24. Anders S, Matschke J, Tsokos M (2001) Internal current mark in a case of suicide by electrocution. Am J Forensic Med Pathol 22:370–373
25. Anders S, Schulz F, Tsokos M (2000) Ausgeprägte intramuskuläre Hämorrhagien vitaler Genese bei letaler suizidaler Strombeibringung. Rechtsmedizin 10:105–109

26. Püschel K, Brinkmann B, Lieske K (1985) Ultrastructural alterations of skeletal muscles after electric shock. Am J Forensic Med Pathol 6:296–300
27. Kristensen S, Tveterås K (1985) Lightning-induced acoustic rupture of the tympanic membrane: (a report of two cases). J Laryngol Otol 99:711–713
28. Cherington M, Kurtzman R, Krider EP, Yarnell PR (2001) Mountain medical mystery. Unwitnessed death of a healthy young man, caused by lightning. Am J Forensic Med Pathol 22:296–298
29. Taylor AJ, McGwin G Jr, Davis GG, Brissie RM, Rue LW III (2002) Occupational electrocutions in Jefferson County, Alabama. Occup Med 52:102–106
30. Taylor AJ, McGwin G Jr, Valent F, Rue LW III (2002) Fatal occupational electrocutions in the United States. Inj Prev 8:306–312
31. Shields LBE, Hunsaker DM, Hunsaker JC III, Wetli CV, Hutchins KD, Holmes RM (2005) Atypical autoerotic death: Part II. Am J Forensic Med Pathol 26:53–62
32. Klintschar M, Grabuschnigg P, Beham A (1998) Death from electrocution during autoerotic practice: case report and review of the literature. Am J Forensic Med Pathol 19:190–193
33. Bligh-Glover WZ, Miller FP, Balraj EK (2004) Two cases of suicidal electrocution. Am J Forensic Pathol 25:255–258
34. Fernando R, Liyanage S (1990) Suicide by electrocution. Med Sci Law 30:219–220
35. Byard RW, Hanson KA, Gilbert JD, James RA, Nadeau J, Blackbourne B, Krous HF (2003) Death due to electrocution in childhood and early adolescence. J Paediatr Child Health 39:46–48

Part III
Forensic Neuropathology

Chapter 5
Central Nervous System Alterations in Alcohol Abuse

Andreas Büttner and Serge Weis

Contents

Abstract Alcohol abuse and dependence is a serious medical and economic problem in the Western countries as its effects on the central nervous system (CNS) are wide-ranging. The main factors contributing to alcohol-induced brain damage are associated with nutritional deficiencies and repeated withdrawal syndrome. CNS lesions associated with alcoholism include brain atrophy and central pontine myelinolysis. At least four distinct conditions leading to dementia, i.e. Wernicke-Korsakoff syndrome, hepatocerebral degeneration, Marchiafava-Bignami disease, and pellagrous encephalopathy, have a close association with chronic alcoholism, whereby the role of alcohol in their causation is secondary. A disproportionate loss of cerebral white matter relative to cerebral cortex suggests that a major neurotoxic effect of chronic alcohol consumption affects the white matter. Brain atrophy in alcoholics has been demonstrated in various studies. There is a regional selectivity, with the frontal lobes being particularly affected,

A. Büttner
Institute of Legal Medicine, University of Munich, Munich, Germany
e-mail: Andreas.Buettner@med.uni-muenchen.de

M. Tsokos (ed.), *Forensic Pathology Reviews, Volume 5,*
doi: 10.1007/978-1-59745-110-9_5, © Humana Press, Totowa, NJ 2008

which might explain the high incidence of cognitive dysfunction observed in alcoholics. In functional genomic studies reported so far, the identity and the number of dysregulated genes, the specific pathways involved and the direction of change show profound interstudy variations and, thus, remain inconclusive.

Keywords Alcohol · Central nervous system · Central pontine myelinolysis · Wernicke-Korsakoff syndrome · Neuropathology · Forensic pathology

5.1 Introduction

Alcohol abuse and dependence are serious medical and economic problems in the Western countries as the effects of alcohol on the central nervous system (CNS) are wide ranging. Direct toxicity of ethanol and its first metabolite acetaldehyde accounts for some of these effects by altering basic physiological and neurochemical functions [1], which ultimately result in structural damage. At the cellular level, alcohol affects brain function primarily by interfering with the action of glutamate, gamma amino butyric acid (GABA), and other neurotransmitters [2].

Similar to other drugs of abuse, the mesolimbic dopaminergic reward pathways are crucial for the reinforcing effects of alcohol and play a central role in alcohol addiction [3, 4, 5, 6, 7, 8, 9]. Recent knowledge of the neurobiological basis of alcoholism suggests that the pharmacological and behavioral effects of alcohol are mediated through its action on neuronal signal transduction pathways and ion channels, G-protein coupled receptors and other receptor systems [10, 11].

Sudden death in alcoholics is nearly equally distributed between trauma, natural causes, acute intoxication and alcohol-related diseases [12]. Upon forensic autopsy, brain abnormalities in alcoholics have been described to occur in up to 70% of the persons [13]. CNS lesions associated with alcoholism include brain atrophy and central pontine myelinolysis. Other frequent findings are myelopathy, neuropathy, subdural hematoma and/or cortical contusions and cerebrovascular lesions [13, 14]. Approximately 10% of alcoholics develop an organic mental disorder/severe cognitive impairments [15]. At least four distinct dementing conditions – Wernicke-Korsakoff syndrome, acquired hepatocerebral degeneration, Marchiafava-Bignami disease, and pellagrous encephalopathy – have a close association with chronic alcoholism; however, the role of alcohol in the causation is secondary [16]. Alcoholic dementia is said to consist of global severe amnesia and intellectual impairment [17, 18, 19]. However, the question whether there is a persistent dementia attributable to the direct toxic effects of alcohol on the brain is still unclear. This is mainly due to the fact that a primary alcoholic dementia lacks a distinctive, well-defined pathology. Therefore, its pathomechanisms must remain ambiguous until its morphologic bases are established [16].

Although a variety of neuropathological changes have been described in the brain of chronic alcoholics, it is difficult to elucidate the exact pathogenetic mechanisms causing the CNS damage since these persons often have concurrent damage to other organs, e.g., liver cirrhosis, repeated traumatic head injuries, malnutrition [20, 21]. The development of brain damage may further be complicated by polysubstance abuse [20]. Moreover, the type and severity of brain damage are influenced by several other factors, such as type and amount of alcoholic beverages, age of onset of drinking, lifetime alcohol consumption and genetic vulnerability [15, 22].

Thus, the neuropathological lesions encountered in chronic alcoholics are most probably the end result of a variety of etiological factors. Increasing evidence indicates that the main factors contributing to alcohol-induced brain damage are associated with nutritional deficiencies and repeated withdrawal syndrome [15]. These two factors may induce neurotoxicity by increased glutamatergic transmission and overactivation of NMDA receptor-induced excitotoxicity [15]. Nevertheless, it is now well established that even uncomplicated alcoholics, who have no specific neurological or hepatic problems, show signs of cognitive dysfunction and brain damage [23].

Some studies suggest that females are more vulnerable to alcohol-induced brain damage than males [24]; however, the evidence remains inconclusive [25, 26, 27].

5.2 Neuroimaging

Neuroradiological studies have demonstrated cerebral atrophy which has occasionally been accompanied by cognitive deficits and was at least partially reversible.

Computed tomography (CT) studies have shown significantly increased ventricular size [28] and cortical atrophy in alcoholics, predominantly of the frontal lobe [29, 30, 31, 32].

Magnetic resonance imaging (MRI) studies confirmed the CT findings in the manner that the frontal lobes are preferentially vulnerable to chronic alcohol abuse [33]. In addition, significant volume deficits have been detected in the anterior hippocampus, the fronto-parietal and temporal gray matter [34, 35] as well as in the brainstem [36], diencephalon, and the caudate nucleus [34]. In chronic alcoholism, smaller hippocampal volumes have been shown to be proportional to the reduction of the brain volume [37]. Quantitative MRI demonstrated that the characteristic memory deficit of Korsakoff's syndrome involves significant bilateral hippocampal volume deficits and diencephalic pathology [38]. The patterns of circuitry disruption identified through structural and functional MRI studies suggest a central role for degradation of fronto-cerebellar neuronal nodes and connecting circuitry affecting widespread brain regions and contributing to the cognitive and motor deficits in alcoholics [39].

Studies with positron emission tomography (PET) have shown a decreased cerebellar and frontal lobe glucose utilization in alcoholics, confirming the preferential involvement of these brain regions in alcohol abuse [40, 41, 42, 43, 44, 45, 46, 47].

Single photon emission computed tomography (SPECT) analyses demonstrated a significant reduction of regional cerebral blood flow (rCBF) in alcoholics as compared to controls [48, 49, 50, 51]. The rCBF ratio was mainly reduced in frontal lobes [50, 52] and the greatest flow reduction was seen in persons with liver cirrhosis [53].

By using proton magnetic resonance spectroscopy (MRS), a reduced N-acetylaspartate (NAA)/choline and NAA/total creatine ratio as compared to age-matched controls has been described. As stated by the authors, the reduction in NAA is consistent with neuronal loss, whereas the reduction in choline suggests significant changes in the membrane lipids of alcoholics [36, 54].

Using magnetic resonance diffusion tensor imaging (MRDTI) to quantify the microstructure of brain tissue, alcoholics showed widespread white matter deficits, which are in contrast to the highly region-specific deficits seen in nutritional deficiency syndromes that can accompany alcoholism [55, 56].

5.3 Acute Intoxication

In acute alcohol intoxication there are no characteristic CNS alterations. Brain edema and vascular congestion (Fig. 5.1) are frequently seen, sometimes in conjunction with focal subarachnoid hemorrhage [57].

5.4 Brain Atrophy

Although the frequency and severity of cerebral atrophy in alcoholics is controversial, several autopsy studies have shown a reduction in brain weight and volume [14, 21, 58, 59]. The greatest reduction in brain weight was seen in

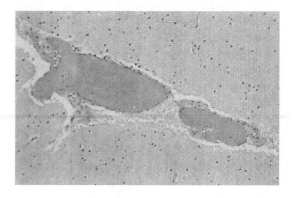

Fig. 5.1 Vascular congestion in acute alcohol intoxication (hematoxylin and eosin, magnification 100×)

alcoholics with additional complications, such as nutritional deficiencies or liver damage [58, 60]. Several studies demonstrated that this brain atrophy, often referred to as "brain shrinkage", is not due to a loss of gray matter but rather due to a reduction in the volume of the white matter [61, 62, 63]. The disproportionate loss of cerebral white matter relative to cerebral cortex suggests that a major neurotoxic effect of chronic alcohol consumption affects the white matter [61, 62, 63]. It has been suggested that the loss of white matter could be caused by changes in hydration [64]. However, postmortem studies could not support this hypothesis [65]. An alcohol-induced degeneration of myelinated fibres in the white matter could not be demonstrated [66]. Interestingly, these abnormalities may be reversed by abstinence from alcohol [21, 58, 59, 67, 68, 69].

In addition to the white matter changes, chronic alcohol consumption is associated with selective neuronal vulnerability, with the frontal lobes more seriously affected than other cortical regions [62, 70, 71]. Within the frontal cortex, this neurodegenerative process was confined to the superior frontal association cortex [60, 62, 63] affecting the non-GABAergic pyramidal neurons [63].

Recent studies have confirmed that the frontal lobe is especially vulnerable to alcohol-related brain damage (Fig. 5.2), whereby shrinkage in this area is largely due to a loss of white matter [71]. Moreover, disruption of fronto-cerebellar circuitry and function has been shown in alcoholism [72]. Since the frontal lobes have extensive connections to different cortical and subcortical areas of the brain, widespread alterations in brain functions result [71]. This might explain the high incidence of cognitive dysfunction observed in alcoholics who often develop frontal lobe symptoms with personality and behavioural changes, disinhibition, social and personal neglect, lack of insight, empathy and emotional control [73]. Such symptoms often increase the risk of engagement in and exposure to acts of violence carrying a risk of physical damage including head trauma and violent death [73].

Neuronal loss has been further shown to occur in the diencephalon, especially in patients with Wernicke-Korsakoff syndrome, and in the cerebellum [57, 59, 60,

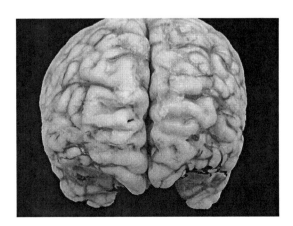

Fig. 5.2 Frontal lobe atrophy in long-term alcohol abuse

74, 75, 76, 77, 78, 79]. It is estimated that almost one half of all severe alcoholics have atrophy of the superior cerebellar vermis, which is clinically characterized by ataxia and incoordination of the lower limbs [79]. Besides a significant loss of Purkinje cells, the cerebellar molecular layer appears to be another vulnerable region in chronic alcoholics [80]. Microscopically, there is also proliferation of Bergmann glia in these cases. However, other groups found no consistent changes in the number of Purkinje cells or the structural volume for any cerebellar region in chronic alcoholics without Wernicke's encephalopathy, thus suggesting that chronic alcohol consumption per se does not necessarily damage the cerebellum [81, 82]. On the other hand, in alcoholics with Wernicke's encephalopathy, there is a significant decrease in Purkinje cell density in the flocculus and vermis as well as decreased volume of the molecular layer of the cerebellar vermis, indicating impairment of spino-cerebellar pathways [82].

The data on neuronal loss in the hippocampus of chronic alcoholics is contradictory. Some authors demonstrated an early neuronal loss [83], whereas others could not find a significant neuronal loss in any subregion of the hippocampus, despite a marked reduction in hippocampal volume which occurred exclusively in the white matter [84, 85].

No significant change was reported for the temporal [63, 70] or motor cortex [63], the basal ganglia [58], nucleus basalis of Meynert, or in the serotonergic raphe nuclei [21, 86]. Within the brainstem, a reduction in the number of serotonergic neurons was described in chronic alcoholics [87], while the number of pigmented cells in the locus coeruleus was unchanged [88].

A significant reduction of the corpus callosum has been detected in older alcoholics compared to age-matched controls [89, 90, 91]. This callosal thinning was even present in chronic alcoholics without clinical symptoms of severe liver disease, amnesia, or alcoholic dementia. The degree of this atrophy seems to correlate with the severity of alcohol intake [89].

In summary, brain atrophy in alcoholics has been demonstrated in various studies. There is a regional selectivity with the frontal lobes being particularly affected. However, the magnitude and topography of the atrophy, and the contributory factors are still not fully resolved [92]. The pathogenetic mechanisms leading to the selected vulnerability of specific brain regions to alcoholism is unknown. It is suggested that differences in the density of glutamatergic innervation or in subunit composition of glutamate receptors among different brain structures may contribute to this selectivity [93].

5.5 Glial Changes

In alcoholics, the morphology of astrocytes is markedly changed by exhibiting enlargement of their cell bodies and beading of the cellular processes [94]. In addition, GFAP-positive astrocytes were seen within and surrounding clusters of magnocellular neurons in the basal forebrain and hypothalamus. A patchy loss of GFAP immunostaining was seen in most severe cases which could not be exclusively related to alcoholics with liver pathology [94].

A statistically significant loss of glial cells was found globally in the hippocampus of alcoholics compared with controls. A reduction of astrocytes and oligodendrocytes and, to a lesser degree, microglial cells accounted for this loss [85].

In animal models and human cell cultures it has been shown that chronic ethanol treatment stimulates astrocytes, upregulating the production and the expression of inflammatory mediators in the brain, and activating signalling pathways and transcription factors [95, 96, 97]. Furthermore, alcohol treatment increased cytochrome P4502E1 and induced oxidative stress in astrocytes [98] which might cause neurotoxicity. In addition, emerging data indicate that alcohol affects microglial cell development and function [96].

5.6 Dendritic and Synaptic Changes

Dendritic and synaptic alterations have been documented in alcoholics and these, together with receptor and neurotransmitter changes, may explain functional changes and cognitive deficits that precede the structural neuronal changes [21]. In "heavy drinkers", synaptic loss has been found in the superior layers of frontal Brodmann area 10, which was not related to liver disease [73].

5.7 Central Pontine Myelinolysis

Central pontine myelinolysis (CPM) is a demyelinating disease of the central portion of the base of the pons (Fig. 5.3A,B) often associated with demyelination of other brain areas [99, 100, 101, 102, 103]. The first cases were described in patients with a history of long-standing alcohol abuse and malnutrition [104],

(A)   (B)

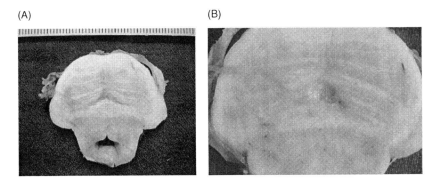

Fig. 5.3A,B Central pontine myelinolysis: destructive lesions in the pons

and chronic alcoholism is still a frequent underlying condition of persons with CPM [105]. However, in subsequent reports, CPM has been shown to occur most frequently in association with rapid correction of hyponatremia [100, 101, 102, 103, 106, 107, 108]. Especially alcoholism and liver diseases make patients more susceptible to the development of CPM.

Other causes include transplant patients, with the development of CPM being attributed to immunosuppressive agents [101, 105, 107, 109] and HIV-1 infection [110].

Depending on the involvement of other CNS structures, the clinical picture can vary considerably. CPM is most often an asymptomatic disorder with small, midline pontine lesions [102]. Destructive lesions in the corticospinal and the corticobulbar tracts in the pons lead to pseudobulbar paralysis with dysphagia, dysarthria, weakness of the tongue, and emotional lability. A large central pontine lesion can cause a locked-in syndrome depriving the patient of speech and the capacity to respond in any way except by vertical gaze and blinking [111]. Lesions involving the descending oculosympathetic tracts can cause bilateral miosis, whereas lesions that involve the lower pons can cause palsy of the sixth cranial nerve [102, 111]. In addition to lesions in the pons, other areas in the CNS can be affected. Such lesions are collectively referred to as extrapontine myelinolysis (EPM) and occur, in order of frequency, in the cerebellum, lateral geniculate body, thalamus, putamen, and cerebral cortex [100, 103, 105, 107]. CPM and EPM are summarized by the term osmotic demyelination disorders [105].

The outcome varies widely, from almost complete recovery to little or no improvement and subsequent death [105, 111, 112]. Since unexplained deaths may occur [113], therefore, a thorough examination of the pons must be performed at autopsy. On neuropathological examination, CPM usually presents as a single large symmetric focus of demyelination in the central part of the base of the pons, with sparing of axis cylinders (Fig. 5.4). No inflammatory changes are seen within the lesion and the blood vessels are unaffected [99, 100, 102, 103, 113, 114]. The etiology and pathogenesis of the myelin loss is still unclear [115].

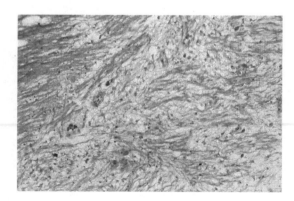

Fig. 5.4 Central pontine myelinolysis: marked demyelination (Luxol Fast Blue, magnification 100×)

5.8 Wernicke-Korsakoff Syndrome

The Wernicke-Korsakoff syndrome (WKS) is one of the most frequently seen neurological disorders associated with long-term and heavy alcohol abuse [15, 116, 117, 118]. Wernicke's encephalopathy is the acute phase of this syndrome and includes mental confusion, ophthalmoplegia (or nystagmus), ataxia, and loss of recent memory [117, 118, 119]. Despite abstinence and the administration of high dose of thiamine, about 25% of the affected persons develop severe memory disorders, the Korsakoff's syndrome which is mainly characterized by memory loss, learning deficits and confabulation [117, 118, 119, 120]. Korsakoff's psychosis is most likely the end-stage resulting from repeated episodes of Wernicke's encephalopathy.

The etiology is a deficiency of vitamin B1 (thiamine), a cofactor of several enzymes implicated in the glucose metabolism, rather than a direct toxic effect of alcohol [120, 121, 122]. The symptoms may be seen in either the acute or the long-term course of alcohol abuse [120]. The WKS can also occur in other conditions associated with vitamin B1 deficiency, e.g., gastrointestinal tract diseases, cerebrovascular disorders, or head trauma [116, 121]. Although the exact pathogenesis of the lesions is not completely understood, the association of vitamin B1 deficiency with intracellular and extracellular edema by glutamate(N-methyl-D-aspartate) receptor-mediated excitotoxicity seems to be an important mechanism [122].

Both conditions appear to have an identical neuropathology characterized by hemorrhages and other lesions around the ventricular system (Figs. 5.5 and 5.6) [117, 122, 123]. The principal structures affected are the mamillary bodies (Fig. 5.6), the walls of the third ventricle, the thalamus, the periaqueductal region of the midbrain and the floor of the fourth ventricle (Fig. 5.7) [116, 117, 122, 124]. The distribution and severity of the CNS lesions varies with the stages of the disease, which are generally considered to be acute, subacute or chronic [124].

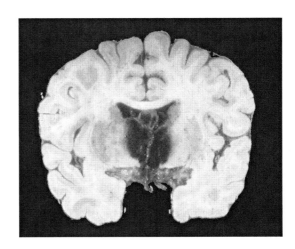

Fig. 5.5 Wernicke encephalopathy: widespread symmetrical hemorrhages around the ventricular system

Fig. 5.6 Wernicke
encephalopathy:
symmetrical hemorrhages
in the mammillary bodies

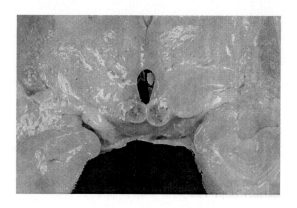

Subjects with acute and subacute disease seem to have more extensive and severe lesions than the chronic ones [122]. Microscopic changes can be related to the duration of the disease [123, 124]. The earliest alterations consist of rarefication of the neuropil by edema formation and petechial hemorrhages. In some instances these extend into the parenchyma to form "ball-like" microhemorrhages. Within 1–2 days there is endothelial hypertrophy and proliferation, which are maximal at about day 7–10. Tissue necrosis is occasionally seen but is more common in the thalamic nuclei. Neurons are relatively spared with the exception of the

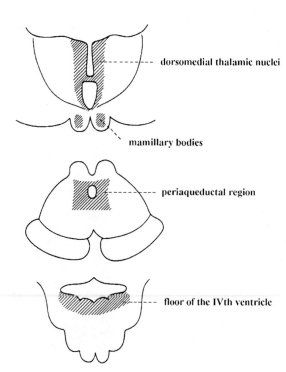

Fig. 5.7 Schematic drawing
of the principal structures
affected in Wernicke-
Korsakoff syndrome

thalamic and olivary neurons. By the third or fourth day, there is an astrocytic reaction with increased numbers of nuclei and eosinophilic cytoplasm. Myelin and axons are often destroyed. There is usually no inflammatory reaction. In contrast to the lesion seen in the mamillary bodies, there is a massive loss of neurons with sparing of the neuropil, and only mild endothelial swelling within the thalamus [122, 123, 124].

The most consistent macroscopic finding in chronic WKS is shrinkage and brown discoloration of the mamillary bodies which varies from barely visible to subtotal destruction of the tissue [122, 123, 124]. Microscopically, there is a loss of myelin and axons, an astrogliosis and an apparent increase in vascularity in the shrunken mamillary bodies, but a relative preservation of neurons. Hemosiderin-laden macrophages are frequently seen and represent the residues of microhemor-rhages (Fig. 5.8). Changes in other hypothalamic nuclei display a similar pattern but the changes are usually much less severe [122, 123, 124].

In the majority of chronic cases, the lesions are restricted to the mamillary bodies and the thalamus. Similar to the alterations within the mamillary bodies, the lesions in the thalamus vary from slight astrogliosis in the dorsomedial nucleus to extensive nerve cell loss in several of its nuclei [122, 123, 124]. While patients with Wernicke's encephalopathy often show neuronal loss in the dorsomedial nucleus of the thalamus, only patients with Korsakoff's psychosis seem to have cell loss in the medial [117] as well as in the anterior thalamic nuclei [125]. Furthermore, in both patient groups, a profound loss of serotonin- and acetylcholine-containing neurons has been found [117]. These observations suggest that cumulative lesions contribute to the amnesia seen in alcoholics with WKS, including deficits in serotonergic, cholinergic, and thalamic pathways.

Despite these apparent lesions, the exact morphological basis of this disorder is still controversial. Autopsy and MRI studies of alcoholic patients with WKS demonstrated gliotic lesions of the mamillary bodies; however, lesions of the mamillary bodies were often present in the absence of the amnestic syndrome [122, 126, 127]. It seems that the thalamus appears to be particularly susceptible to

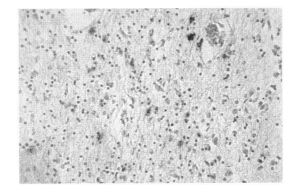

Fig. 5.8 Wernicke encephalopathy: hemosiderin-laden macro-phages in the mammillary bodies representing residues of microhemorrhages (Iron stain, magnification 200×)

damage in WKS [122, 128]. Subsequent studies demonstrated that lesions of the mediodorsal nucleus of the thalamus correlated with the amnestic syndrome [118, 119, 122, 127] and the role of the mamillary bodies in this memory disorder was largely, although not entirely, dispelled [128].

Autopsy studies have shown that up to 80% of patients with the WKS were not diagnosed as such during life [129, 130, 131, 132, 133, 134]. Therefore, in cases with coma of unidentified cause or patients found dead who might have been alcoholics, a thorough neuropathologic examination is of utmost importance.

5.9 Hepatic Encephalopathy

Hepatic encephalopathy may arise as a complication of liver disease in alcoholics, particularly in the course of liver cirrhosis, which results in cognitive, psychiatric, and motor impairments [135, 136, 137]. The damaged liver can no longer clear neurotoxic substances from the blood which subsequently enter the brain and damage neurons and astrocytes. The clinical picture consists of a deterioration in the level of consciousness accompanied by decreased (or occasionally increased) psychomotor activity that, if left untreated, progresses to increasing drowsiness, stupor and eventual coma [135, 136, 137]. As the encephalopathy progresses, signs of pyramidal tract dysfunction such as hypertonia, hyperreflexia are common, eventually being replaced by hypotonia as coma develops. Treatment is largely supportive. The prognosis of patients who develop hepatic encephalopathy is poor. Following the first episode of overt hepatic encephalopathy, the 1-year survival is about 40%, falling to about 15% after 3 years [136]. The major causes of death in hepatic encephalopathy are brain edema and intracranial hypertension [138].

Although the pathogenesis of hepatic encephalopathy is not fully understood, there is considerable evidence that an ammonia-induced dysfunction of astrocytes is the major contributory factor [136, 139, 140]. Deficits in the uptake of glutamate by astrocytes from the extracellular space may lead to abnormal glutamatergic and GABAergic-mediated neurotransmission and subsequent neuronal excitotoxicity [139, 141]. In addition, an altered blood-brain barrier permeability [141, 142] and a combined derangement of cellular osmolarity coupled with cerebral hyperemia [138] appear to be involved in the generation of the edema.

In fulminant hepatic failure where hepatic encephalopathy develops within 8 weeks of the onset of liver disease, autopsy reveals brain edema and astrocyte swelling [139, 142]. In patients with liver cirrhosis and portal-systemic shunts, the typical finding is the Alzheimer type II astrocyte, which is the pathological hallmark of hepatic encephalopathy [140]. These cells show a characteristic swollen shape with a large, pale nucleus, prominent nucleolus and margination of chromatin, and are found in widespread regions of the brain including the cortex and the lenticular, lateral thalamic, dentate and red nuclei [140, 141]. The majority of these cells show prominent immunoreactivity for S100P but not for GFAP, especially in the grey matter [143, 144]. Thus, this glial reaction with a rather selective deficit of GFAP metabolism has been termed "gliofibrillary dystrophy" [143].

5.10 Marchiafava-Bignami Syndrome

Marchiafava-Bignami disease is an extremely rare, severe and usually fatal neurological disorder associated with chronic alcoholism [145]. It is characterized by primary demyelination/necrosis and subsequent atrophy of the corpus callosum [124, 145, 146]. However, this lesion is not only limited to the corpus callosum but also affects the cortico-cortical and cortico-subcortical projections due to disconnection, and causes frontal lobe syndromes and dementia [145, 146].

Macroscopically, necrotizing, often cystic lesions of the corpus callosum are seen. Microscopically, there is prominent demyelination with relative sparing of the axons. Oligodendrocytes are reduced in number and there are numerous lipid-laden macrophages. Astrocytes show only mild reactive changes, but are more prominent in and around necrotizing lesions. Blood vessels often show proliferation and hyalinization of their walls [124, 146].

5.11 Pellagra Encephalopathy

Nicotinamide deficiency may result in a rare condition, alcoholic pellagra encephalopathy, which often has a similar clinical presentation to Wernicke-Korsakoff syndrome which includes confusion and/or clouding of consciousness, marked oppositional hypertonus and myoclonus [147, 148]. On neuropathological examination, no gross macroscopic changes are usually visible. Microscopically, the major finding is a central chromatolysis of neurons, predominantly in the brainstem and in the cerebellar dentate nuclei. The affected neurons are ballooned with a loss of Nissl substance and eccentrically located nuclei. Nuclei of cranial nerves, the reticular nuclei, arcuate nuclei and posterior horn cells, may also be involved. Glial cells, myelin or blood vessels are not affected [149, 150].

5.12 Stroke

Recent heavy alcohol intake seems to be an independent risk factor for all major subtypes of stroke [151] and to be associated with cerebral infarcts localized in the putamen and superior anterior cerebral artery area [152]. The ultimate mechanisms leading to this increased risk are unclear [151].

Concerning the relation between moderate alcohol consumption and the risk of stroke, there is insufficient epidemiologic evidence to conclude whether recent alcohol use affects the risk of either ischemic or hemorrhagic stroke [153]. Both occasional ethanol intoxication and regular heavy drinking seem to carry an increased risk of subarachnoid hemorrhage [154].

5.13 Functional Genomic Alterations

Although functional genomic studies have failed to identify a single alcoholism gene, they have demonstrated important pathways and gene products that may contribute to the risk of alcohol abuse and alcoholism [155, 156, 157, 158]. Several research groups have searched for alcohol-responsive genes using microarrays. It could be shown that the alteration in expression of genes involved in DNA repair, myelination, signal transduction, ubiquitination as well as proteasome-related genes represent common changes seen in the various studies performed in alcohol abusers. However, the identity and number of dysregulated genes reported so far, the specific pathways involved, and the direction of change differs profoundly between the reports and thus remains inconclusive [11, 158].

Acknowledgment   The help of Ida C. Llenos, MD in correcting the manuscript is highly appreciated. We thank Ms. Susanne Ring for her skillful technical assistance.

References

1. Zimatkin SM, Deitrich RA (1997) Ethanol metabolism in the brain. Addiction Biol 2:387–399
2. Oscar-Berman M, Shagrin B, Evert DL, Epstein C (1997) Impairments of brain and behavior: the neurological effects of alcohol. Alcohol Health Res World 21:65–75
3. Appel SB, McBride WJ, Diana M, Diamond I, Bonci A, Brodie MS (2004) Ethanol effects on dopaminergic "reward" neurons in the ventral tegmental area and the mesolimbic pathway. Alcohol Clin Exp Res 28:1768–1778
4. Boileau I, Assaad J-M, Pihl RO, Benkelfat C, Leyton M, Diksic M et al. (2003) Alcohol promotes dopamine release in the human nucleus accumbens. Synapse 49:226–231
5. Diana M, Brodie M, Muntoni A, Puddu MC, Pillolla G, Steffensen S et al. (2003) Enduring effects of chronic ethanol in the CNS: basis for alcoholism. Alcohol Clin Exp Res 27:354–361
6. Herz A (1997) Endogenous opioid systems and alcohol addiction. Psychopharmacology 129:99–111
7. Lê AD, Kiianmaa K, Cunningham CL, Engel JA, Ericson M, Soderpalm B et al. (2001) Neurobiological processes in alcohol addiction. Alcohol Clin Exp Res 25: 144S–151S
8. Noble EP (1996) Alcoholism and the dopaminergic system: a review. Addict Biol 1:333–348
9. Tupala E, Tiihonen J (2004) Dopamine and alcoholism: neurobiological basis of ethanol abuse. Prog Neuropsychopharmacol Biol Psychiatry 28:1221–1247

10. Basavarajappa BS, Hungund BL (2005) Role of the endocannabinoid system in the development of tolerance to alcohol. Alcohol Alcohol 40:15–24
11. Flatscher-Bader T, van der Brug MP, Landis N, Hwang JW, Harrison E, Wilce PA (2006) Comparative gene expression in brain regions of human alcoholics. Genes Brain Behav 5(Suppl 1):78–84
12. Clark JC (1988) Sudden death in the chronic alcoholic. Forensic Sci Int 36:105–111
13. Skullerud K, Andersen SN, Lundevall J (1991) Cerebral lesions and causes of death in male alcoholics. A forensic autopsy study. Int J Legal Med 104:209–213
14. Torvik A (1987) Brain lesions in alcoholics: neuropathological observations. Acta Med Scand Suppl 717:47–54
15. Fadda F, Rossetti ZL (1998) Chronic ethanol consumption: from neuroadaptation to neurodegeneration. Prog Neurobiol 56:385–431
16. Victor M (1994) Alcoholic dementia. Can J Neurol Sci 21:88–99
17. Cutting J (1978) The relationship between Korsakoff's syndrome and "alcoholic dementia". Br J Psychiat 132:240–251
18. Martin PR, Adinoff B, Weingartner H, Mukherjee AB, Eckardt MJ (1986) Alcoholic organic brain disease: nosology and pathophysiologic mechanisms. Prog Neuropsychopharmacol Biol Psychiatry 10:147–164
19. Willenbring ML (1988) Organic mental disorders associated with heavy drinking and alcohol dependence. Clin Geriatr Med 4:869–887
20. Butterworth RF (1995) Pathophysiology of alcoholic brain damage: synergistic effects of ethanol, thiamine deficiency and alcoholic liver disease. Metab Brain Dis 10:1–8
21. Harper C (1998) The neuropathology of alcohol-specific brain damage, or does alcohol damage the brain? J Neuropathol Exp Neurol 57:101–110
22. Harper C, Dixon G, Sheedy D, Garrick T (2003) Neuropathological alterations in alcoholic brains. Studies arising from the New South Wales Tissue Resource Centre. Prog Neuropsychopharmacol Biol Psychiatry 27:951–961
23. Harper C, Matsumoto I (2005) Ethanol and brain damage. Curr Opin Pharmacol 5:73–78
24. Wuethrich B (2001) Does alcohol damage female brains more? Science 291:2077–2079
25. Harper CG, Smith NA, Kril JJ (1990) The effects of alcohol on the female brain – a neuropathological study. Alcohol Alcohol 25:445–448
26. Hommer DW (2003) Male and female sensitivity to alcohol-induced brain damage. Alcohol Res Health 27:181–185
27. Rosenbloom M, Sullivan EV, Pfefferbaum A (2003) Using magnetic resonance imaging and diffusion tensor imaging to assess brain damage in alcoholics. Alcohol Res Health 27:146–152
28. Fox JH, Ramsey RG, Huckman MS, Broske AE (1976) Cerebral ventricular enlargement. Chronic alcoholics examined by computerized tomography. JAMA 236:365–368
29. Carlen PL, Wortzman G, Holgate RC, Wilkinson DA, Rankin JG (1978) Reversible cerebral atrophy in recently abstinent chronic alcoholics measured by computed tomographic scans. Science 200:1076–1078
30. Ron MA (1977) Brain damage in chronic alcoholism: a neuropathological, neuroradiological and psychological review. Psychol Med 7:103–112
31. Rosse RB, Riggs RL, Dietrich AM, Schwartz BL, Deutsch SI (1997) Frontal cortical atrophy and negative symptoms in patients with chronic alcohol dependence. J Neuropsychiatry Clin Neurosci 9:280–282
32. Wilkinson DA (1982) Examination of alcoholics by computed tomographic (CT) scans. A critical reviews. Alcohol Clin Exp Res 6:31–45
33. Pfefferbaum A, Sullivan EV, Mathalon DH, Lim KO (1997) Frontal lobe volume loss observed with magnetic resonance imaging in older chronic alcoholics. Alcohol Clin Exp Res 21:521–529

34. Jernigan TL, Butters N, DiTraglia G, Schafer K, Smith T, Irwin M et al. (1991) Reduced cerebral grey matter observed in alcoholics using magnetic resonance imaging. Alcohol Clin Exp Res 15:418–427
35. Sullivan EV, Marsh L, Mathalon DH, Lim KO, Pfefferbaum A (1996) Relationship between alcohol withdrawal seizures and temporal lobe white matter volume deficits. Alcohol Clin Exp Res 20:348–354
36. Bloomer CW, Langleben DD, Meyerhoff DJ (2004) Magnetic resonance detects brainstem changes in chronic, active heavy drinkers. Psychiatr Res 132:209–218
37. Agartz I, Momenan R, Rawlings RR, Kerich MJ, Hommer DW (1999) Hippocampal volume in patients with alcohol dependence. Arch Gen Psychiatry 56:356–363
38. Sullivan EV, Marsh L (2003) Hippocampal volume deficits in alcoholic Korsakoff's syndrome. Neurology 61:1716–1719
39. Sullivan EV, Pfefferbaum A (2005) Neurocircuitry in alcoholism: a substrate of disruption and repair. Psychopharmacology (Berlin) 180:583–594
40. Adams KM, Gilman S, Koeppe RA, Kluin KJ, Brunberg JA, Dede D et al. (1993) Neuropsychological deficits are correlated with frontal hypometabolism in positron emission tomography studies of older alcoholic patients. Alcohol Clin Exp Res 17:205–210
41. Dao-Castellana MH, Samson Y, Legault F, Martinot JL, Aubin HJ, Crouzel C et al. (1998) Frontal dysfunction in neurologically normal chronic alcoholic subjects: metabolic and neuropsychological findings. Psychol Med 28:1039–1048
42. Gilman S, Koeppe RA, Adams K, Johnson-Greene D, Junck L, Kluin KJ et al. (1996) Positron emission tomographic studies of cerebral benzodiazepine-receptor binding in chronic alcoholics. Ann Neurol 40:163–171
43. Gilman S, Adams K, Koeppe RA, Berent S, Kluin KJ, Modell JG et al. (1990) Cerebellar and frontal hypometabolism in alcoholic cerebellar degeneration studied with position emission tomography. Ann Neurol 28:775–785
44. Sachs H, Russell JA, Christman DR, Cook B (1987) Alteration of regional cerebral glucose metabolic rate in non-Korsakoff chronic alcoholism. Arch Neurol 44:1242–1251
45. Samson Y, Baron JC, Feline A, Bories J, Crouzel C (1986) Local cerebral glucose utilisation in chronic alcoholics: a positron tomographic study. J Neurol Neurosurg Psychiatr 49:1165–1170
46. Volkow ND, Wang GJ, Hitzemann R, Fowler JS, Wolf AP, Pappas N et al. (1993) Decreased cerebral response to inhibitory neurotransmission in alcoholics. Am J Psychiatr 150:417–422
47. Wik G, Borg S, Sjogren I, Wiesel FA, Blomqvist G, Borg J et al. (1988) PET determination of regional cerebral glucose metabolism in alcohol-dependent men and healthy controls using 11C-glucose. Acta Psychiat Scand 78:234–241
48. Gansler DA, Harris GJ, Oscar-Berman M, Streeter C, Lewis RF, Ahmed I et al. (2000) Hypoperfusion of inferior frontal brain regions in abstinent alcoholics: a pilot SPECT study. J Stud Alcohol 61:32–37
49. Melgaard B, Henriksen L, Ahlgren P, Danielsen UT, Sorensen H, Paulson OB (1990) Regional cerebral blood flow in chronic alcoholics measured by single photon emission computerized tomography. Acta Neurol Scand 82:87–93
50. Nicolas JM, Catafau AM, Estruch R, Lomena FJ, Salamero M, Herranz R et al. (1993) Regional cerebral blood flow-SPECT in chronic alcoholism: relation to neuropsychological testing. J Nucl Med 34:1452–1459
51. Valmier J, Touchon J, Zanca M, Fauchere V, Bories P, Baldy-Moulinier M (1986) Correlations between cerebral grey matter flow and hepatic histology in alcoholism. Eur Neurol 25:428–435
52. Hunter R, McLuskie R, Wyper D, Patterson J, Christie JE, Brooks DN et al. (1989) The pattern of function-related regional cerebral blood flow investigated by single photon

emission tomography with 99 mTc-HMPAO in patients with presenile Alzheimer's disease and Korsakoff's psychosis. Psychol Med 19:847–855

53. Shimojyo S, Scheinberg P, Reinmuth D (1967) Cerebral blood flow and metabolism in the Wernicke-Korsakoff Syndrome. J Clin Invest 46:849–854

54. Jagannathan NR, Desai NG, Raghunathan P (1996) Brain metabolite changes in alcoholism: an in vivo proton magnetic resonance spectroscopy (MRS) study. Magn Reson Imaging 14:553–557

55. Pfefferbaum A, Adalsteinsson E, Sullivan EV (2006) Supratentorial profile of white matter microstructural integrity in recovering alcoholic men and women. Biol Psychiatry 59:364–372

56. Pfefferbaum A, Sullivan EV (2005) Disruption of brain white matter microstructure by excessive intracellular and extracellular fluid in alcoholism: evidence from diffusion tensor imaging. Neuropsychopharmacology 30:423–432

57. Courville CB (1964) Forensic neuropathology. XII. The alcohols. J Forensic Sci 9:209–235

58. Harper CG, Kril J (1985) Brain atrophy in chronic alcoholic patients: a quantitative pathological study. J Neurol Neurosurg Psychiatr 48:211–217

59. Harper CG, Kril JL (1990) The neuropathology of alcoholism. Alcohol Alcohol 25:207–216

60. Krill JJ (1995) The contribution of alcohol, thiamine deficiency and cirrhosis of the liver to cerebral cortical damage in alcoholics. Metab Brain Dis 10:9–16

61. Harper CG, Kril JJ, Holloway RL (1985) Brain shrinkage in chronic alcoholics: a pathological study. Br Med J 290:501–504

62. Kril JL, Halliday GM (1999) Brain shrinkage in alcoholics: a decade on and what have we learned? Prog Neurobiol 58:381–387

63. Kril JJ, Halliday GM, Svoboda MD, Cartwright H (1997) The cerebral cortex is damaged in chronic alcoholics. Neuroscience 79:983–998

64. Eisenhofer G, Johnson RH (1982) Effects of ethanol ingestion on plasma vasopressin and water balance in humans. Am J Physiol 242:522–527

65. Harper CG, Kril J, Daly JM (1988) Brain shrinkage in alcoholics is not caused by changes in hydration: a pathological study. J Neurol Neurosurg Psychiatry 51:124–127

66. Tang Y, Pakkenberg B, Nyengaard JR (2004) Myelinated nerve fibres in the subcortical white matter of cerebral hemispheres are preserved in alcoholic subjects. Brain Res 1029:162–167

67. de la Monte SM (1988) Disproportionate atrophy of cerebral white matter in chronic alcoholics. Arch Neurol 45:990–992

68. Jensen GB, Pakkenberg B (1993) Do alcoholics drink their neurons away? Lancet 342:1201–1204

69. Trabert W, Betz T, Niewald M, Huber G (1995) Significant reversibility of alcoholic brain shrinkage within 3 weeks of abstinence. Acta Psychiatr Scand 92:87–90

70. Kril JJ, Harper CG (1989) Neuronal counts from four cortical regions of alcoholic brains. Acta Neuropathol 41:67–80

71. Moselhy HF, Georgiou G, Kahn A (2001) Frontal lobe changes in alcoholism: a review of the literature. Alcohol Alcohol 36:357–368

72. Sullivan EV, Harding AJ, Pentney R, Dlugos C, Martin PR, Parks MH et al. (2003) Disruption of frontocerebellar circuitry and function in alcoholism. Alcohol Clin Exp Res 27:301–309

73. Brun A, Andersson J (2001) Frontal dysfunction and frontal cortical synapse loss in alcoholism – the main cause of alcohol dementia? Dement Geriatr Cogn Disord 12:289–294

74. Cavanagh JB, Holton JL, Nolan CC (1997) Selective damage to the cerebellar vermis in chronic alcoholism: a contribution from neurotoxicology to an old problem of selective vulnerability. Neuropathol Appl Neurobiol 23:355–363

75. Courville CB (1964) Cerebellar degeneration as a consequence of chronic alcoholism. Bull Los Angeles Neurol Soc 29:198–207
76. Karhune PJ, Erkinjuntti T, Laippala P (1994) Moderate alcohol consumption and loss of cerebellar Purkinje cells. Br Med J 308:1663–1667
77. Nicolás JM, Fernández-Solà J, Robert J, Antúnez E, Cofán M, Cardenal C et al. (2000) High ethanol intake and malnutrition in alcoholic cerebellar shrinkage. QJM 93:449–456
78. Pfefferbaum A, Sullivan EV, Rosenbloom MJ, Mathalon DH, Lim KO (1998) A controlled study of cortical gray matter and ventricular changes in alcoholic men over a 5-year interval. Arch Gen Psychiatry 55:905–912
79. Torvik A, Torp S (1986) The prevalence of alcoholic cerebellar atrophy. A morphometric and histological study of an autopsy material. J Neurol Sci 75:43–51
80. Phillips SG, Harper CG, Kril J (1987) A quantitative histological study of the cerebellar vermis in alcoholic patients. Brain 110:301–314
81. Andersen BB (2004) Reduction of Purkinje cell volume in cerebellum of alcoholics. Brain Res 1007:10–18
82. Baker KG, Harding AJ, Halliday GM, Kril JJ, Harper CG (1999) Neuronal loss in functional zones of the cerebellum of chronic alcoholics with and without Wernicke's encephalopathy. Neuroscience 91:429–438
83. Bengochea O, Gonzalo LM (1990) Effect of chronic alcoholism on the human hippocampus. Histol Histopathol 5:349–357
84. Harding AJ, Wong A, Svoboda MD, Kril JL, Halliday GM (1997) Chronic alcohol consumption does not cause hippocampal neuron loss in humans. Hippocampus 7:78–87
85. Korbo L (1999) Glial cell loss in the hippocampus of alcoholics. Alcohol Clin Exp Res 23:164–168
86. Baker KG, Halliday GM, Kril JJ, Harper CG (1996) Chronic alcoholics without Wernicke-Korsakoff syndrome or cirrhosis do not lose serotonergic neurons in the dorsal raphe nucleus. Alcohol Clin Exp Res 20:61–66
87. Halliday G, Ellis J, Heard R, Caine D, Harper C (1993) Brainstem serotonergic neurons in chronic alcoholics with and without the memory impairment of Korsakoff's psychosis. J Neuropathol Exp Neurol 52:567–579
88. Halliday G, Ellis J, Harper C (1992) The locus coeruleus and memory: a study of chronic alcoholics with and without the memory impairment of Korsakoff's psychosis. Brain Res 598:33–37
89. Estruch R, Nicolas JM, Salamero M, Aragon C, Sacanella E, Fernandez-Sola J, Urbano-Marquez A (1997) Atrophy of the corpus callosum in chronic alcoholism. J Neurol Sci 146:145–151
90. Pfefferbaum A, Lim KO, Desmond J, Sullivan EV (1996) Thinning of the corpus callosum in older alcoholic men. A magnetic resonance imaging study. Alcohol Clin Exp Res 20:752–757
91. Pfefferbaum A, Adalsteinsson E, Sullivan EV (2006) Dysmorphology and microstructural degradation of the corpus callosum: Interaction of age and alcoholism. Neurobiol Aging 27:994–1009
92. Crews FT, Collins MA, Dlugos C, Littleton J, Wilkins L, Neafsey EJ et al. (2004) Alcohol-induced neurodegeneration: when, where and why? Alcohol Clin Exp Res 28:350–364
93. Randoll LA, Wilson WR, Weaver MS, Spuhler-Phillips K, Leslie SW (1996) N-Methyl-D-aspartate-stimulated increases in intracellular calcium exhibit brain regional differences in sensitivity to inhibition by ethanol. Alcohol Clin Exp Res 20:197–200
94. Cullen KM, Halliday GM (1994) Chronic alcoholics have substantial glial pathology in the forebrain and diencephalon. Alcohol Alcohol Suppl 2:253–257

95. Davis RL, Syapin PJ (2004) Ethanol increases nuclear factor-kappa B activity in human astroglial cells. Neurosci Lett 371:128–132
96. Syapin PJ, Hickey WF, Kane CJM (2005) Alcohol brain damage and neuroinflammation: Is there a connection? Alcohol Clin Exp Res 29:1080–1089
97. Vallés SL, Blanco AM, Pascual M, Guerri C (2004) Chronic ethanol treatment enhances inflammatory mediators and cell death in the brain and in astrocytes. Brain Pathol 14:365–371
98. Montoliu C, Sancho-Tello M, Azorin I, Burgal M, Vallés SL, Renau-Piqueras J et al. (1995) Ethanol increases cytochrome P4502E1 and induces oxidative stress in astrocytes. J Neurochem 65:2561–2570
99. Gocht A, Colmant HJ (1987) Central pontine and extrapontine myelinolysis: a report of 58 cases. Clin Neuropathol 6:262–270
100. Kleinschmidt-DeMasters BK, Rojiani AM, Filley CM (2006) Central and extrapontine myelinolysis: then ... and now. J Neuropathol Exp Neurol 65:1–11
101. Lampl C, Yazdi K (2002) Central pontine myelinolysis. Eur Neurol 47:3–10
102. Newell KL, Kleinschmidt-DeMasters BK (1996) Central pontine myelinolysis at autopsy; a twelve year retrospective analysis. J Neurol Sci 142:134–139
103. Wright DG, Laureno R, Victor M (1979) Pontine and extrapontine myelinolysis. Brain 102:361–385
104. Adams R, Victor M, Mancall E (1959) Central pontine myelinolysis. A hitherto undescribed disease occurring in alcoholic and malnourished patients. Arch Neurol Psychiatr 81:154–172
105. Brown WD (2000) Osmotic demyelination disorders: central pontine and extrapontine myelinolysis. Curr Opin Neurol 13:691–697
106. Norenberg MD, Leslie KO, Robertson AS (1982) Association between rise in serum sodium and central pontine myelinolysis. Ann Neurol 11:128–135
107. Kumar S, Fowler M, Gonzalez-Toledo E, Jaffe SL (2006) Central pontine myelinolysis, an update. Neurol Res 28:360–366
108. Sterns RH, Riggs JE, Schochet SS (1986) Osmotic demyelination syndrome following correction of hyponatremia. N Engl J Med 314:1535–1542
109. Haibach H, Ansbacher LE, Dix JD (1987) Central pontine myelinolysis: a complication of hyponatremia or of therapeutic intervention? J Forensic Sci 32:441–451
110. Miller RF, Harrison MJG, Hall-Craggs MA, Scaravilli F (1998) Central pontine myelinolysis in AIDS. Acta Neuropathol 96:537–540
111. Messert B, Orrison WW, Hawkins MJ, Quaglieri CE (1979) Central pontine myelinolysis: considerations on etiology, diagnosis and treatment. Neurology 29:147–160
112. Menger H, Jörg J (1999) Outcome of central pontine and extrapontine myelinolysis. J Neurol 246:700–705
113. Wilske J, Henn R (1983) Zentrale pontine Myelinolyse - Ursache unklarer Todesfälle. In: Barz J, Bösche J, Frohberg H, Joachim H, Käppner R, Mattern R (eds) Fortschritte der Rechtsmedizin. Festschrift für Georg Schmidt. Springer, Berlin Heidelberg New York, pp 123–128
114. Endo Y, Oda M, Hara M (1981) Central pontine myelinolysis. A study of 37 cases in 1,000 consecutive autopsies. Acta Neuropathol 53:145–153
115. Ashrafian H, Davey P (2001) A review of the causes of central pontine myelinosis: yet another apoptotic illness? Eur J Neurol 8:103–109
116. Cravioto H, Korein J, Silberman J (1961) Wernicke's encephalopathy. A clinical and pathological study of 28 autopsied cases. Arch Neurol 4:510–519
117. Halliday G, Cullen K, Harding A (1994) Neuropathological correlates of memory dysfunction in the Wernicke-Korsakoff syndrome. Alcohol Alcohol Suppl 2:245–251
118. Victor M, Adams RD, Collins GH (1971) The Wernicke-Korsakoff syndrome: a clinical and pathological study of 245 patients, 82 with post-mortem examinations. Contemp Neurol Ser 7:1–206

119. Malamud N, Skillicorn SA (1956) Relationship between the Wernicke and the Korsakoff syndrome: a clinicopathologic study of seventy cases. Arch Neurol Psychiatr 76:585–596
120. Kopelman MD (1995) The Korsakoff syndrome. Br J Psychiatr 166:154–173
121. Berger JR (2004) Memory and the mammillothalamic tract. AJNR Am J Neuroradiol 25:906–907
122. Torvik A (1987) Topographic distribution and severity of brain lesions in Wernicke's encephalopathy. Clin Neuropathol 6:25–29
123. Torvik A (1985) Two types of brain lesions in Wernicke's encephalopathy. Neuropathol Appl Neurobiol 11:179–190
124. Harper C, Butterworth R (2002) Nutritional and metabolic disorders. In: Graham DI, Lantos PL (eds) Greenfield's neuropathology, 7th edn. Arnold Publishers, London, pp 607–652
125. Harding A, Halliday G, Caine D, Kril J (2000) Degeneration of anterior thalamic nuclei differentiates alcoholics with amnesia. Brain 123:141–154
126. Shear PK, Sullivan EV, Lane B, Pfefferbaum A (1996) Mammillary body and cerebellar shrinkage in chronic alcoholics with and without amnesia. Alcohol Clin Exp Res 20:1489–1495
127. Visser PJ, Krabbendam L, Verhey FRJ, Hofman PAM, Verhoeven WMA, Tuinier S et al. (1999) Brain correlates of memory dysfunction in alcoholic Korsakoff's syndrome. J Neurol Neurosurg Psychiatr 67:774–778
128. Victor M (1987) The irrelevance of mammillary body lesions in the causation of the Korsakoff amnesic state. Int J Neurol 21/22:51–57
129. Harper C (1983) The incidence of Wernicke's encephalopathy in Australia – a neuropathological study of 131 cases. J Neurol Neurosurg Psychiatr 46:593–598
130. Harper CG, Giles M, Finlay-Jones R (1986) Clinical signs in the Wernicke-Korsakoff complex: a retrospective analysis of 131 cases diagnosed at necropsy. J Neurol Neurosurg Psychiatr 49:341–345
131. Naidoo DP, Bramdev A, Cooper K (1996) Autopsy prevalence of Wernicke's encephalopathy in alcohol-related disease. S Afr Med J 86:1110–1112
132. Thomson AD (2000) Mechanisms of vitamin deficiency in chronic alcohol misusers and the development of the Wernicke-Korsakoff syndrome. Alcohol Alcohol Suppl. 35:2–7
133. Charness ME (1993) Brain lesions in alcoholics. Alcohol Clin Exp Res 17:2–11
134. Rodda R, Cummings R, Milligens KS (1978) Wernicke-Korsakov syndrome lesions in coronial necropsies. Clin Exp Neurol 15:114–126
135. Butterworth RF (2003) Hepatic encephalopathy. Alcohol Res Health 27:240–246
136. Lewis M, Howdle PD (2003) The neurology of liver failure. QJM 96:623–633
137. Lizardi-Cervera J, Almeda P, Guevara L, Uribe M (2003) Hepatic encephalopathy: a review. Ann Hepatol 2:122–130
138. Vaquero J, Chung C, Cahill ME, Blei AT (2003) Pathogenesis of hepatic encephalopathy in acute liver failure. Semin Liver Dis 23:259–269
139. Blei AT, Larsen FS (1999) Pathophysiology of cerebral edema in fulminant hepatic failure. J Hepatol 31:771–776
140. Norenberg MD (1998) Astroglial dysfunction in hepatic encephalopathy. Metab Brain Dis 13:319–335
141. Häussinger D, Kircheis G, Fischer R, Schliess F, vom Dahl S (2000) Hepatic encephalopathy in chronic liver disease: a clinical manifestation of astrocyte swelling and low-grade cerebral edema? J Hepatol 32:1035–1038
142. Kato M, Hughes RD, Keays RT, Williams R (1992) Electron microscopic study of brain capillaries in cerebral edema from fulminant hepatic failure. Hepatology 15:1060–1066
143. Kimura T, Budka H (1986) Glial fibrillary acidic protein and S-100 protein in human hepatic encephalopathy: immunoyctochemical demonstration of dissociation of two glia-associated proteins. Acta Neuropathol 70:17–21

144. Sobel RA, De Armond SJ, Forno LS, Eng LF (1981) Glial fibrillary acidic protein in hepatic encephalopathy. An immunohistochemical study. J Neuropathol Exp Neurol 40:625–632
145. Kohler CG, Ances BM, Coleman AR, Ragland JD, Lazarev M, Gur RC (2000) Marchiafava-Bignami disease: literature review and case report. Neuropsychiatr Neuropsychol Behav Neurol 13:67–76
146. Jellinger K (1961) Marchiafava-Bignami-Syndrom. Acta Neuropathol 1:101–104
147. Cook CC, Hallwood PM, Thomson AD (1998) B Vitamin deficiency and neuropsychiatric syndromes in alcohol misuse. Alcohol Alcohol 33:317–336
148. Serdaru M, Hausser-Hauw C, Laplane D, Buge A, Castaigne P, Goulon M et al. (1988) The clinical spectrum of alcoholic pellagra encephalopathy. A retrospective analysis of 22 cases studied pathologically. Brain 111:829–842
149. Hauw JJ, De Baecque C, Hausser-Hauw C, Serdaru M (1988) Chromatolysis in alcoholic encephalopathies. Pellagra-like changes in 22 cases. Brain 111:843–857
150. Ishii N, Nishihara Y (1981) Pellagra among chronic alcoholics: clinical and pathological study of 20 necropsy cases. J Neurol Neurosurg Psychiatr 44:209–215
151. Hillbom M, Juvela S, Numminen H (1999) Alcohol intake and the risk of stroke. J Cardiovasc Risk 6:223–228
152. Leppävuori A, Vataja R, Pohjasvaara T, Kaste M, Mäntylä R, Erkinjuntti T (2003) Alcohol misuse: a risk factor for putaminal damage by ischemic brain infarct? Eur Neurol 50:69–72
153. Camargo CA Jr (1989) Moderate alcohol consumption and stroke. The epidemiologic evidence. Stroke 20:1611–1626
154. Hillbom M, Kaste M (1982) Alcohol intoxication: a risk factor for primary subarachnoid hemorrhage. Neurology 32:706–711
155. Dick DM, Foroud T (2003) Candidate genes for alcohol dependence: a review of genetic evidence from human studies. Alcohol Clin Exp Res 27:868–879
156. Dodd PR, Foley PF, Buckley ST, Eckert AL, Innes DJ (2004) Genes and gene expression in the brain of the alcoholic. Addict Behav 29:1295–1309
157. Worst TJ, Vrana KE (2005) Alcohol and gene expression in the central nervous system. Alcohol Alcohol 40:63–75
158. Anni H, Israel Y (2002) Proteomics in alcohol research. Alcohol Res Health 26:219–232

Chapter 6
The Medicolegal Evaluation of Excited Delirium

James R. Gill

Contents

Abstract   Excited delirium is a life-threatening syndrome that may be initiated by a variety of causes including drug intoxications and psychiatric illnesses. People in an excited delirium may demonstrate paranoid, aggressive, and incoherent behavior. Due to their actions, people in an excited delirium may come to the attention of law enforcement. The challenge for the forensic pathologist arises when these deaths occur during or shortly following a violent struggle, often involving law enforcement agents. Three instances of excited delirium are described to demonstrate further the syndrome and to serve as a basis for the discussion of the medicolegal aspects of excited delirium. There are several theories for this syndrome and much attention has been given to the role of restraint and struggle. In addition to asphyxial mechanisms,

J.R. Gill
Office of Chief Medical Examiner, New York, NY 10016
e-mail: jgill@ocme.nyc.gov

M. Tsokos (ed.), *Forensic Pathology Reviews, Volume 5*,
doi: 10.1007/978-1-59745-110-9_6, © Humana Press, Totowa, NJ 2008

other neurochemical abnormalities involving dopamine, elevated potassium concentrations, lactic acidosis, and increased catecholamine effects on the heart have been examined. Cocaine and amphetamine are two of many substances that may cause the syndrome of excited delirium. The goal of the autopsy in suspected excited delirium deaths is to identify (or exclude) a disease or injury sufficient to explain a sudden death in the context of the investigated circumstances. In deaths due to excited delirium, there is no pathognomonic autopsy finding and minor injuries (abrasions, contusions, cuts) are typical. Due to the complex physiologic, chemical, environmental, and traumatic interactions that occur, there is perhaps no other type of death in which it is so important to apply the forensic maxim that each death must be evaluated "one at a time". The roles of restraint, electromuscular disruption devices (e g , Tasers®), mechanical trauma, stress, and natural disease must be considered in the certification of death.

Keywords Forensic pathology · Agitated delirium · Excited delirium · Taser® · Cocaine psychosis · Restraint

6.1 Introduction

Delirium is an acute, confusional syndrome with a transient disturbance in consciousness and cognition that has a variety of causes (Table 6.1) [6.1]. There is a subset of patients with delirium that involves marked agitation and violent behavior. In recent years, studies have examined individuals with delirium who present in a highly agitated state and die suddenly [2, 3, 4, 5, 6, 7, 8, 9, 10, 11, 12, 13]. Excited delirium is a type of delirium involving violent behavior. Delirium and excited delirium are not synonyms.

Excited (agitated) delirium is a life-threatening syndrome that may be initiated by a variety of causes. Presently, the syndrome is largely associated with drug intoxications (cocaine, methamphetamine) and psychiatric illness [2, 3]. It is characterized by sudden death during or following an episode of excited delirium in which an autopsy fails to detect a disease or physical injury that has an extent or severity to explain the death and the circumstances are consistent with the syndrome [3]. It is a clinicopathologic diagnosis based upon the autopsy and toxicologic results evaluated in the context of the history and circumstances.

Excited delirium is characterized by a sudden onset of bizarre and violent behavior and may be accompanied by combativeness, confusion, hyperactivity, paranoid delusions, incoherent shouting, hallucinations, hyperthermia, and sudden death [4, 5, 6, 7, 8, 9, 10, 11, 12, 13]. If these individuals come to the attention of others (usually law enforcement), they are often restrained in an attempt to prevent them from injuring themselves or others. During this attempt at restraint, a violent struggle often ensues. Shortly after the struggle ends, the individual abruptly becomes unresponsive and is found in cardiopulmonary arrest [5, 6, 12]. The syndrome is more common when the weather is warm and humid [6, 11].

Table 6.1 Causes of delirium/psychosis (according to [1, 10, 67])

Drug intoxications/withdrawals
Acute functional psychosis (schizophrenia, acute mania)
Endocrine/Metabolic disease
Hyperthyroidism, hypothyroidism ("myxedema madness")
Hypoglycemia
Pituitary disease with secondary endocrine effects
Postpartum psychosis
Porphyria
Liver and kidney failure (uremia)
Electrolyte disorders
Acid base imbalance,
Nutritional disorders
Thiamin/vitamin B12 deficiency ("megaloblastic madness")
Infections
Meningitis, encephalitis, sepsis
Neoplasia (brain tumors)
Seizure disorders
Complex partial seizures ("temporal lobe" or "psychomotor" epilepsy), postictal state
Vascular disorders
Hypertensive encephalopathy/cerebral infarcts
Systemic lupus erythematosus
Disseminated intravascular coagulation
Trauma
Concussion
Subdural, epidural, subarachnoid hematoma
Hypothermia/Hyperthermia
Hypoxia
Factitious psychosis/malingering

The challenge for the forensic pathologist arises when these deaths occur during or shortly following a violent struggle, often involving law enforcement agents. If death occurs during the ensuing struggle and restraint, the differential diagnosis of the cause of death is invariably expanded to include possible physical trauma including neck or chest compression (from choke holds or restraint), blunt impact injury, electrical injury from the use of electromuscular disruption devices (e.g., Tasers®), or chemical injury from pepper sprays [14, 15]. Others have noted that virtually all of these episodes are terminated by a struggle with police or medical personnel [3]. This observation, however, has a selection bias since most people in a state of excited delirium who come to the attention of others, will usually result in police or medical notification.

There are deaths due to cocaine-induced excited delirium, however, that do not come to the attention of the police or medical personnel [11]. Without a careful scene investigation, these deaths may not be recognized as an instance of excited delirium. Instead, they are simply certified, for example, as acute cocaine intoxication. Therefore, some deaths with an excited delirium mechanism may not be recognized by the medical examiner/coroner and simply be certified as the underlying intoxication. The only evidence of an unwitnessed excited delirium may be a broken-up apartment where the decedent was found, or unexplained non-lethal injuries.

The evaluation and certification of these deaths can be a challenge for the medical examiner/coroner [2, 3, 16, 17, 18]. Not only can the determination of the cause of death be demanding, but also are the invariable challenges by family, the press, and other legal agencies that believe that the police caused the death.

6.2 Pathogenesis and Pathophysiology

There are several theories for this syndrome [2, 3, 6, 12, 19]. Historically it has been described in psychiatric patients as acute exhaustive mania (Bell's mania) [2, 3]. Much attention has been given to the role of restraint and struggle [7, 9, 20, 21, 22, 23, 24, 25, 26]. In addition to asphyxial mechanisms, other neuro-chemical abnormalities involving dopamine, elevated potassium concentrations, lactic acidosis, autonomic dysfunction, and increased catecholamine effects on the heart have been examined [3, 12, 27, 28, 29]. Cocaine and amphetamine are two of many substances that may cause the syndrome of excited delirium. Chemically, cocaine affects the dopamine and catecholamine systems of the body. Some have linked the syndrome to the neuroleptic malignant syndrome (NMS) [6]. Medications involved with dopamine activity also play a role in the NMS. It is postulated that abnormalities in the number and type of dopamine receptors result in the syndrome. Elevated environmental temperature creates a further risk for morbidity and mortality with cocaine abuse [30]. Deaths from excited delirium have been reported to occur more often in the summer (June to September) than in any other season [6, 11].

6.3 Case Studies

Three instances of excited delirium are described in the following to further demonstrate the syndrome and to serve as a basis for the discussion of the medicolegal aspects of excited delirium.

Case #1: Classic Excited Delirium A 37-year-old man assaulted a woman on the street and was found running around with his pants down when police arrived. He resisted arrest and ran back and forth, slammed his head on the sidewalk, and ate dirt out of a planter. The emergency service unit was called to help restrain him. He bit an officer's shoe and holster. It took over ten people to restrain and cuff him. When the emergency medical services arrived, they found him prone and combative. He was placed on a stretcher. Since he was still combative, he was placed on his left side and strapped to the stretcher by his shoulders, pelvis, and lower legs. The emergency medical technicians stated that they needed to restrain his arms and that they had seen the police restrain him only by holding his extremities. No police officer was seen to restrain him by the neck, head, or by standing or sitting on him. His initial vitals signs were pulse of 220 and respiratory rate of 22. He was diaphoretic and "hot to touch". His temperature was not recorded. He had a patent airway. After loading him into the ambulance, he became apneic and pulseless. Cardiopulmonary resuscitation was started. He was pronounced dead in the Emergency Department. Neither pepper spray (oleresin capsicum) nor electromuscular disruption devices were used.

At autopsy, he measured 5′11″ and weighed 195 lbs. He had a rectal temperature of 91°F obtained 11.5 h after death. He had numerous blunt injuries of the head, neck, trunk, and extremities. There were numerous recent contusions of the head with a focal area of subarachnoid hemorrhage. There was no skull fracture, epidural/subdural hemorrhage, or cerebral contusion. There was slight cardiac hypertrophy and steatosis of the liver. There was hemorrhage in both sternocleidomastoid muscles and the posterior neck muscles. There were no petechiae. There were numerous contusions and abrasions of the chest, back, and buttocks (0.5–1.5″). There were numerous contusions/abrasions of the upper and lower extremities including band-like contusions/abrasions of the wrists (consistent with handcuffs). There were no fractures or visceral injuries. His blood cocaine concentration was 0.16 mg/L. In addition, ethanol (0.04 gm%), pseudoephedrine (<0.1 mg/L), and bupropion (<0.1 mg/L) were detected. His cause of death was certified as being due to acute intoxication due to the combined effects of cocaine, ethanol, bupropion, and pseudoephedrine with agitated delirium. The manner of death was certified as an accident.

Case #2: Excited Delirium Without Restraint A 31-year-old man was found dead in his locked and secured apartment on a June afternoon in New York City. The previous night he was with his wife and cousin who stated that the decedent had been on a three day cocaine binge and "was acting crazy". At one point, he picked up a kitchen knife and threatened them. He began breaking up the apartment and stabbing the walls and doors. The wife and cousin left the apartment. The wife shortly returned to the apartment for her slippers but the decedent would not let her enter. The wife could hear the decedent still breaking things in the apartment. The wife returned the next day and could not gain entrance to the apartment. She went up the fire escape and could see the decedent on the bedroom floor with blood around him. The window and window gate were forced open and 911 was called. He was pronounced dead at the scene at 1 pm. There was blood spatter on the floor, furniture, and ceiling. The bed frame was broken and a knife (with a broken handle) was recovered on the bed. The bloody decedent had a plastic bag with white powder protruding from his mouth. At the scene, 7 h after he was initially found, he was in full rigor with a body temperature of 96°F (room temperature 88°F).

At autopsy, he had superficial cuts of his right palm, fingers, and forearm without injury of major blood vessels. He had scattered contusions of his upper extremities and no other injuries of the body including the neck. There were no petechiae. His blood cocaine concentration was 6.2 mg/L. The powder residue in the plastic bag was cocaine. His death was certified as a cocaine-induced excited delirium with an accidental manner. The sharp injuries did not contribute to his death.

Case #3: Excited Delirium with Restraint, Videotaped in the Emergency Department An excited 40-year-old man was screaming and behaving in a paranoid manner on a sidewalk in New York City. He had a long history of substance abuse. According to his wife, he had recently started using drugs again and so she had put him out of the house a few days earlier. Two police officers arrived and spoke with him. He walked freely on his own to the ambulance. He was transported by emergency medical services to the hospital. In the emergency department, he continued screaming and stated that "people are following him". He became uncooperative and more agitated. Security and police officers brought him to the floor and handcuffed him. The treating physician, who was present for this, stated that he continued to be verbally and physically aggressive while on the floor.

He was placed on a gurney face down while a physician was in attendance. He was immediately rolled into an examination room. The patient was still shouting and moving while on the gurney. An IV was started and the patient vomited. He was turned over and, as he was being undressed, was noted to be apneic. He had pulseless electrical activity and advanced cardiac life support was started. Attempts at resuscitation were unsuccessful. His body temperature was reported to be normal. The events in the emergency department were recorded by security cameras and confirmed the verbal descriptions given by the physician and security officers. The struggle and placement on the gurney before being wheeled to the examination room lasted less than 2 min.

At autopsy, he weighed 218 lbs and was 65″ tall. There were scattered superficial abrasions and contusions of the upper extremities and chest. There was a 0.25″ laceration of the upper lip. There were no petechiae, neck injury, or blockage of the airway. He had no underlying heart, liver, lung, or kidney disease. Toxicology was positive for cocaine (0.10 mg/L), benzoylecgonine (1.2 mg/L), and methadone (1.2 mg/L). His death was certified as a cocaine-induced excited delirium with an accidental manner.

6.4 Dissection and Toxicology

The goal of the autopsy in suspected excited delirium deaths is to identify (or exclude) a disease or injury sufficient to explain a sudden death in the context of the investigated circumstances. To make the diagnosis of excited delirium, one must search for the cause of the delirium, have circumstances consistent with the syndrome, and exclude other intervening causes. The diagnosis is made through a complete case investigation, an autopsy, and toxicology studies.

6.4.1 Gross Pathology

In deaths due to excited delirium, there is no pathognomonic autopsy finding, and minor injuries (abrasions, contusions, cuts) are typical. It is common for people in an excited delirium to have numerous blunt and/or sharp injuries even without attempts at restraint or intervention by police or medical personnel. There are case reports of people in an excited delirium who have slammed their head against a brick wall, jumped down a flight of stairs, dived through a window, and crashed a car [5, 10, 31, 32]. In these instances, one must carefully document the injuries and search for other potential mechanisms of death. For example, are the sharp injuries and the amount of blood at the scene sufficient to produce exsanguination or another mechanism (air embolism)? An expanding subdural hematoma or a large hemoperitoneum due to a splenic laceration are examples of potential efficient intervening causes in an instance of excited delirium.

At autopsy, full body photographs demonstrating all positive and negative findings must be done. The presence, or absence, of petechiae (conjunctival, facial, and oral mucosa) and strap muscle hemorrhage of the neck should be documented. Postmortem radiographs and subcutaneous dissection for occult contusions, particularly in darkly pigmented individuals, also can be of benefit. Some patients who are successfully resuscitated succumb later in the hospital due to rhabdomyolysis, acute renal failure, and disseminated intravascular coagulation. One may see evidence of these mechanisms including extensive gastrointestinal mucosal hemorrhages or myoglobin casts in the renal tubules.

6.4.2 Toxicology

Toxicologic analysis must be performed in these deaths. Common and uncommon drugs of abuse (cocaine, methamphetamine, PCP, and other hallucinogens) should be investigated, in addition to various psychiatric medications and anticholinergic medications. Vitreous electrolyte studies can detect hyperglycemia and uremia.

Cocaine and amphetamines are often detected in instances of the syndrome of excited delirium. They are commonly abused drugs and so it is not surprising that they have become a common cause of excited delirium [2, 4, 11]. Although the most common antecedent for excited delirium is a recent cocaine binge, the concentrations of cocaine in people who die of excited delirium are not always high [5, 20, 33]. Cocaine and amphetamine, however, are not the only toxicologic causes for the syndrome. Other illicit and therapeutic drugs (e.g., psychotropic medications) are associated with excited delirium and/or can cause delirium and acute psychosis (Table 6.2). Sometimes, a cause of the excited delirium is undetermined [10]. In delayed hospital deaths due to suspected excited delirium, an admission blood sample may be retrieved for forensic toxicology testing.

Table 6.2 Drugs associated with acute psychosis

Ethanol
Ethanol intoxication
Ethanol withdrawal
Sympathomimetic drugs
Cocaine
Amphetamines
Tricyclic antidepressants
Monoamine oxidase inhibitors
Methylphenidates
Sedative drugs
Sedative drug withdrawal
Hallucinogens
Lysergic acid diethylamide (LSD)
Mescaline
Phencyclidine (PCP)
Psilocybin
Anticholinergic drugs
Includes drugs with anticholinergic side-effects, antipsychotic agents, antihistamine, etc.
Corticosteroids

6.4.3 Neuropathology

There is no gross or microscopic neuropathologic finding that is diagnostic of death caused by excited delirium. Postmortem neurochemical examination of the brain (dopamine synaptic markers/receptors in the striatum and hypothalamus) has been suggested by some to diagnose excited delirium [6, 12]. These examinations require the brain to be frozen and sent on dry ice to a special laboratory for testing. These tests may lend support to the diagnosis of excited delirium but they do not diagnose the proximate cause of death. In addition, they will not determine if there was an efficient intervening cause of death that occurred in a person in an excited delirium. The circumstances and autopsy findings are usually more important than this neurochemical analysis. It is analogous to finding a seizure focus in the brain of an epileptic. Such a finding may support that the person was an epileptic but, by itself, does not prove that the person died of a seizure.

Serious (but non-life threatening) craniocerebral trauma has been reported in instances of excited delirium [32]. These *incidental* head injuries do not cause or contribute to death. There are reports of people who die due to excited delirium but also have head injuries (e.g., a skull fracture) [32]. These must be carefully evaluated in the context of the circumstances and with regard to mechanisms of death. For example, a small subarachnoid hemorrhage or limited cerebral contusion, under ordinary circumstances, are insufficient to explain death [32]. One must not overestimate these findings, particularly without placing them in the context of the circumstances. Before one invokes an injury as the cause of death, the injury must mechanistically and circumstantially fit with the death. Is the head injury consistent with a delayed death with a lucid interval (expanding subdural hematoma) or an immediate incapacitation (traumatic diffuse axonal injury)? This requires a thorough understanding of craniocerebral trauma including its interpretation, mechanisms of death, and secondary changes. As Karch stated, "attributing a death to a trivial head injury is still another temptation best avoided" [12].

6.5 Medicolegal Aspects of Excited Delirium

The role of the medical examiner/coroner in these deaths is ultimately to certify the cause and manner of death. Due to the complex physiologic, chemical, environmental, and traumatic interactions that occur, this can be a challenge. There is perhaps no other type of death in which it is so important to apply the forensic maxim that each death must be evaluated "one at a time". Certain guidelines, however, need to be understood in order to maintain consistency and objectivity. Consistency is crucial if the medical examiner/coroner is to be an unbiased, objective participant in the judicial system [34].

In these fatalities, the circumstances supply important information for proper certification. Investigators should go directly to the primary sources of information (witnesses) and not rely on an emergency department physician who received the information from the medical resident who received it from the emergency medical service (EMS). A step-by-step, freeze frame analysis of the events as suggested by Luke and Reay [18], should be carried out. One needs to ask the witnesses "what did you see and hear? Was there neck or chest compression? If so, for how long? Was the person speaking, yelling, or making noises? Was it continuous, and if so for how long? When did the person become unresponsive?" These questions are very important when trying to include or exclude certain causes of death. For example, it does not make physiologic sense for a cause of death to be electrocution in a person who becomes unresponsive 10 min after an electromuscular disruption device (EMDD) shock. When cocaine users with excited delirium die, the cocaine intoxication should be considered the cause of death, unless there is clear evidence that death is due to some mechanism other than cocaine intoxication, such as mechanical asphyxia [6].

6.5.1 The Role of Restraint/Positional Asphyxia and Cause of Death

Several studies on excited delirium report that all of their fatalities were restrained prior to death [7, 9, 20, 21]. This is not surprising since these are instances of excited delirium that have come to the attention of the police/EMS. Restraint is commonly employed in emotionally disturbed people in an attempt to prevent them from injuring themselves or others. There are, however, reports of deaths due to excited delirium that did not occur in police custody and/or with hobble restraint [7, 11].

Restraint asphyxia is one proposed cause of death that has been considered in these fatalities [21, 31, 35]. Initial studies of hobble restraint in the prone position examined peripheral oxygen saturations and heart rates following exercise. The authors concluded that the results showed that positional restraint can prolong recovery from exercise as determined by changes in peripheral oxygen saturation and heart rate [36]. This study was followed by three case reports describing positional asphyxia [37]. Later studies that have used more sophisticated monitoring and examination have come to varying conclusions [38, 39, 40, 41]. Authors of the initial study subsequently acknowledged that the hobble position should be viewed as an inherently neutral position with no significant physiologic consequence in normal people [42].

These later studies by Chan and others examined the role that hobble restraint has on pulmonary function [38, 41, 43]. In one study, they sought to determine the effect on respiratory function of 25 and 50 lbs of weight placed on the backs of human volunteers in this prone restraint position. They measured pulse oximetry, end-tidal CO_2 concentrations, forced vital capacity (FVC), and forced expiratory volume in 1 s (FEV1). They concluded that prone restraint with and without 25 and 50 lbs of weight resulted in a restrictive pulmonary function pattern but there was no evidence of hypoxia or hypoventilation [39].

One may reasonably question whether is it valid to equate studies on normal subjects to the effect of prone restraint on a struggling (exhausted) person in excited delirium. Attempts have been made in the laboratory to reproduce some of these factors as well. Chan examined the effects of strenuous exercise followed by prone restraint on respiratory function on 15 healthy men ages 18 through 40 years [38]. Pulmonary function tests were obtained with subjects in the sitting, supine, prone, and restraint positions. After a 4-min exercise period, subjects rested in the sitting position while pulse, oxygen saturation, and arterial blood gases were monitored. The subjects repeated the exercise and then were placed in the restraint position. There was a statistically significant decline in the mean FVC and FEV1 comparing the sitting with the restraint position. There was no evidence of hypoxia in either position and the mean carbon dioxide tension (PCO_2) for both groups was not different after 15 min of rest in the sitting vs the restraint position. In their study population of healthy subjects, the restraint position resulted in a restrictive pulmonary function pattern but did not result in clinically relevant changes in oxygenation or ventilation [38].

At autopsy, the differentiation of death due to intoxication versus asphyxia may be difficult. Usually the question is not answered solely by the autopsy. Facial plethora with florid conjunctival petechiae are supportive of neck or chest compression and can be powerful evidence in the proper context. But their absence does not exclude neck compression and they may be caused in other ways [44]. Witness statements can be particularly helpful to assess if chest compression caused death. In order for people to speak, yell, or moan, they must be able to move air through their larynx. If they can move air, they can breath. In order to be asphyxiated by chest compression, one must have a prolonged interference with ventilation. During this time, one would expect to hear no vocalization.

Rarely, positional asphyxia may play a role in these deaths. Some individuals, typically those morbidly obese, may have respiratory compromise if for example, they are placed in hobble restraint on the floor of a car with their abdomen over the transmission hump [45, 46].

6.5.2 The Role of Mechanical Injury and the Cause of Death

Excited delirium is a competent immediate cause of death and other non-fatal injuries need not be invoked to explain the death. As Wetli et al. noted in regard to cocaine-induced excited delirium: "it is often tempting to attribute the cause of death to one of the minor injuries, such as minor head injury. Needless litigation is often the result" [6]. Nonlethal injuries sustained in the process of subduing an individual should not be overinterpreted [32]. One must evaluate the death in the context of the entire event with consideration of mechanisms of death to avoid the trap of ascribing the death to scant subarachnoid hemorrhage or linear skull fracture even when the circumstances are inconsistent with death from a head injury. There is a temptation to focus on the readily demonstrable injury which is much easier to show and explain than the "invisible" functional mechanism of a drug intoxication death.

In the study by Stratton et al., all 18 decedents struggled with law enforcement personnel and had abrasions and contusions of the body including the head [9]. External injuries from the struggle may appear striking and difficult to ignore with regard to the cause of death. However, as a forensic pathologist, one must identify a pathophysiologic mechanism to link the often impressive external injuries with death. One must look for corresponding internal injuries that are sufficient to explain death (e.g., lacerated spleen with hemoperitoneum). Without a mechanistic link, these external injuries usually are incidental and not the cause of death. This interpretation can be difficult for the family to understand.

6.5.3 The Role of an Electromuscular Disruption Device (EMDD) and the Cause of Death

Electromuscular disruption devices (EMDD) may be used on people in a state of excited delirium. Law enforcement agents have a continuum of use of force at their disposal to employ as violence (or the risk of violence or injury) escalates. These start with verbal commands and progress to physical contact, chemical agents (pepper spray), EMDDs, and firearms. EMDDs are battery powered electrical devices used by law enforcement to temporarily incapacitate people with a short duration, high voltage, and low amperage electric current. The current is not limited to the path between the two electrodes and will find low resistance routes within the body (e.g., blood vessel and nerve pathways) which results in an incapacitating effect on the whole body [47].

With EMDDs the question arises, what, if any, role did it play in the fatality? If it did cause or contribute to the death, what was the mechanism? Did it cause a direct electrical disturbance in the heart or did the stress from its application result in a cardiac arrhythmia?

The risk of an EMDD directly causing a cardiac arrhythmia through an electrical mechanism appears extremely rare [17, 28, 48]. In one study, 32 resting adults received a 5-s EMDD application [28]. EKGs and blood testing were done before and after the application. There was no affect on cardiac electrical activity after receiving the application. A study by Levine et al. used continuous electrocardiographic monitoring before, during, and after an EMDD application. They found no cardiac dysrhythmias or EKG changes in human subjects who received an EMDD shock [48].

People die of excited delirium without having been struck by an EMDD. In a study of fatalities of 18 people with signs of excited delirium (all witnessed by emergency medical technicians), EMDDs were used in 28%. In another study of 61 excited delirium deaths, EMDDs were used in 5% of the deaths [7]. EMDDs are not required for death to occur in a person in an excited delirium. Therefore, should it be invoked in the cause of death? Could a person who was in an excited delirium die from direct EMDD electrical effects on the heart causing a lethal cardiac arrhythmia? This is essentially asking if the EMDD is capable of causing death by electrocution. Over the years, training classes conducted on EMDDs by their manufacturer have delivered more than 100,000 EMDD applications to participants with no reported cardiac arrests or deaths [28]. Even though this population may not be representative of an individual in excited delirium, it is compelling evidence that EMDDs rarely, if ever, cause death by an electrocution mechanism.

Some may argue that these studies are not a valid comparison because these populations are different to people in an excited delirium. Patients in an excited delirium have increased heart rates, high concentrations of adrenalin, and possibly other "arrythmogenic" chemicals in their system. Would these factors lower the arrhythmia "threshold" in this group so their hearts are susceptible to this electrical current that, in a "normal" person, would not cause a problem? This may be possible (and impossible to exclude) but the lack of any cardiac electrical changes in the above studies and analysis of strength-duration thresholds for myocyte excitation and induction of ventricular fibrillation support that EMDDs do not generate currents in the heart that are high enough to excite myocytes or trigger VF [49]. A study on sheep in which the skin and subcutaneous tissues were reflected, however, was able to trigger VF if the dart was implanted within 2.3 cm of the heart [50, 51]. A recent report of a man with an implanted pacemaker, who survived an EMDD application, described ventricular myocardial capture at a high rate corresponding to the exact time of the barb application as determined by subsequent interrogation of the pacemaker [52].

Electrocution causes death by two mechanisms. The first is a non-cardiac contraction of muscles (including respiratory) that may cause death by an asphyxial mechanism if the current application is continuous and prolonged (on the order of minutes). The second mechanism is passage of the electricity through a vital organ that is susceptible to disruption by the flow of electricity (e.g., the brain and heart) [53]. Fatal cardiac arrhythmias typically are caused by higher currents (50 mA for 2 s) than those that are reported to occur with EMDDs (Tasers's® manufacturer reported average 2.1 mA and other reported ranges: 3.3–10.9 mA) [17, 47, 54]. In addition to the current magnitude, one also must consider the body weight, duration, current frequency, and whether it is continuous [54]. A recent study has reported that an EMDD produces considerably more power and current than claimed by the manufacturer [55]. Analysis of this study by others (including the manufacturer) have pointed out several errors and the inability to reproduce certain results [56, 57].

Witness statements may assist to clarify further the role, if any, that EMDDs played in causing the death. If the death (unresponsiveness) does not occur until minutes after the EMDD was discharged then the pathophysiology of an electrocution or sudden cardiac arrhythmia has been excluded [58]. A prolonged application of an EMDD could potentially cause problems with respiration; however, if the person is conscious after the cessation of the shock, this mechanism of electrocution can be excluded. EMDDs cause pain and the role of this stress also should be considered.

6.5.4 The Role of Stress and the Cause of Death

Stress has been invoked to explain certain deaths. The classic example is "homicide by heart attack" [59, 60]. Homicide by heart attack is a well-accepted certification of death involving non-life-threatening, physical injury or assault (act that threatens physical harm). In these instances, death is typically due to underlying ischemic heart disease that is acutely stressed by the assault and/or battery. The stress of the illegal, hostile activity contributes to the cause of death and such fatalities are certified as homicides. The important components of this determination are the illegal, threatening nature of the altercation. Stress from this threat is the implied link between the illegal action, the heart disease, and the resultant cardiac arrhythmia.

Stress, from restraint or struggle, may also occur in deaths due to excited delirium. The person in an excited delirium, however, is already experiencing stress. They are in the midst of an acute, independently efficient syndrome that can cause death, with or without restraint. A person with stable ischemic heart disease also carries a risk of sudden death but with a homicide by heart attack, the temporal relationship between the assault and the death is so compelling that it links the two resulting in the homicide certification. This temporal relationship of a struggle also may be present in some excited delirium deaths but the struggle is not the major instigating factor and is not required for death to occur. But for the assault, it is unlikely that a person with ischemic heart disease would happen to die at that precise moment. However, a person in an excited delirium, even without struggle, EMDD injury, or hobble restraint, is already at increased risk to die at that particular time [7].

Pudiak and Bozarth [61] examined the fatal effects of cocaine and stress on laboratory rats. Rats were injected with cocaine or saline and then either returned to their cages or subjected to 30 min of restraint stress. The restraint stress consisted of putting the rat into a plastic cylinder that confined the rat but did not prohibit all movement or interfere with respiration (so-called confinement stress). Fatalities were recorded at the end of 30 min and the test was repeated for 5 consecutive days. At the end of the 5-day injection series, 58% of the cocaine-plus-restraint group died (25% died after the first exposure) and 17% of the cocaine-without-restraint died. None of the animals that received saline injection-plus-confinement died. Significantly ($p < 0.025$) more fatalities occurred in the cocaine-plus-restraint group [61]. Some rats, however, died even without the confinement stress. It is unknown whether any of the rats were in an excited delirium, or what the mortality rates would have been with and without restraint in those rats. Cocaine and stress, from any cause, are not a good mix. Veterinary studies also have reported the phenomenon of unexpected death following the chase and capture of big game animals due to "capture myopathy" (or "exertional myopathy") [7, 62].

Clinical studies have demonstrated the effects of stress ("myocardial stunning") on the heart [63, 64]. Elevated plasma catecholamines have been reported and an exaggerated sympathetic stimulation is a proposed mechanism [63]. People who are restrained against their will may experience stress. For example, a patient with dementia may become agitated and needs to be restrained. What if, during the struggle to restrain the patient, the patient dies and marked coronary disease is found at autopsy? There is restraint and struggle, yet would this be certified as a homicide? The treatment was appropriate and legal. This is similar to the excited delirium patient who struggles with police or medical personnel and is restrained. Did that struggle result in stress? Probably, but the primary trigger of the stress is not the restraint and struggle. If there is an independent, initiating cause for the stress, this underlying cause should dictate the manner of death and not any potential additional stress from the restraint.

Invariably, the person in an excited delirium is already experiencing an elevated degree of stress even before contact with law enforcement or medical personnel. Did the subsequent struggle and restraint contribute to death through the addition of more stress? The added stress certainly did not help, but does it need to be invoked? People in a state of excited delirium may die (or survive) with or without police restraint [11]. Since the excited delirium is the initiating and primary source of stress, the subsequent legal restraint is not considered in the certification of death.

6.5.5 Certification of Death

These deaths must be examined on a case by case basis. Some have stated that, because a violent struggle has occurred between two or more individuals, the best classification of the manner of death is probably homicide [45]. Others have certified them as accidents (with or without physical restraint) [7, 21]. Some have noted considerable variability, even in the same medical examiner's office, in the determination of the manner of death (accident vs homicide vs undetermined) and the wording of the cause of death [17, 21]. Before certifying the manner, one must first determine the cause of death since it will, in part, dictate the manner. The potential causes of death must be evaluated in the context of the circumstances of the death. Since these deaths are potential homicides, one must have a higher degree of certainty (reasonable degree of medical certainty) than for a natural death. To a reasonable degree of medical certainty, did the physical contact cause or contribute pathologically to the death? Physical restraint, violent struggle, or use of EMDDs or pepper spray, in and of themselves, should not automatically make the manner of death a homicide.

The syndrome of excited delirium is potentially lethal all by itself, as are a ruptured cerebral artery aneurysm and pulmonary embolism [65]. Even though excited delirium is a clinicopathologic diagnosis, once it is made, it has a potency similar to pulmonary embolism and should be treated as such. Due to the lack of compelling autopsy findings, however, it is usually not given the same standing. A descriptive or situational statement that encompasses identified factors in the death has been proposed to certify these deaths [42]. In fact, in some deaths, medical examiners/coroners may not be able to distinguish associations from causality or separate or assign percentages of causality. In deaths in which there is no single factor that is convincing enough to stand alone as the undisputed cause of death, it is reasonable to "cover the waterfront" [42]. A well-investigated, excited delirium diagnosis, however, is convincing enough to stand alone. The addition to the death certificate of other factors in such a death has the potential to obfuscate the proximate cause of death and turn associations into poorly supported causes [66].

Generally, death at the hand of another person, or due to the hostile or illegal actions (or inaction) of another person, are certified as homicide. Exceptions exist, however, including most motor vehicle collisions and contact sporting events. One must recognize that murder and homicide are not interchangeable and that certifying a death as a homicide does not always involve criminal activity. An armed bank robber who is fatally shot by the police (whether justified or not) is also certified as a homicide (as are judicial executions).

If physical restraint is to the extent that it causes lethal injury (e.g., asphyxia from chest compression or choke holds), then the manner of death is homicide [34]. If there is restraint/struggle, however, without lethal physiologic compromise, the manner should be dictated by the underlying pathology of the excited delirium. Any struggle/restraint, per se, should not automatically result in a homicide certification.

The physical confrontation ("struggle") causes some to conclude that these deaths are certified as homicide. But are these deaths caused by the hand of another or are they deaths caused by the syndrome of excited delirium with incidental contact? Violent physical contact with another is not required for a person to die from excited delirium. The physical contact reported in most instances of fatal excited delirium is a consequence of the excited delirium. This is an example of the *post hoc, ergo propter hoc* ("after this, therefore because of this") fallacy in which the temporal proximity of an action is confused with causality.

What most studies on excited delirium lack, are descriptions of all deaths due to excited delirium, not just those that occur during or following police action. Unfortunately, police custody deaths are usually the only ones that are reported as excited delirium fatalities. Forensic pathologists and medical examiners see not only the high profile fatalities in which law enforcement is involved but others that do not come to public attention. These include the excited delirium deaths in which the person dies alone in an apartment or in the emergency department during medically-applied restraint. Surveillance cameras have recorded some of these events which confirm the absence of neck or chest compression.

For example, a partially nude man is found in his secured apartment with empty crack cocaine vials, a few acute contusions, and an apartment in disarray with a smashed mirror. At autopsy there are no injuries or disease that explain his death. Cocaine is later detected in the blood and the death is certified as acute cocaine intoxication. Is this a missed instance of cocaine-induced excited delirium? It may be, but the medical examiner/coroner has no need to pursue this mechanism because even if it were, the proximate cause is still the cocaine intoxication. So it becomes another acute cocaine intoxication death and is not captured when someone retrospectively reviews all excited delirium deaths that were investigated by that office. In a study of cocaine-related deaths, Ruttenber et al. found that 45.6% of the deaths certified as acute cocaine toxicity were found dead at the scene [8].

Underlying natural disease may result in delirium. Patients with marked hypoxia, diabetic ketoacidosis, or intracerebral hemorrhage may have mental status changes (acute confusional states) and some may become agitated [1, 67, 68]. In an attempt to prevent such patients from hurting themselves, they may be restrained [69]. Depending upon the underlying cause of the delirium, they may die. What if, at autopsy, a pulmonary embolism (or a ruptured cerebral artery aneurysm or diabetic ketoacidosis) were found? Most pathologists would have little difficulty in determining the cause of death as due to the underlying pathology without any need to invoke the restraint or struggle. One reason for this degree of comfort is that there is a compelling anatomic finding in which the lethal mechanism is structurally demonstrable as opposed to a purely functional cause. Interestingly, in a review of 20 EMS-witnessed, restrained patients in a state of "excited delirium" who then died suddenly, one death was excluded from the study because a pulmonary embolism had been diagnosed at autopsy [9]. One suspects that the cause of death in this instance was not certified as pulmonary thromboembolism due to chronic phlebothrombosis during police restraint.

Efficient intervening causes must always be considered. A person in an excited delirium may still die from a choke hold. The investigation of the circumstances, including witness statements, may help include or exclude these possibilities. If there is unexplained injury of the neck or poor witness corroboration of events, then homicide or an undetermined certification of death should be considered.

The use of EMDDs and pepper spray may complicate the manner determination (homicide vs non-homicide) of these deaths. Pepper spray causes discomfort and irritation but rarely causes death. It has been described, however, to cause bronchospasm as evidenced by florid bronchiolitis and the rapid onset of dyspnea following exposure to the spray [14]. This would be an efficient intervening cause and so the cause and manner of death statement should reflect this (homicide). More recent laboratory studies on the pulmonary effects of oleresin capsicum, however, have not demonstrated abnormal spirometry, hypoxemia, or hypoventilation [70]. Similarly, EMDDs rarely, if ever, cause death by electrocution. But they certainly cause pain and stress. In a decedent with advanced heart disease, it is reasonable to invoke these external stressors in the cause of death if the circumstances and time sequence of events supports it. Once these external violent stressors are included in the cause of death, the manner of death is best certified as a homicide.

Absent any advanced underlying disease or efficient intervening cause, these external stressors usually do not need to be invoked since the person is already in the midst of an acute, independently-efficient-lethal syndrome that may cause death with or without additional stress. If, however, the EMDD or pepper spray causes death by its own independent mechanism, then it is an efficient intervening cause, and the manner of death is certified as homicide.

6.5.6 Family, Press, and Prosecutors

Discussions with family members in suspected excited delirium deaths need to include explanations of the procedures and issues involved with these deaths. A death due to excited delirium is not usually certified on the day of the autopsy. It will take time for the investigation to proceed, toxicology testing, and other ancillary studies. It should be made clear to the family that it may take weeks before a final determination is made. Some families may want to retain a forensic pathologist to view the autopsy or conduct a second autopsy. Requests by the family for second autopsies are usually of little value if a properly conducted forensic autopsy has been done; however, it is not up to the medical examiner/coroner to allow or prohibit one. Once the family claims the body, they may have another autopsy performed at their expense. Some offices may even allow the second autopsy to take place in their facility. Of course, if it is performed in your facility, you may watch it. This avoids some of the problems that may occur when a second autopsy is performed after the body has been embalmed.

Embalming makes contusions appear worse (larger, darker) than they did before embalming. This is because of the embalming fluid's effects on blood and the way that embalming is done. Typically, the embalming fluid is injected into the arterial system which pushes the remaining intravascular blood through and out of the body. If there are damaged blood vessels (e.g., a contusion), blood will be pushed out of these defects. This will result in a larger bruise. If the contusions of an embalmed body are compared to the contusions described in the pre-embalmed body, there will be a clear disparity. This discrepancy is an artifact of the embalming but it may appear to the lay person that the forensic pathologist is downplaying the injuries or trying to cover them up. The value of full body photographs (even if there are no or minimal external findings) cannot be overstated. Photographs that show "negative" findings (e.g., the absence of an injury) can sometimes be just as important as the photographs that demonstrate the injury.

Once the investigation is completed including appropriate laboratory studies, clear communication of the cause and manner of death to the family and appropriate law enforcement agencies is done.

References

1. Brown TM, Boyle MF (2002) Delirium. BMJ 325:644–647
2. Wetli C (2005) Excited delirium. In: Payne-James J, Byard RW, Corey TS, Henderson C (eds) Encyclopedia of forensic and legal medicine. Elsevier Academic Press, Amsterdam, pp 276–281
3. DiMaio TG, DiMaio JM (2006) Excited delirium syndrome, 1st edn. CRC, Boca Raton, FL
4. Raval MP, Welti CV (1995) Sudden death from cocaine induced excited delirium: 45 cases (abstract). Am J Clin Pathol 104:329
5. Wetli CV, Fishbain DA (1985) Cocaine-induced psychosis and sudden death in recreational cocaine users. J Forensic Sci 30:873–880
6. Wetli CV, Mash D, Karch SB (1996) Cocaine-associated agitated delirium and the neuroleptic malignant syndrome. Am J Emerg Med 14:425–428
7. Ross D (1998) Factors associated with excited delirium deaths in police custody. Mod Pathol 11:1127–1137

8. Ruttenber AJ, McAnally HB, Wetli CV (1999) Cocaine-associated rhabdomyolysis and excited delirium: different stages of the same syndrome. Am J Forensic Med Pathol 20:120–127
9. Stratton SJ, Rogers C, Brickett K, Gruzinski G (2001) Factors associated with sudden death of individuals requiring restraint for excited delirium. Am J Emerg Med 19:187–191
10. Hayes J (1991) Sudden death during excited delirium, etiology unknown. ASCP Check Sample 91-5 (FP-178), pp 1–7
11. Ruttenber AJ, Lawler-Heavner J, Yin M et al. (1997) Fatal excited delirium following cocaine use: epidemiologic findings provide new evidence for mechanisms of cocaine toxicity. J Forensic Sci 42:25–31
12. Karch S (2002) The pathology of drug abuse, 3rd edn. CRC Press, Boca Raton, FL
13. Fishbain DA, Wetli CV (1981) Cocaine intoxication, delirium, and death in a body packer. Ann Emerg Med 10:531–532
14. Steffee CH, Lantz PE, Flannagan LM, Thompson RL, Jason DR (1995) Oleoresin capsicum (pepper) spray and "in-custody deaths". Am J Forensic Med Pathol 16:185–192
15. Reay DT, Eisele JW (1982) Death from law enforcement neck holds. Am J Forensic Med Pathol 3:253–258
16. Lifschultz BD, Donoghue ER (1991) Deaths in custody. Leg Med 45–71
17. Kornblum RN, Reddy SK (1991) Effects of the Taser in fatalities involving police confrontation. J Forensic Sci 36:434–438
18. Luke J, Reay D (1992) The perils of investigating and certifying deaths in police custody. Am J Forensic Med Pathol 13:98–100
19. Allam S, Noble JS (2001) Cocaine-excited delirium and severe acidosis. Anaesthesia 56:385–386
20. Pollanen MS, Chiasson DA, Cairns JT, Young JG (1998) Unexpected death related to restraint for excited delirium: a retrospective study of deaths in police custody and in the community. CMAJ 158:1603–1607
21. O'Halloran RL, Lewman LV (1993) Restraint asphyxiation in excited delirium. Am J Forensic Med Pathol 14:289–295
22. Karch SB, Wetli CV (1995) Agitated delirium versus positional asphyxia. Ann Emerg Med 26:760–761
23. Laposata EA (1993) Positional asphyxia during law enforcement transport. Am J Forensic Med Pathol 14:86–87
24. Farnham FR, Kennedy HG (1997) Acute excited states and sudden death. BMJ 315:1107–1108
25. Pounder D (1998) Acute excited states and sudden death. Death after restraint can be avoided. BMJ 316:1171
26. Stratton SJ, Rogers C, Green K (1995) Sudden death in individuals in hobble restraints during paramedic transport. Ann Emerg Med 25:710–712
27. Jauchem J, Sherry C, Fines D, Cook M (2006) Acidosis, lactate, electrolytes, muscle enzymes, and other factors in the blood of Sus scrofa following repeated Taser exposures. Forensic Sci Int 161:20–30
28. Ho JD, Miner JR, Lakireddy DR, Bultman LL, Heegaard WG (2006) Cardiovascular and physiologic effects of conducted electrical weapon discharge in resting adults. Acad Emerg Med 13:589–595
29. Rosh A, Sampson BA, Hirsch CS (2003) Schizophrenia as a cause of death. J Forensic Sci 48:164–167
30. Marzuk P, Tardiff K, Leon A et al. (1998) Ambient temperature and mortality from unintentional cocaine overdose. JAMA 279:1795–1800
31. Park KS, Korn CS, Henderson SO (2001) Agitated delirium and sudden death: two case reports. Prehosp Emerg Care 5:214–216

32. Mirchandani HG, Rorke LB, Sekula-Perlman A, Hood IC (1994) Cocaine-induced agitated delirium, forceful struggle, and minor head injury. A further definition of sudden death during restraint. Am J Forensic Med Pathol 15:95–99
33. Karch SB, Stephens BG (1998) Acute excited states and sudden death. Acute excited states are not caused by high blood concentrations of cocaine. BMJ 316:1171
34. Hirsch CS (1994) Restraint asphyxiation [letter]. Am J Forensic Med Pathol 15:266
35. O'Halloran RL, Frank JG (2000) Asphyxial death during prone restraint revisited: a report of 21 cases. Am J Forensic Med Pathol 21:39–52
36. Reay DT, Howard JD, Fligner CL, Ward RJ (1988) Effects of positional restraint on oxygen saturation and heart rate following exercise. Am J Forensic Med Pathol 9:16–18
37. Reay D, Fligner C, Stilwell A, Arnold J (1992) Positional asphyxia during law enforcement transport. Am J Forensic Med Pathol 13:90–97
38. Chan TC, Vilke GM, Neuman T, Clausen JL (1997) Restraint position and positional asphyxia. Ann Emerg Med 30:578–586
39. Chan TC, Neuman T, Clausen J, Eisele J, Vilke GM (2004) Weight force during prone restraint and respiratory function. Am J Forensic Med Pathol 25:185–189
40. Schmidt P, Snowden T (1999) The effects of positional restraint on heart rate and oxygen saturation. J Emerg Med 17:777–782
41. Roeggla M, Wagner A, Muellner M et al. (1997) Cardiorespiratory consequences to hobble restraint. Wein Klin Wochenschr 109:359–361
42. Reay DT, Howard JD (1999) Restraint position and positional asphyxia. Am J Forensic Med Pathol 20:300–301
43. Chan TC, Vilke GM, Neuman T (1998) Reexamination of custody restraint position and positional asphyxia. Am J Forensic Med Pathol 19:201–205
44. Ely SF, Hirsch CS (2000) Asphyxial deaths and petechiae: a review. J Forensic Sci 45:1274–1277
45. DiMaio V, DiMaio D (2001) Forensic pathology, 2nd edn. CRC Press, Boca Raton, FL
46. Adelson L (1974) Pathology of homicide. Charles C Thomas, Springfield
47. Robinson MN, Brooks CG, Renshaw GD (1990) Electric shock devices and their effects on the human body. Med Sci Law 30:285–300
48. Levine S, Sloane C, Chan T, Vilke G (2006) Cardiac monitoring of human subjects exposed to the Taser (abstract). Acad Emerg Med 13:S47
49. Stratbucker R, Kroll M, McDaniel W, Panescu D (2006) Cardiac current density distribution by electrical pulses from Taser devices. Conf Proc IEEE Eng MED Biol Soc 1:6305–6307
50. Wu JY, Sun H, O'Rourke AP et al. (2007) Taser dart-to-heart distance that causes ventricular fibrillation in pigs. IEEE Trans Biomed Eng 54:503–508
51. Nanthakumar K, Masse S, Umapathy K et al. (2008) Cardiac stimulation with high voltage discharge from stun guns. CMAJ 178(II):1451–1457
52. Cao M, Shinbane JS, Gillberg JM, Saxon LA (2007) Taser-induced rapid ventricular myocardial capture demonstrated by pacemaker intracardiac electrograms. J Cardiovasc Electrophysiol 18:876–879
53. Spitz W (2006) Spitz and Fisher's medicolegal investigation of death, 4th edn. Charles C Thomas, Springfield
54. O'Brien DJ (1991) Electronic weaponry – a question of safety. Ann Emerg Med 20:583–587
55. Ruggieri J (2005) Forensic engineering analysis of electro-shock weapon safety. J Nat Acad Forensic Eng 23:19–48
56. Anglen R (2006) Study raises concerns over Taser's safety, The Arizona Republic, Phoenix, AZ
57. Yamaguchi G (2006) Letter on preliminary testing results on Taser M18, 2/3/06

58. Ordog GJ, Wasserberger J, Schlater T, Balasubramanium S (1987) Electronic gun (Taser) injuries. Ann Emerg Med 16:73–78
59. Davis JH (1978) Can sudden cardiac death be murder? J Forensic Sci 23:384–387
60. Turner SA, Barnard JJ, Spotswood SD, Prahlow JA (2004) "Homicide by heart attack" revisited. J Forensic Sci 49:598–600
61. Pudiak CM, Bozarth MA (1994) Cocaine fatalities increased by restraint stress. Life Sci 55:PL379–382
62. Kock MD, Jessup DA, Clark RK, Franti CE, Weaver RA (1987) Capture methods in five subspecies of free-ranging bighorn sheep: an evaluation of drop-net, drive-net, chemical immobilization and the net-gun. J Wildl Dis 23:634–640
63. Wittstein IS, Thiemann DR, Lima JA et al. (2005) Neurohumoral features of myocardial stunning due to sudden emotional stress. N Engl J Med 352:539–548
64. Cebelin M, Hirsch C (1980) Human stress cardiomyopathy: myocardial lesions in victims of homicidal assaults without internal injuries. Hum Pathol 11:123–132
65. Carson JL, Kelley MA, Duff A et al. (1992) Clinical course of pulmonary embolism. N Engl J Med 326:1240–1245
66. Amnesty International (2004) United States of America: excessive and lethal force? Amnesty International's concerns about deaths and ill-treatment involving police use of Tasers. 1-94 (report)
67. Kasper D, Braunwald E, Fauci A et al. (2004) Harrison's principles of internal medicine, 16th edn. McGraw-Hill Professional, New York
68. Meagher DJ (2001) Delirium: optimising management. BMJ 322:144–149
69. Zun LS (2003) A prospective study of the complication rate of use of patient restraint in the emergency department. J Emerg Med 24:119–124
70. Chan TC, Vilke GM, Clausen J et al. (2002) The effect of oleoresin capsicum "pepper" spray inhalation on respiratory function. J Forensic Sci 47:299–304

Part IV
Death from Natural Causes

Chapter 7
Myocardial Bridging: Is it Really a Cause of Sudden Cardiac Death?

Michael J.P. Biggs, Benjamin Swift and Mary N. Sheppard

Contents

Abstract Myocardial bridges are described as myocardial muscle fibre bundles covering an epicardial coronary artery for a variable distance. They are a relatively common finding, with incidence changing on the basis of the study method used (angiographic/necropsy). Although myocardial bridges are usually associated with a benign prognosis, being in many cases asymptomatic and found only by chance, their presence has also been considered a cause of angina, malignant arrhythmia, myocardial infarction and sudden death. They are diagnosed by angiography in vivo when systolic compression of a segment of coronary artery that remains patent during diastole is observed. Whether or not myocardial bridges are benign or of pathological significance is the subject of ongoing controversy. Arguments and evidence for and against this phenomenon are discussed here, and a potential solution is offered in an attempt to clarify the situation.

Keywords Myocardial bridging · Sudden death · Forensic pathology · Cardiac pathology

B. Swift
Forensic Pathology Services, Culham Science Centre, Oxfordshire, United Kingdom
e-mail: forensicpathology@hotmail.co.uk

M. Tsokos (ed.), *Forensic Pathology Reviews, Volume 5*,
doi: 10.1007/978-1-59745-110-9_7, © Humana Press, Totowa, NJ 2008

7.1 Introduction

The coronary arteries are arguably some of the most important blood vessels in the body (Table 7.1). For this reason they have been examined in great detail resulting in well documented normal anatomical parameters. Many deviations from this accepted standard have been described. The incidence of significant coronary artery anomalies within the general population ranges from 0.3 to

Table 7.1 Causes of sudden cardiac death

Coronary artery disease and ischaemic heart disease
  Atherosclerosis
  Structural/congenital malformation (including anomalous origin)
  Kawasaki's disease
  Myocardial bridging
  Coronary artery dissection
  Aortitis and secondary atherosclerosis
  Embolism into coronary arteries
  Fibromuscular dysplasia of intramyocardial artery
  Coronary artery spasm (regional infarction in absence of coronary lesion)
Valve disease
  Aortic stenosis
  Mitral valve prolapse
  Infective endocarditis
Myocardial disease
  Myocarditis (including myocardial sarcoidosis)
  Cardiomyopathies
  LV hypertrophy and hypertension
  Idiopathic myocardial fibrosis
  Amyloidosis
  Cardiac tumour – primary (myxoma) or metastatic
Structural conduction system abnormalities
  Absence of atrial portion of AV node
  Bundle of His damage
  Nodal mesothelioma
  Atrioventricular nodal artery stenosis
  Anomalous conduction pathways (e.g., Wolf-Parkinson-White syndrome)
Drug toxicity
  Cocaine
  Amphetamine and ecstasy
  Solvent abuse
  Marijuana
  Antidepressants and antipsychotics
No morphological abnormalities (sudden adult death syndrome)
  Functional conduction system abnormalities (long QT, Brugada syndrome)
  Catecholaminergic polymorphic ventricular tachycardia
  Idiopathic ventricular fibrillation
  Blunt chest trauma (commotio cordis)

5.6% [1]. Whilst serious congenital defects can understandably have adverse effects in terms of morbidity and mortality, many slight alterations do not produce any discernable effect, and controversy exists over whether these are truly pathological entities or simply variations of normal. One of the more common examples of the latter is *myocardial bridging*. When a portion of a major epicardial coronary artery tunnels into the substance of the muscle for part of its course, it appears in cross sections to be traversed by a bridge of myocardium. Numerous synonyms have been used to describe this; "muscular bridge", "intramural coronary artery", "mural coronary", "tunnelled coronary artery", "myocardial loop" and "coronary artery overbridging". The earliest known record of this phenomenon was in 1737 by Reyman [2]. Although subsequently alluded to in the literature from time to time, it was not until 1951 that a thorough analysis was reported by Geiringer [3]. Technological advances allowed the radiological appearances to be described by Porstmann and Iwig in 1960 [4]. For a long time considered to be a benign anatomical variant, myocardial bridging began to be investigated as an entity of potential clinicopathological significance.

Figure 7.1 demonstrates the radiographic features of myocardial bridging in a segment of proximal left anterior descending artery during both diastole and systole. Segments of intramyocardial major coronary artery are thought to be congenital abnormalities due to incomplete exteriorisation of the primitive coronary intra-trabecular arterial network [5]. It has been postulated after comparison with animal species that human coronary bridges may represent evolutionary genetic remnants [6]. Both the site and the number of myocardial bridges present vary from individual to individual. A number of studies provide relative incidences of locations among the major coronary vessels. Figure 7.2 illustrates the range of distributions quoted for myocardial bridges of the left anterior descending (LAD), circumflex and right coronary arteries [7, 8, 9].

(A)   (B)

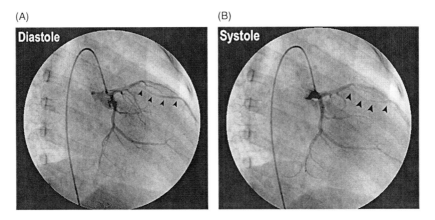

Fig. 7.1 Radiographic features of myocardial bridging in a segment of proximal left anterior descending artery during: **A** diastole; **B** systole

Fig. 7.2 Range of distribution of myocardial bridge location

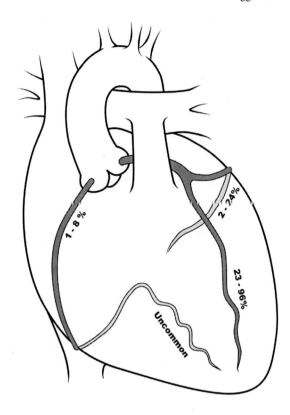

Involvement of the diagonal, obtuse marginal or posterior descending arteries is regarded as uncommon. Despite the notable discrepancy between studies, the consensus is that the mid portion of the LAD artery is by far the most common site for a bridged segment. Figure 7.3 shows the macroscopic appearance of a typical myocardial bridge, whereas Fig. 7.4 presents the microscopic appearances.

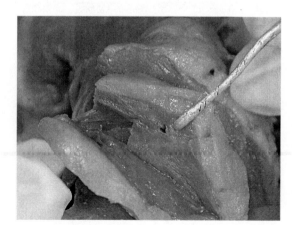

Fig. 7.3 Typical autopsy appearance of a myocardial bridge

(A)   (B)

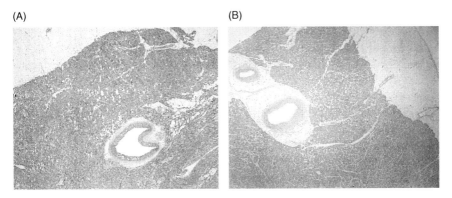

Fig. 7.4 Microscopic appearances of myocardial bridging

7.2 Myocardial Bridging

7.2.1 Incidence

It is difficult to determine the true prevalence of myocardial bridges within the general population. Observation rates as diverse as 5% and 86% have been quoted in autopsy studies [10]. Fluctuations in autopsy rates and practice, inter-observer variability with regard to examination technique, differing methods of data collection and inconsistency over what constitutes a myocardial bridge are potential factors that could in part be responsible for this disparity. Angio-graphic studies exhibit a narrower spread (0.5% to 12%) than that seen in autopsy series [11]. It could be argued that selection bias in angiographic studies might render them unrepresentative of the general population. In addition, not all myocardial bridges are necessarily seen on angiography. As with autopsy data, inter-observer variation and other factors make precise figures complex to evaluate. Cardiothoracic surgeons have noted an incidence of approximately 15% in patients undergoing coronary artery bypass procedures [11]. Patients undergoing investigations for hypertrophic obstructive cardiomyopathy have a reported myocardial bridging incidence of 40% [12]. Again, selected patient groups may not be representative of the population as a whole, and extrapola-tion of their data outside of the defined context may not be valid. Vast differ-ences in myocardial bridge incidence have been observed between continents. Whether this is a true representation of genetic variation or merely a reflection of inherent differences between geographically distant studies is unclear. Despite the apparent limitations of these seemingly inconsistent data, it is clear that myocardial bridging is far from uncommon within the general population.

7.2.2 Clinical Significance

Most authors agree that myocardial bridging is rather frequent and seldom generates ischaemia. However, while most cases appear to be asymptomatic, there are numerous reports linking myocardial bridging with myocardial ischaemia [13] and infarction [14, 15, 16, 17], coronary thrombosis and infarction [18], acute left ventricular dysfunction [19], arrhythmias [20], abnormal ventricular repolarisation [21], ventricular septal rupture [22] and sudden death [23, 24]. Angiographic investigations have identified myocardial bridge segments of coronary artery that undergo marked compression during systole [4, 25]. Furthermore, direct measurement of pressure and flow using sophisticated Doppler ultrasound techniques has shown that pressure within the bridged segment is increased, causing impediment or even temporary reversal of blood flow [25, 26]. This concurs with logical reasoning that an artery surrounded by contracting muscle will be compressed with inevitable consequences on the contents of its lumen. However, it is also known that only 15% of coronary perfusion occurs during systole; the majority occurs during diastole [7, 12]. There is also the conundrum of the intramural coronary arteries. All the branches of coronary arteries that are *normally* found within the substance of the myocardium are surrounded by muscle. For the heart to function effectively, sufficient blood flow must be taking place within these intramural vessels. Such "everyday" intramural vessels undoubtedly endure similar pressure and flow constraints to myocardial bridges without apparent detriment, so why should these intramural segments of epicardial vessels cause symptoms?

Ischaemia in the context of myocardial bridging is most likely multifactorial in origin. Altered coronary vasoreactivity has been detected in patients with myocardial bridging [27]. It has been suggested that this may contribute to a dynamic obstruction greater than would be expected for a mechanical obstruction alone. Coronary artery spasm is a known cause of myocardial ischaemic symptoms [28]. It has the potential to mimic other cardiac pathology both clinically and angiographically. Griffet et al. [29] report a case of acute coronary syndrome in a 45-year-old man where two separate myocardial bridges were detected on angiography. These were deemed insufficient to explain his symptoms and a second angiogram revealed diffuse coronary artery spasm. Thus, two pathologies can occur together, and bridged coronary arteries are more prone to spasms.

In periods of increased heart rate the length of time spent in diastole is shortened. Coronary perfusion is therefore less, in addition to myocardial oxygen demand being increased, and so any occult flow deficit should manifest itself during periods of exercise. There is a strong association between strenuous exercise and sudden cardiac death in the young [30, 31, 32], and sudden death has also been linked with myocardial bridging [33]. Acute coronary syndrome linked to coronary spasm during exercise is also described [29]. There may be obstruction as well as or instead of flow disturbance. The bridged segment is usually described as being free from coronary atheroma, but reports have shown atheroma within the affected segment [34], as well as thrombosis, intimal fibrosis and adventitial fibrosis [23]. This could explain the ischaemic symptoms in certain cases.

Myocardial bridges are believed to be a congenital malformation, but are not linked to symptoms until later in life [7, 10]. If the flow disturbances caused by myocardial bridging are significant then logical reasoning might predict effects to be seen in patients of all ages. Also, with myocardial bridging being so prevalent, higher incidences of adverse outcome might be expected. Neither of these assumptions is borne out in practice, however. The possibility that myocardial bridges may be acquired should be considered since the growth spurt seen in adolescence is responsible for marked hypertrophy of the myocardium in hypertrophic cardiomyopathy, and may also be responsible for growth over the epicardial vessels which can give rise to scarring and even fatal infarction [35]. As an aside, chimpanzees have a coronary circulation that is predominantly intramural [3] and yet they do not apparently suffer ill effects as a result of this.

It seems to be the general consensus that myocardial bridges, whilst usually harmless, might become pathologically important in a subset of patients, perhaps with additional confounding factors. In a study of compression of both epicardial and intramural coronary arteries Mohiddin and Fananapazir [36] found (albeit within the specific context of hypertrophic cardiomyopathy) no evidence that myocardial bridging was an important cause of cardiac perfusion abnormalities, morbidity or mortality. They state that, in normal hearts, a myocardial bridge "most often of the mid LAD artery, should possibly be considered a (frequent) coronary variant rather than a coronary anomaly." When Virmani et al. advise that "pathologists must exercise caution in attributing myocardial bridging as a cause of myocardial ischaemia and sudden death as the prevalence of myocardial bridging is high ($\geq$30%) in the normal population" [37], they are warning of a potential possibility for over-diagnosis of pathological myocardial bridges. Möhlenkamp and co-workers concede that whilst "myocardial bridging can occasionally generate clinically important complications," it is usually "a benign condition" [38]. Whilst the vast majority of case reports involving myocardial bridging exist to highlight associations with adverse clinical events, numerous review articles exist which put the significance of such occurrences into perspective. Gow concludes that "there is no strong evidence to support the role of myocardial bridging in sudden death in the general population" [39]. Kramer et al. state that "myocardial bridges, as an isolated finding, are benign" [10].

7.3 Sudden Cardiac Death

7.3.1 Background

Sudden cardiac death is death occurring within 6 h of the onset of symptoms in a previously symptom-free individual. The Royal College of Pathologists lists a multitude of possible causes of sudden cardiac death, including myocardial bridging (Table 7.1) [40]. If no cause can be found for the death, but myocardial bridging is present, then there may be a temptation to blame the sudden death on the presence of the myocardial bridge. To avoid erroneous overuse, this should be accepted by pathologists only in the context of a deep, long bridge in the LAD artery, preferably associated with ischaemic changes in the myocardium.

There have been numerous documented cases of sudden cardiac death in young, previously healthy adults with coronary artery anomalies [1, 30]. There is repeated mention of an association with exercise and sudden death [30, 31]. In such cases, the cause is often attributed to hypertrophic cardio-myopathy, idiopathic left ventricular hypertrophy or congenital coronary abnormalities [30]. There have been several reports linking myocardial bridging with sudden death. Data found in the literature are prone to bias since all studies published are retrospective and the populations studied are limited and highly selective. In the case of sudden death, we think that to consider myocardial bridging as a cause there has to be more than a simple necropsy finding of a myocardial bridge. Myocardial bridging can be proved to be an isolated, independent risk factor for sudden cardiac death only when there is a history of clinical and/or electrocardiographically confirmed ischaemia, or the presence of histological abnormalities indicating myocardial ischaemia in the area supplied by the bridged coronary artery where there is no other explanation for the ischaemia [41].

7.3.2 Pathological Significance of Myocardial Bridging

Most series emphasise that it is bridging of the left anterior descending coronary artery that is usually linked with clinical and pathological complications. It can be straightforward to attribute death to a bridge in the LAD coronary artery when ischaemic changes or infarction are seen in the anteroseptal wall of the left ventricle. However, in the absence of such changes it can be difficult or even impossible to establish the role of the myocardial bridge in the sudden death. Whilst originally considered to be a benign variant of normal, likely patholo-gical significance has been said to occur when a length of 20 mm and a depth of 2 mm are exceeded [42]. Distinction between "superficial" and "deep" variants of myocardial bridge has been made by Ferreira et al. [43]. This important pathological study emphasised that myocardial bridges, either single or multi-ple, were seen in 50 (55.6%) out of 90 hearts in a specialist centre. The LAD artery was the most commonly affected artery. Just 35 of the 50 hearts, which contained 41 muscle bridges in total, were dissected further under magnifica-tion. Two different types of muscle bridges could be identified. Of these 41 myocardial bridges, 31 were "superficial": they crossed the artery transver-sely towards the apex of the heart at an acute angle, or perpendicularly. The remaining 10 "deep" myocardial bridges crossed the LAD coronary artery and surrounded it with a muscle bundle that arose from the right ventricular apical trabeculae, crossing the artery transversely, obliquely, or helically before terminating in the interventricular septum. The superficial type of myocardial bridge does not seem to constrict the artery during systole but the deep muscle bridges, by virtue of their relation with the LAD coronary artery, can twist the vessel and thus compromise its diastolic flow resulting in ischaemia [43].

The idea that different types of myocardial bridge exist was reinforced by Morales et al., who found that adverse clinical events and myocardial changes were seen only with deep intramural LAD arteries [24]. This is an important issue which must be emphasised. The size and location of the bridging muscle is often not described in sufficient detail, especially in autopsy studies. The majority of bridges described are short and superficial, with perhaps only a millimetre of muscle crossing over the vessel. These probably represent the benign bridges described as a common finding in many studies. Pathologists now accept that longer lesions (a minimum of 15–20 mm) lying deeper within the muscle (at a minimum depth of 2–5 mm) and involving the proximal LAD vessel, not the distal vessel towards the apex, are more likely to contribute to clinical symptoms and sudden death. In a recent study of sudden death carried out in the United Kingdom by Fabre and Sheppard, myocardial bridges fulfilling these criteria were found in six out of four hundred cases in young patients under the age of 35 [44].

In a report detailing with two cases of fatal outcome associated with myocardial bridging of the LAD artery, one patient is said to have died as a result of acute cerebral emboli from thrombus within a left ventricular aneurysm and the other was found to have marked left ventricular hypertrophy [45]. The coexistent pathology cannot be ignored in such cases simply because myocardial bridging has been found. An autopsy study of 19 cases of myocardial bridging of the LAD artery in a series of 930 medicolegal autopsy studies highlights this [23]. The patients were 15 men and 4 women with an average age of 39.2 years. A potentially lethal cardiac abnormality (ischaemic lesion, cardiomyopathy, conduction tissue lesion) was found in addition to the myocardial bridge in 11 cases. Of the other 8 cases, 7 had minor abnormalities and 1 heart was absolutely normal. All of the hearts had fresh, microscopic, ischaemic lesions in the territory of the LAD artery. The anatomical lesions of the coronary arteries at the site of bridging were varied: 11 had dense collagen fibrosis of the adventitia, 16 showed intimal fibrosis of varying degrees of thickness (10 circumferential), 2 contained atherosclerotic plaques (a 40- and a 54-year-old man), 2 contained recent thromboses (1 at the site of the bridge in a 50-year-old man, and the other just distal to the bridge in a 25-year-old man). Only one case (a 39-year-old woman) displayed no microscopic changes of the LAD artery at the site of the myocardial bridge. This study demonstrates that pathology within the bridged segment of the coronary artery (either intimal thickening, thrombotic or spastic phenomena) may act to cause sudden death However, at the same time it draws attention to potentially significant associated cardiac pathology (conduction tissue lesions remain uncertain in sudden death cases). It is thus argued that in cases where more than one cardiac pathology exists, it cannot be reliably stated that the myocardial bridge was itself solely responsible for the death.

Sudden cardiac death is reported in young, healthy individuals where there is an absence of any cardiac pathology, including myocardial bridges [46]. The cause of such deaths with morphologically normal hearts has been linked to genetic diseases: the channelopathies [47]. It is best in these sudden cardiac deaths due to an unknown cause, that might have coincidental small myocardial bridges, not to implicate the bridge in the cause of death. Obviously when there are other pathological cardiac conditions, the underlying cause of death is usually attributed to this, unless there is myocardial ischaemia associated with the bridge.

7.4 Conclusions

Myocardial bridging is a relatively common finding. There is a wide spectrum of abnormality, the vast majority of which is benign. Many review articles conclude that there is insufficient evidence for myocardial bridging as a cause of sudden cardiac death. However, this needs to be assessed in view of the significant finding of a deep bridge with ischaemic changes as described above. Geiringer describes the entire vascular system as "notoriously variable" [3]. A potential strategy is to regard myocardial bridging not as a phenomenon that is either present or absent, but as a continuum. It would be simplistic to state that myocardial bridging is either entirely benign or always associated with increased morbidity and mortality. At one end of the scale are people with no myocardial bridging whatsoever. At the opposite extreme there are people with grossly aberrant coronary arteries, which can have detrimental effects on the individual under certain conditions. Schwarz et al. draw this conclusion, supporting "the concept of a haemodynamically significant obstruction to coronary flow due to myocardial bridging in a selected subset of patients" [48].

Multiple reports indicate there are extreme circumstances in which the most severe myocardial bridges are capable of causing adverse clinical events and sudden death. The recommendations of this review are that the presence of myocardial bridging should continue to be looked for and recorded in detail. To certify isolated myocardial bridging as causative in a case of sudden cardiac death, it must be a deep bridge as described, involving the proximal LAD coronary artery and preferably with ischaemic damage in the myocardium. Superficial bridges are very common and attributing sudden death to them is erroneous. In such a case, there is the possibility that another cause of death might be overlooked.

Acknowledgments Many thanks to Prof. James L. Wilkinson, Royal Children's Hospital, Melbourne, Australia for providing the radiographic images for Fig. 7.1.

References

1. Angelini P, Velasco JA, Flamm S (2002) Coronary anomalies: incidence, pathophysiology, and clinical relevance. Circulation 105:2449–2454
2. Reyman HC (1737) Disertatio de vasis cordis propriis. Haller Bibl Anat 2:359–379
3. Geiringer E (1951) The mural coronary. Am Heart J 41:359–368
4. Porstmann W, Iwig J (1960) Intramural coronary vessels in the angiogram [Article in German] Fortschr Geb Rontgenstr Nuklearmed 92:129–133
5. Chen J, Lin C (2003) Myocardial bridging. Tzu Chi Med J 15:357–361
6. Möhlenkamp S, Hort W, Ge J, Erbel R (2002) Update on myocardial bridging. Circulation 106:2616–2622
7. Alegria JR, Herrmann J, Holmes DR, Lerman A, Rihal CS (2005) Myocardial bridging. Eur Heart J 26:1159–1168
8. Rozenberg VD, Nepomnyashchikh LM (2004) Pathomorphology and pathogenic role of myocardial bridges in sudden cardiac death. Bull Exp Biol Med 138:87–92
9. Çay S, Öztürk S, Cihan G, Kisacik HL, Korkmaz S (2006) Angiographic prevalence of myocardial bridging. Anadolu Kardiyol Derg 6:9–12
10. Kramer JR, Kitazume H, Proudfit WL, Sones FM (1982) Clinical significance of isolated coronary bridges: benign and frequent condition involving the left anterior descending artery. Am Heart J 103:283–288
11. Tauth J, Sullebarger T (1997) Myocardial infarction associated with myocardial bridging: case history and review of the literature. Cathet Cardiovasc Diagn 40:364–367
12. Mohiddin SA, Begley D, Shih J, Fananapazir L (2000) Myocardial bridging does not predict sudden death in children with hypertrophic cardiomyopathy but is associated with more severe cardiac disease. J Am Coll Cardiol 36:2270–2278
13. Elyounassi B, Kendoussi M, Khatouri A, Fall PD, Mouyopa C, Nazzi M et al. (1998) Muscle bridge and myocardial ischemia. Study of 6 cases. Ann Cardiol Angeiol (Paris) 47:459–463
14. Çay S, Biyikoglu F, Korkmaz S (2006) Myocardial bridging as a cause of acute anterior myocardial infarction. Acta Cardiol 61:111–113
15. Bashour TT, Espinosa E, Blumenthal J, Wong T, Mason DT (1997) Myocardial infarction caused by coronary artery myocardial bridge. Am Heart J 133:473–477
16. Diaz-Widmann J, Cox SL, Roongsritong C (2003) Unappreciable myocardial bridge causing anterior myocardial infarction and postinfarction angina. South Med J 96:400–402
17. Nayar PG, Nyamu P, Venkitachalam L, Ajit SM (2002) Myocardial infarction due to myocardial bridging. Indian Heart J 54:711–712
18. Cheng TO (1998) Myocardial bridge as a cause of thrombus formation and myocardial infarction in a young athlete. Clin Cardiol 21:151, 231
19. Roul G, Sens P, Germain P, Bareiss P (1999) Myocardial bridging as a cause of acute transient left heart dysfunction. Chest 116:574–580
20. Feld H, Guadanino V, Hollander G, Greengart A, Lichstein E, Shani J (1991) Exercise-induced ventricular tachycardia in association with a myocardial bridge. Chest 99:1295–1296
21. Dean JW, Mills PG (1994) Abnormal ventricular repolarisation in association with myocardial bridging. Br Heart J 71:366–367

22. Tio RA, Ebels T (2001) Ventricular septal rupture caused by myocardial bridging. Ann Thorac Surg 72:1369–1370

23. Desseigne P, Tabib A, Loire R (1991) Myocardial bridging on the left anterior descending coronary artery and sudden death. Apropos of 19 cases with autopsy. Arch Mal Coeur Vaiss 84:511–516

24. Morales AR, Romanelli R, Tate LG, Boucek RJ, de Marchena E (1993) Intramural left anterior descending coronary artery: significance of the depth of the muscular tunnel. Hum Pathol 24:693–701

25. Noble J, Bourassa MG, Petitclerc R, Dyrda I (1976) Myocardial bridging and milking effect of the left anterior descending coronary artery: normal variant or obstruction? Am J Cardiol 37:993–999

26. Ge J, Jeremias A, Rupp A, Abels M, Baumgart D, Liu F et al. (1999) New signs characteristic of myocardial bridging demonstrated by intracoronary ultrasound and Doppler. Eur Heart J 20:1707–1716

27. Herrmann J, Higano ST, Lenon RJ, Rihal CS, Lerman A (2004) Myocardial bridging is associated with alteration in coronary vasoreactivity. Eur Heart J 25:2134–2142

28. El Menyar AA (2006) Drug-induced myocardial infarction secondary to coronary artery spasm in teenagers and young adults. J Postgrad Med 52:51–56

29. Griffet V, Finet G, Rioufol G, Chartron J, Caignault JR, Guerard S et al. (2006) Myocardial bridging and coronary spasm on effort. Arch Mal Coeur Vaiss 99:65–67

30. Drezner JA (2000) Sudden cardiac death in young athletes. Causes, athlete's heart, and screening guidelines. Postgrad Med 108:37–50

31. Lesauskaite V, Valanciute A (1998) Causes of sudden cardiac death in young athletes: the role of hypoperfusion. Am J Forensic Med Pathol 19:157–161

32. Shotar A, Bsuttil A (1994) Myocardial bars and bridges and sudden death. Forensic Sci Int 68:143–147

33. Chiappa E, Vineis C (1993) Sudden death during a game of soccer in a young adolescent with a myocardial muscle bridge. G Ital Cardiol 23:473–477

34. de Winter RJ, Kok WE, Piek JJ (1998) Coronary atherosclerosis within a myocardial bridge, not a benign condition. Heart 80:91–93

35. Cheng MF, Wu YW, Liu YB, Huang PJ, Tzen KY, Yen RF (2007) Extensive scar myocardium in hypertrophic cardiomyopathy with severe myocardial bridge. Int J Cardiol 115:105–107

36. Mohiddin SA, Fananapazir L (2002) Systolic compression of epicardial coronary and intramural arteries in children with hypertrophic cardiomyopathy. Tex Heart Inst J 29:290–298

37. Virmani R, Farb A, Burke AP (1993) Ischemia from myocardial coronary bridging: fact or fancy? Hum Pathol 24:687–688

38. Möhlenkamp S, Eggebrecht H, Ebralidze T, Munzberger S, Schweizer T, Quast B et al. (2005) Normal coronary angiography with myocardial bridging: a variant possibly relevant for ischemia. Herz 30:37–47

39. Gow RM (2002) Myocardial bridging: does it cause sudden death? Card Electrophysiol Rev 6:112–114

40. Lucas S, Burnett R, Corbishley C, Leadbeatter S, MacKenzie J, Moore I, Start R (The Royal College of Pathologists Working Party on the Autopsy) (2005) Guidelines on autopsy practice – Scenario1: sudden death with likely cardiac disease. Royal College of Pathologists, London

41. Grigoriu C, Astarastoae V, Grigoriu B (2001) Myocardial bridging and sudden death. Rev Med Chir Soc Med Nat Iasi 105.77–82

42. Silver MD, Gottleib AI, Schoen FJ (2001) Cardiovascular pathology, 3rd edn. Churchill Livingstone, Philadelphia, PA

43. Ferreira AG, Trotter SE, Konig B, Decourt LV, Fox K, Olsen EG (1991) Myocardial bridges: morphological and functional aspects. Br Heart J 66:364–367

44. Fabre A, Sheppard MN (2006) Sudden adult death syndrome and other non-ischaemic causes of sudden cardiac death. Heart 92:316–320
45. Bestetti RB, Costa RS, Zucolotto S, Oliveira JS (1989) Fatal outcome associated with autopsy proven myocardial bridging of the left anterior descending coronary artery. Eur Heart J 10:573–576
46. Behr ER, Casey A, Sheppard M, Wright M, Bowker TJ, Davies MJ, McKenna WJ, Wood DA (2007) Sudden arrhythmic death syndrome: a national survey of sudden unexplained cardiac death. Heart 93:547–548
47. Behr E, Wood DA, Wright M, Syrris P, Sheppard MN, Casey A et al. (2003) Cardiological assessment of first-degree relatives in sudden arrhythmic death syndrome. Lancet 362:1457–1459
48. Schwarz ER, Klues HG, vom Dahl J, Klein I, Krebs W, Hanrath P (1997) Functional characteristics of myocardial bridging. A combined angiographic and intracoronary Doppler flow study. Eur Heart J 18:434–442

Chapter 8
Nontraumatic Intramuscular Hemorrhages Associated with Death Caused by Internal Diseases

Friedrich Schulz, Holger Lach and Klaus Püschel

Contents

Abstract Nine cases of death from natural causes that showed agonal intramuscular hemorrhages in the region of the shoulder girdle, the back, the neck as well as partly on the arms are presented. In each case, a medicolegal autopsy had been performed. The appearance and pattern of this muscular damage is reminiscent of convulsive breathing in dyspnea with subsequent ruptures of the auxiliary respiratory muscles. Such bleedings are a long- and well-known phenomenon associated with asphyxia (especially drowning deaths). The appearance of such bleedings originating from internal disease has to be carefully differentiated from those bleedings with a traumatic origin.

Keywords Intramuscular hemorrhages · Alterations of muscle fibers · Vital reactions · Natural death

8.1 Introduction

During medicolegal autopsies, special attention has to be paid to intramuscular hemorrhages appearing in the region of the shoulder girdle and upper posterior dorsal region. As possible signs of blunt trauma, these lesions are of special forensic importance. They can indicate the occurrence of blows or kicks, or be seen as evidence of force having been applied from the front (abutment injuries).

F. Schulz
Institute of Legal Medicine, University of Hamburg, Hamburg, Germany

M. Tsokos (ed.), *Forensic Pathology Reviews, Volume 5*,
doi: 10.1007/978-1-59745-110-9_8, © Humana Press, Totowa, NJ 2008

A separate class are intramuscular bleedings in the pectoral girdle, including the cervical region and the thoracic posterior, that originate in the muscle itself without an external cause. There have been repeated descriptions of such bleedings connected with death caused by drowning since the late nineteenth century [1, 2, 3, 4, 5, 6, 7], first described by Paltauf in his famous book in 1888 [8]. They are regarded as vital signs as they are caused by the extreme strain of the accessory respiratory musculature under the strong forced breathing in the phase of dyspnea as well as by the clonicotonic seizures of the subsequent phase of asphyxia under cerebral oxygen deprivation.

Though intramuscular hemorrhages are not specific signs of drowning deaths, they still prove a hypoxic or asphyctic mechanism in death as described by Reuter in 1922 [6]. Thus, such lesions are being considered in connection with death by strangulation [9]. The general theme of intramuscular hemorrhages is increasingly being studied; such studies include the use of modern micromorphologic methods [1, 10, 11]. Interestingly, this happens regularly in cases of violent deaths [9, 12]. Until recently, there were no such studies in connection with death from natural causes [13], though from clinical experience, in many cases strong dyspnea has to be expected. It appears that until now, from the medicolegal point of view, the recognition of such phenomena has been limited to the examination of unnatural deaths.

8.2 Nine Case Reports

Here, we report nine cases with intramuscular hemorrhages of the shoulder girdle and the posterior of the body, all observed at autopsies carried out in the Institute of Legal Medicine in Hamburg, Germany (Table 8.1). In all cases, a legal autopsy had been ordered by the prosecutor. In each case, the discovery of intramuscular hemorrhages lead to forensically meaningful differential diagnostic considerations.

Case #1: A 35-year-old female; died unnoticed in front of a cash machine. Myocarditis and a chronic bronchitis were found at autopsy. There were marked hemorrhages on both sides in the muscles originating from below the scapular spine, in the right supraspinatus muscle and the erector spinae muscle on the left side of the upper thoracic vertebral column.

Case #2: An 88-year-old female, single; found dead on her garden path with the front door of the house wide open. Acute left ventricular heart failure associated with chronic cardiac insufficiency. Intramuscular hemorrhages in part with blood-filled caverns at the height of both shoulders, on both sides of the infraspinatus muscles, in the intercostal muscles, in the flexor and extensor muscles of both upper arms as well as on the extensor side of the left lower arm.

Table 8.1 Summary of cases with intramuscular hemorrhages

No.	Age (years)	Gender[a]	Cause of death	Localization of bleedings
1	35	f	Myocarditis	Muscles originating from below the scapular spine on both sides/right supraspinatus muscles/erector spinae muscle on left side of upper thoracic vertebral column
2	88	f	Acute left ventricular heart failure	At height of both shoulders/ infraspinatus muscles on both sides/ intercostal muscles/flexor and extensor muscles of both upper arms/ extensor muscles of left lower arm
3	36	m	Acute right heart failure	Muscles originating from below the scapular spine on both sides/on inward surface of left scapula/both trapezius muscles (cervical parts)/ erector spinae muscle on both sides of upper thoracic vertebral column/ right sternocleidomastoid muscle
4	66	f	Heart failure by myocardial hypertrophy	Muscles below both scapular spines/on inward surfaces of both scapulas/ erector spinae muscle on both sides of upper thoracic vertebral column
5	75	m	Acute right heart failure	Muscles originating from below the scapular spine on both sides/on inward surface of right scapula/ erector spinae muscle on both sides of upper thoracic vertebral column/ flexor muscles of both upper arms/ extensor muscles of right upper arm/ extensor and flexor muscles of right lower arm
6	89	m	Recurrent myocardial infarction	Left infraspinatus muscle/on inward surface of left scapula/erector spinae muscle beside upper right thoracic vertebral column
7	62	m	Recurrent myocardial infarction	Dorsal, at height of both shoulders
8	77	m	Recurrent myocardial infarction	Above both shoulder levels/erector spinae muscle on right side of upper thoracic vertebral column
9	9	m	Acute right heart failure due to bronchial asthma	Infraspinatus muscles on both sides/ right supraspinatus muscle

[a]f = female, m = male.

Case #3: A 36-year-old truck driver, suffering from bronchial asthma and chronic bronchitis. Found dead in the cab of his parked truck in a parking lot. His death was caused by acute right heart failure in association with hypertrophy of the right heart and lipomatosis cordis destruens. There were intramuscular hemorrhages in the muscles originating from below the scapular spine on both sides, on the inward surface of the left scapula, in the cervical parts of both trapezius muscles, in the erector spinae muscle on both sides of the upper thoracic vertebral column as well as in the right sternocleidomastoid muscle.

Case #4: A 66-year-old female; died unnoticed in a park from a decompensated heart failure with predominantly left sided hypertrophy of the heart and severe sclerosis of the coronary vessels. At the time of death she was under light influence of alcohol (66 mg/dL). Erosions found in the gastric mucosa were interpreted as possible signs of hypothermia. There were intramuscular hemorrhages in the muscles below both scapular spines, on the inward surfaces of both scapulas and in the erector spinae muscle on both sides of the upper thoracic vertebral column, partly accompanied with muscular ruptures.

Case #5: A 75-year-old male, died at home. Death was caused by a combination of chronic insufficiency of the heart (cardiac weight 540 g) and acute right heart failure due to pneumonia. There were intramuscular hemorrhages in the muscles originating from below the scapular spine, as well as on the inward surface of the right scapula, in the erector spinae muscle on both sides of the upper thoracic vertebral column, in the flexor muscles of both upper arms, in the extensor muscles of the right upper arm and the extensor and flexor muscles of the right lower arm.

Case #6: An 89-year-old single male; found dead under suspicious circumstances in his flat. Death was caused by a recurrent heart attack associated with hypertrophy of the myocardium (cardiac weight 485 g) and severe sclerosis of the coronary arteries. Intramuscular hemorrhages in the left infraspinatus muscle, on the inward surface of the left scapula as well as in the erector spinae muscle beside the upper thoracic vertebral column on the right were present.

Case #7: A 62-year-old male; died in a shelter for the homeless from a recurrent ischemic heart attack associated with high-grade hypertrophy of the myocardium (cardiac weight 750 g). An emergency physician, called by the deceased's roommates, undertook an unsuccessful attempt to reanimate the patient. There were intramuscular hemorrhages dorsal at the height of both shoulders.

Case #8: A 77-year-old male; died in a shrubbery in front of his home from a recurrent myocardial infarction associated with a high-grade hypertrophy of the myocardium (cardiac weight 740 g). Unsuccessful resuscitation attempts were carried out by emergency personnel and had caused a fracture of the fifth to seventh rib on the right at the insertion into the sternum. Intramuscular hemorrhages were seen above both shoulders, as well as in the erector spinae muscle on the right of the upper thoracic vertebral column.

Case #9: A 9-year-old boy, known to suffer from severe asthma. He had collapsed in the presence of his mother in the street during a severe asthma attack. There had been an unsuccessful resuscitation attempt by an emergency physician. Autopsy showed an acute failure of the remarkably dilated heart accompanied by a fulminant bronchial asthma. There were intramuscular hemorrhages in the infraspinatus muscle on both sides as well as in the right supraspinatus muscle.

8.3 Discussion

A common finding in all the cases reported above was the discovery of intramuscular hemorrhages in typical localizations, such as the shoulder girdle and dorsum, and in some cases beyond this into the arm area (cases 2 and 5), in the intercostal muscles (case 2), or in the sternocleidomastoid muscle (case 3). In three cases (cases 1, 2 and 3), the circumstances made a murder in combination with robbery appear possible. In the other cases, murder by family members (case 5) or roommates (case 7), or an act of violence by unknown persons (cases 4, 6 and 8) could not initially be ruled out.

Thus, in every case the differential diagnosis whether the intramuscular hemorrhages discovered at autopsy were a sign of external blunt force or if the destruction of tissue was caused by force developed by the muscle itself (as a sequel of different kinds of internal diseases) had to be answered. In cases 7, 8, and 9 resuscitation attempts had to be considered as possible causes of the muscle lesions, whereas in the other cases presented, reanimation attempts could definitely be ruled out as possible causes.

In all the cases described here, hemorrhages were exclusively limited to muscle tissue. They never appeared anywhere beyond the covering muscle fascia and the subcutaneous adipose tissue was never affected. In addition, there was never a hematoma or an abrasion found on the covering skin area. In the cases of attempted resuscitation (cases 7, 8, and 9), the difference between two types of lesions in the same individual was conspicuous. Naturally, a force applied (to tissue) upsets the order of anatomical structures. Thus, lesions combined with destruction of tissue extending beyond the boundaries of skin, fat, and muscle tissue caused by resuscitation attempts were observed. In contrast, the described intramuscular hemorrhages in the muscles of the shoulder and back were principally confined to the area of the affected muscular structure (Fig. 8.1). They concurred with the architecture of the muscles: an aspect investigated further in the microscopic observation (see below).

Concerning the localization of these hemorrhages, a similar pattern of distribution has long been known and demonstrated in cases of drowning [2, 4, 5, 6, 8]. As already pointed out by von Hoffmann in 1903 [2], some authors

Fig. 8.1 Case #1. **A** Fresh intramuscular bleedings in the erector spinae muscle on the left side of the upper thoracic vertebral column. **B** Fresh intramuscular bleedings in infraspinatus muscle on the right side

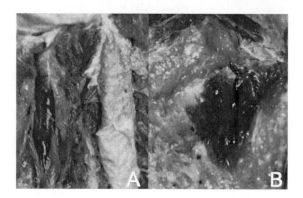

believe the influence of hypothermia to be at least partially responsible for the formation of intramuscular hemorrhages [14, 15]. In one of the cases described here (case 4), evidence for hypothermia could indeed be found. More significant is the fact that the affected muscles in all nine cases were so-called auxiliary respiratory muscles. This implies an increased muscle activity in dyspnea, as seen in cases of drowning and strangulation. As first described by von Hofmann and Haberda [3], during panic inhalation, the extreme strain can cause cavernous ruptures in the muscle tissue, a picture of lesions that presented itself here in two cases (cases 2 and 4). In the cases described here, no connection with other phenomenological aspects such as age, gender, alcoholization, or influence of drugs could be ascertained.

In addition, the histological examination showed a picture familiar from the description of lesions of the auxiliary respiratory muscles in cases of drowning and strangulation [4, 9, 16, 17]. Under loss of the cross-striation typical for skeletal muscles, a clear longitudinal striation emerged. So-called hypercontraction bands indicated the enormous overexertion of the contractile tissue (Fig. 8.2). Complete ruptures of fibers showed a disintegration of the sarcolemma with discoid

Fig. 8.2 Histologic appearance of fresh hemorrhages in a hypercontracted muscle, with cross-striation disappearing, ruptures and pre-ruptures, and bleedings in between individual muscle fibers

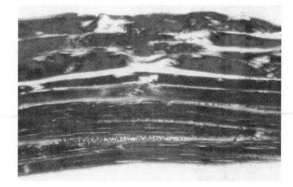

protuberances at the ruptures' endings. This does not appear to be a change resulting from autolytic disintegration in postmortal tissue [4, 16].

Pre-ruptures in which muscle membranes remained as empty sarcolemmal tubes could also be found; when located on the inside, the arrangement of over-exerted muscle fibers disintegrated. Hemorrhages in between the lesioned muscle fibers spread the fibers, causing star- or cobweb-like dispersal around small hemorrhagic centers. This argues against hemorrhages in tissue caused by trauma and against postmortem bleedings, which usually disperse evenly into the entire tissue [4, 16, 17, 18]. Furthermore, the absence of clear cellular reactions by leukocytes – a typical vital sign – has to be considered. Thus, these changes in muscle-fiber structure have to be regarded as being agonal, developing in tissue affected by hypoxia.

8.4 Conclusions

In all nine cases reported here, a natural death could be ascertained. Obviously, there have been agonal spasmodic attempts to breathe, causing intramuscular hemorrhages in the auxiliary respiratory muscles, a phenomenon otherwise known from asphyxia in cases of drowning or strangulation.

However, if natural death could not have been absolutely established, due to their localization, a less accurate evaluation might have led to the interpretation of the hemorrhages as being of traumatic origin. Forensic pathologists and medical examiners, respectively, should therefore always consider the possibility of intramuscular hemorrhages caused by internal diseases. During the autopsy, the extension of the lesions regarding the muscles' fascias and the surrounding tissue must be carefully established. Combined with a subsequent histological examination of the muscle tissue, differentiation between hemorrhages with an internal cause and those with a blunt traumatic origin should not cause any fundamental problems.

References

1. Bajanowski T, Brinkmann B, Stefanec AM, Barckhaus RH, Fechner G (1998) Detection and analysis of tracers in experimental drowning. Int J Legal Med 111:57–61
2. von Hofmann ER (1903) Lehrbuch der gerichtlichen Medizin. Urban und Schwarzenberg, Wien
3. von Hofmann ER, Haberda A (1927) Lehrbuch der gerichtlichen Medizin, 11th edn. Urban und Schwarzenberg, Berlin, Wien
4. Püschel K, Schulz F, Darrmann I, Tsokos M (1999) Macromorphology and histology of intramuscular hemorrhages in cases of drowning. Int J Legal Med 112:101–106
5. Reuter F (1907) Die anatomische Diagnose des Ertrinkungstodes. Vjschr Gerichtl Med (Suppl.) 33:20–28
6. Reuter F (1922) Über das Vorkommen, die Entstehung und Bedeutung von Muskelblutungen beim Erstickungstode. Beitr Gerichtl Med 5:137–156

7. Sigrist T, Schulz F, Koops E (1994) Irreführende Muskelblutungen bei einer Wasserleiche. Ein Beitrag zur Differenzierung zwischen intravitaler und postmortaler Entstehung. Arch Kriminol 193:90–96

8. Paltauf A (1888) Über den Tod durch Ertrinken. Urban und Schwarzenberg, Wien, Leipzig

9. Keil W, Forster A, Meyer HJ, Peschel O (1995) Characterization of haemorrhages at the origin of the sternocleidomastoid muscles in hanging. Int J Legal Med 108:140–144

10. Fechner G, Hauser R, Sepulchre MA, Brinkmann B (1991) Immunhistochemical investigations to demonstrate vital direct traumatic damage of skeletal muscle. Int J Legal Med 104:215–219

11. Fechner G, Petkovits T, Brinkmann B (1990) Zur Ultrastruktur-Pathologie mechanischer Skelettmuskelschädigungen. Rechtsmedizin 103:291–299

12. Walcher K (1926) Die vitale Reaktion bei der Beurteilung des gewaltsamen Todes. Dtsch Z Gerichtl Med 26:193–211

13. Lach H, Püschel K, Schulz F (2005) Intramuskuläre Blutungen beim Tod aus innerer Ursache. Arch Kriminol 216:97–107

14. Dirnhofer R, Sigrist T (1979) Muskelblutungen im Körperkern – ein Zeichen vitaler Reaktion beim Tod durch Unterkühlung? Beitr Gerichtl Med 37:159–166

15. Sigrist T, Markwalder C, Dirnhofer R (1990) Veränderung der Skelettmuskulatur beim Tod durch Unterkühlung. Rechtsmedizin 103:463–472

16. Sigrist T (1987) Untersuchungen zur vitalen Reaktion der Skelettmuskulatur. Beitr Gerichtl Med 45:87–101

17. Sigrist T, Rabl W (1993) Skelettmuskelblutungen – vital oder postmortal? Rechtsmedizin 3:94–96

18. Hauser R, Fechner G, Brinkmann B (1989) Zur Unterscheidung zwischen intravitalen und postmortalen Blutungen. Beitr Gerichtl Med 48:437–441

Part V
Ballistics

Chapter 9
Forensic Ballistics

Bernd Karger

Contents

Abstract Forensic ballistics is the application of ballistics for forensic purposes. The basis is formed by wound ballistics. Two main mechanisms of injury are differentiated: the crush-mechanism resulting in the permanent cavity and the stretch-mechanism resulting in the temporary cavity. The missile-tissue interactions such as yawing, deformation, fragmentation, and bone contact are explained here and it is shown why the energy deposit or the missile velocity are not the sole or primary factors in determining the severity of a wound. The special wound ballistics of the head including indirect ("remote") injuries in the

B. Karger
Institute of Legal Medicine, University of Münster, Münster, Germany
e-mail: karger@uni-muenster.de

M. Tsokos (ed.), *Forensic Pathology Reviews, Volume 5*,
doi: 10.1007/978-1-59745-110-9_9, © Humana Press, Totowa, NJ 2008

brain and skull are discussed. Incapacitation is a necessarily occuring inability to perform complex movements and is therefore based on physiological effects independent of psychological mechanisms such as pain or surprise. Immediate incapacitation can only be caused by direct disruption of brain tissue and thus by penetrating gunshots to the head. Ballistic parameters and intracranial trajectories where sustained capability to act is possible are discussed. Rapid incapacitation is produced by massive blood loss via acute cerebral hypoxemia and subsequent unconsciousness. Targets of rapid incapacitation are the heart, aorta, and the truncus of the pulmonary artery. In cases of considerable ballistic injury to the lungs, liver, kidneys, spleen, large arteries or central veins, the latent period until incapacitation will be in the range of one or several minutes (*delayed incapacitation*). This potential for physical activity is not always exhausted due to psychological factors. Backspatter is biological material propelled retrogradely out of the entrance wound towards the firearm/the hand of the person shooting. Blood and tissue particles are accelerated by the subcutaneous gas effect, temporary cavitation, and tail splashing. Backspatter therefore is common in close-range gunshots to the head where blood and tissue can travel for several meters. The number of bloodstains can vary greatly and the stains are located in a semicircle of almost 180° in front of the entrance wound. Characteristic for backspatter are small or tiny droplet or splashing stains with the elongated shapes roughly aiming at the entrance wound. Magnification and appropriate lightning are necessary for investigating backspatter. DNA-analysis of stains can establish a clear link between a person or object and a clearly defined gunshot. Contact of a bullet with an intermediate target can alter the trajectory and stability of the bullet. Contact with fragile materials such as concrete, glass, asphalt, or gypsum-board regularly results in abundant deposits on the bullet, which can be visualized by SEM (scanning electron microscopy) and determined by X-ray microanalysis. Ductile materials such as wood and car body parts only transfer scarce deposits to the bullet which can be indicative of the intermediate target. This important trace evidence is not eliminated by subsequent perforation of tissue. Individualisation of deposits on FMJ bullets after perforation of a human body can be successfully carried out by PCR-typing of STRs and mitochondrial DNA. In cases of gunfights, this makes it possible to determine who was killed or injured by which bullet. The person shooting can be identified by additional comparison of rifling marks. Cellular material is recovered by swabbing the bullet, which should be protected against contamination and loss of material.

Keywords Backspatter · Capability to act · Cross sectional area · Deformation · Deposits on bullets · DNA-analysis · Energy deposit · Fragmentation · Gunshots to the head · Incapacitation · Intermediate target · Transfer of trace evidence · Wound ballistics

9.1 Introduction

Forensic ballistics can be briefly defined as the application of ballistics for forensic purposes. The major task of this heterogenous discipline is the reconstruction of the events that produced a gunshot injury, fatal or not. So the very basis is formed by wound ballistics, i.e. the science of the penetration of a biological target. Every forensic pathologist should know how a gunshot injury is produced and wound ballistics therefore is the first field considered here. Although the principles of wound ballistics are not so complicated, bullets take a special position among the objects relevant in traumatology due to their physical characteristics: compared to other wounding agents, the mass is very small and the velocity is high. Unlike other blunt accelerated objects, this allows per se a deep penetration of tissue. But unlike sharp force, a dynamic penetration mechanism is effective which has not ended by the time the bullet exits. The resulting phenomena such as temporary cavitation can be misinterpretated and have given rise to myths and half-truths, which are discussed briefly later.

The second part on incapacitation is closely related to wound ballistics. It deals with the possible reaction of those being injured by a bullet, which can also be an integral part of reconstruction efforts.

A large variety of additional findings and evidence can be utilized for reconstructing the events leading to a gunshot injury such as gunshot residue or the geometry of the bullet tract. Since a complete presentation of all these aspects would clearly go beyond the scope of this chapter, a selection of topics was made. The third part is dedicated to blood and tissue particles exiting via the entrance wound: backspatter. The direction against the line of fire is the reason for the high evidential value of this phenomenon. The firearm and the body, especially the hand of the person shooting, are within the reach of the biological particles in cases of close-range gunshots and individualisation of backspatter stains can connect the person or gun to the gunshot injury at hand.

Trace evidence on spent bullets is the topic of the last part of this chapter. Contact of bullets with intermediate targets is an important field in exterior ballistics but also has wound ballistic and legal implications. A method for identifying deposits from intermediate targets on spent bullets is presented together with our experience in DNA-analysis of tissue deposits on bullets after perforation of a body.

9.2 Wound Ballistics

9.2.1 Mechanisms of Injury

Wound ballistics can be defined as missile-tissue-interaction [1]. The biological effect is therefore determined by:

– Parameters of the missile such as mass, caliber, velocity, shape, material or construction
– Parameters of the tissue such as density, elasticity, viscosity, and anatomical structure

Two different mechanisms of injury can be distinguished when a projectile penetrates a dense medium such as tissue [2, 3, 4]. Both represent distinct aspects of the same rapid fluiddynamic process and can therefore be regarded as theoretical abstractions essential for the understanding of wound ballistics.

9.2.1.1 Crush-mechanism and Permanent Tract

Tissue located in line with the trajectory is crushed by excessive pressures build-up directly in front of the tip of the moving projectile. The tissue is completely disintegrated, resulting morphologically in the permanent tract [2, 3, 5].

9.2.1.2 Stretch-mechanism and Temporary Cavity

Tissue located at the side of the trajectory is temporarily accelerated radially. This radial displacement of tissue creates a fusiform or conical cavity reaching a maximum 2–4 ms after the projectile has passed [3, 6, 7]. Tissue elasticity causes the cavity to collapse immediately, hence the name temporary cavity. The kinetic energy transferred to the tissue is expended after several cycles of expansion and contraction comparable to a pendulum: the temporary cavity is said to pulsate or "breathe" [3, 8, 9, 10].

During the formation of the temporary cavity, tissue is injured in three distinct modes (Fig. 9.1A–C), summarized as stretch-mechanism [2, 5] according to the predominating factor. Radial tissue displacement stretches the circumference of tubular areas of tissue around the permanent tract from $2\pi r$ to $2\pi(r+x)$ [3, 11]. Simultaneously, the thickness of these tubes is reduced resulting in compression of tissue. Moreover, the formation of the temporary cavity is a dynamic phenomenon. The whole process of temporary cavitation takes about 10 ms [7] during which the shape of the cavity changes continuously. Because of inhomogenities and interfaces within the tissue, the cavity will push out along lines of least resistance such as fascial planes. This "principle of nonconfinement of the cavity" [3] produces an asymmetrical temporary cavity and consequently shear forces inside adjacent layers of tissue. The radial displacement of tissue and associated overpressures in the tissue around the expanding cavity gradually decrease with increasing distance from the tract like waves in calm water [3, 9].

So the stretch-mechanism of ballistic trauma is essentially nothing more than a localized blunt trauma analogous to a fist displacing tissue [1, 12, 13]. The maximum speed of moving tissue forming the boundary of the temporary cavity has been reported to be in the range of 40–100 m/s for so-called high-velocity missiles [14, 15, 16]. The structural integrity of tissue displaced by cavitation will generally

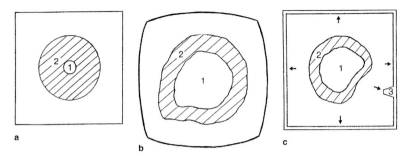

Fig. 9.1 Schematic illustration of the sectional area of soft tissue before and after a projectile has passed: temporary cavitation and stretch-mechanism. **A** Tubular tissue portions *before* the projectile has passed (1 = future trajectory; 2 = tubular tissue portion around the trajectory). **B** Tubular tissue portions *after* the projectile has passed at the moment of maximum temporary cavitation (1 = maximum) temporary cavity including future permanent tract; 2 = same tubular tissue portion as in **A**). The diameter of the tube has increased, resulting in stretching of tissue. Tissue inhomogenities are causing an asymmetrical shape of the tube (principle of nonconfinement), resulting in shearing of tissue. The thickness of the tube's wall has decreased, resulting in compression of tissue. **C** Tubular tissue portions *after* the projectile has passed at the moment of maximum temporary cavitation, tissue confined in a rigid *casing* such as the head 1: the diameter of the temporary cavity is smaller compared to one in tissue not confined in a casing; 2: compared to **B**, the diameter of the tubular tissue circle is smaller, resulting in less stretching of tissue. The thickness of the wall of the tube is smaller, resulting in increased compression of tissue. Additionally, the surface of the tissue is pushed against the rigid casing (arrows), resulting in contusion of tissue remote from the tract analogous to blunt trauma; 3: prominent part of the casing (rim, edge, etc.). The prominence results in additional regional shearing and especially compression and contusion of tissue

not be completely destroyed [1, 5, 17, 18]. Therefore, the stretch-mechanism is not a reliable factor in wounding. The severity of injury decreases with increasing distance from the permanent tract, a zone of extravasation being located next to the permanent tract [3, 9]. Thus, the term "Seitenstoßkraft" (= sideways force) used in the past by German speaking experts in ballistics (e.g., [19]) probably illustrates the effect of the temporary cavity more vividly than the term cavitation, although the latter is perhaps more correct in terms of physics.

The sonic pressure wave ("shock wave") originating from the impact of the projectile plays no part in wounding. Despite extremely high pressures, the duration of the amplitude is too brief (2 ms) to move or injure tissue [4, 20].

9.2.2 *Missile-tissue-interactions*

It becomes apparent by distinguishing two mechanisms of injury that the striking energy or the energy transferred to tissue only determines the potential of a given projectile for tissue disruption [2, 5, 12]. There are three crucial points for the realization of this wounding potential. The first is the ratio of distribution of the energy between the crush- and the stretch-mechanism. The portion of the transferred energy used up in cavitation and stretching depends on ballistic parameters such as striking velocity, mass, and construction and generally increases with increasing velocity and decreasing mass [5, 21]. Therefore, bullets having the same striking energy made up of different velocities and masses (Fig. 9.2A,B) or even bullets with identical velocity and mass but different construction will produce very different injuries in identical tissue [2, 5, 22]. The second crucial point is the location of energy-transfer along the shot channel, considering the spatial aspect of a gunshot injury, and the third is the degree of elasticity of the tissues involved because tissue characteristics also determine the severity of a wound. In terms of the analogy used before: it does make a difference what kind of tissue is hit by a fist. The more flexible and elastic the tissue is, the less damage will be caused by the same amount of energy transferred to the stretch-mechanism [3, 5, 22]. Most soft tissues such as muscle, lung, skin, and bowel wall have the physical characteristics of a good energy or shock absorber, keeping the zone of

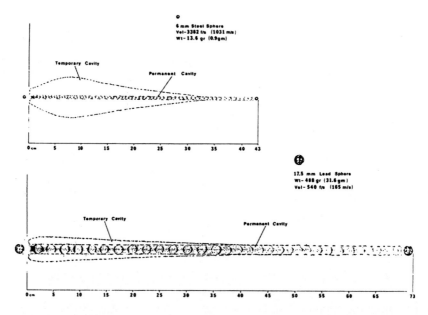

Fig. 9.2 Wound profiles according to Fackler [1, 2, 21] of two stable spheres depositing roughly the same amount of energy in gelatine blocks but producing strikingly different wound cavities. In the case of the fast, small and light-weight steel sphere (478 J), most of the kinetic energy is used up in the stretch mechanism, producing a large temporary cavity and a small permanent tract. In contrast to this, most of the large and heavy but slow sphere's energy (430 J) is used up in crushing of tissue, thus producing a large permanent tract but a small temporary cavity. This sharp contrast already demonstrates that gunshot injuries cannot be adequately described by terms like energy or energy deposit. The energy transfer of the fast sphere is also higher than that of the slow one

extravasation small [1, 5]. In contrast, in inelastic tissue such as the liver, spleen, or brain, the cavitation and resulting stretch-mechanism can produce devastating wounds up to a complete laceration or dispersion of the organ [8, 17, 22, 23, 24].

The general principles of wound ballistics outlined above are modified by yawing, deformation, and fragmentation of a projectile and by bone contact, all of which increase the missile's cross sectional area, i.e., the frontal surface of the bullet coming into contact with tissue.

In contrast to spheres, bullets commonly *yaw* or rotate around a lateral axis when moving in a dense medium such as tissue (Fig. 9.3). The angle between the trajectory and the long axis of the bullet increases due to destabilising forces until it reaches 90°, i.e., the bullet's long axis is perpendicular to the trajectory. The yawing motion then continues until 180° and the bullet will remain in this stable position where the base is the leading part. Increasing the cross sectional area of a bullet produces enhanced deceleration, reduced penetration depth and larger diameters of the wound cavities [2, 5, 9, 21]. The path of a projectile in a dense medium therefore shows three distinct sections, depending on the respective cross sectional area: narrow channel, increased cavities, and tail end (Figs. 9.3 and 9.4A).

Deformation will increase the missile's cross sectional area due to expansion (Fig. 9.4A,B) and a *fragmenting bullet* will also increase its cross sectional area (Fig. 9.5A,B), although distributed among multiple missiles of smaller mass and reduced penetration depth [16]. These so-called secondary missiles will produce multiple secondary shot channels, which, apart from their direct wounding effect, represent points of least resistance and will thus increase the

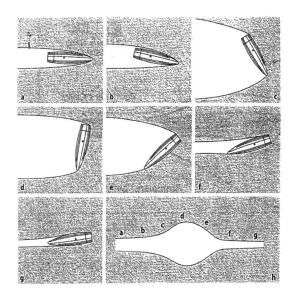

Fig. 9.3 Schematic illustration of the typical motion of a stable bullet during penetration of tissue ("yawing"). **a,b** The "narrow channel", no yawing. **c–e** Rotation around a lateral axis. This yawing motion considerably increases the cross sectional area of the bullet, thus increasing the diameters of the resulting wound cavities but decreasing penetration depth. **f,g** The "tail end". **h**: Schematic illustration of the resulting wound cavities in soap. The orientation of the bullet is indicated by the letters

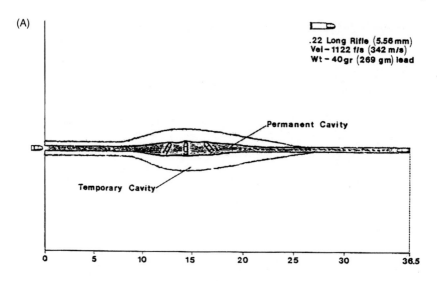

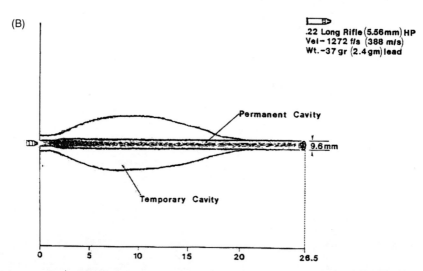

Fig. 9.4 Wound profiles according to Fackler [1, 2, 21] of two .22 lr bullets. **A** The stable lead bullet produces a long narrow channel and rather small wound cavities. **B** The deforming hollow point bullet, however, produces a short narrow channel and rather large wound cavities while the penetration depth is reduced. This difference is solely caused by the differing constructions since not only energy but also mass and velocity of the two bullets are almost identical

(A)

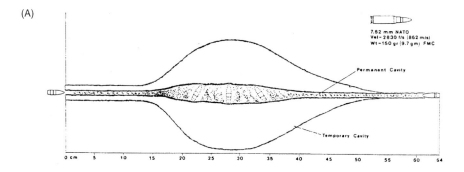

(B)

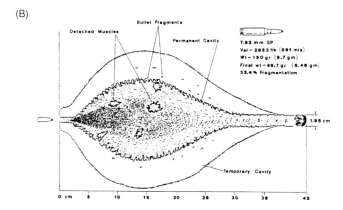

Fig. 9.5 Wound profiles according to Fackler [1, 2, 21] of two 7.62×51mm NATO (.308 Winchester) bullets. **A** The stable FMJ bullet causes the typical wound morphology including a long narrow channel. **B** The soft point bullet possessing the same mass and velocity does deform and fragment due to the differing construction. This results in a non-existent narrow channel and in huge wound cavities

susceptibility for the subsequent stretching of tissue. There is a synergistic effect of secondary missiles and cavitation [2, 16, 23, 25].

Compared to soft tissue, bone is a hard and dense material, reducing the penetration depth of bullets that strike it. Depending on the construction, material, and velocity of the projectile, bone contact favors deformation, fragmentation, and increased yaw [26, 27] with the above-mentioned effects. Frequently, bone contact causes additional secondary missiles in the form of bone fragments [7, 23, 26, 28, 29]. The accelerated bone fragments travel in different directions in the vicinity of the bone, to a small extent even against the line of fire [28, 30]. The effect of secondary bone fragment missiles is analogous to bullet fragments including secondary shot channels (Fig. 9.6), enhancing the severity of the wound [5, 7, 23, 28].

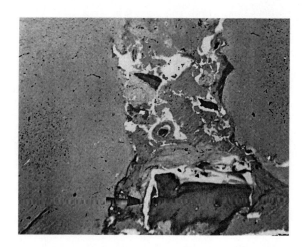

Fig. 9.6 Microscopical
appearance of intracerebral
bone fragment (arrow) at the
end of a retracted secondary
shot channel 3 cm in length
(Hematoxylin & Eosin)

9.2.3 *Energy Deposit, Energy Transfer, and High-velocity Missiles*

The energy deposit concept states that the kinetic energy ($E = mv^2/2$) used up in
the production of a gunshot wound determines the severity of the wound [35].
The energy transfer concept additionally considers the distribution along the
shot channel [35]. In both concepts, the missile-tissue interaction is considered
a black box and can therefore be reduced to an abstract physical value.
However, the kinetic energy is only secondarily derived from two basic ballistic
parameters, mass and velocity. Since the velocity is squared in this equation, the
popular thesis about the primacy of velocity over mass for the wounding
potential appears consistent but nevertheless is based on an oversimplifying
approach. Therefore, the popular differentiation of high-velocity and low-
velocity missiles should be dropped – the lack of a reasonable border velocity
has even led to the introduction of medium-velocity [32]. So-called high-velocity
missiles do not necessarily carry a high wounding potential and extremity
amputations produced by tangential high-velocity gunshot wounds are nothing
more than abstruse legends.

The differentiation of two ideal penetration mechanisms and the dynamics
and variability of the missile-tissue interactions clearly demonstrate that a
secondary ballistic parameter such as kinetic energy cannot adequately describe
a gunshot wound. Instead, basic parameters such as mass, velocity, caliber,
degree of deformation and fragmentation, length of the narrow channel, and
penetration depth are decisive in determining the severity of a gunshot wound
[33]. As a consequence, studies investigating the mass of non-vital tissue as a
function of energy transfer [34, 35, 36, 37, 38, 39, 40] were not successful in
establishing a close relationship but only found a tendency, which is not
surprising considering the abstract relationship between energy transfer and
the possible destruction work.

9.2.4 Special Wound Ballistics of the Head

In intracranial gunshot wounds, several of the above-mentioned factors enhance the degree of tissue disruption. The inelastic quality and the high water content of brain tissue make it per se very vulnerable to cavitation and stretch-mechanism. The penetration of the skull can imply the generation of secondary missiles in the form of bone (Fig. 9.7) or bullet fragments [28, 41, 42, 43, 44] and a tendency towards early tumbling or deformation of the bullet. Kirkpatrick and DiMaio [44], for example, were able to demonstrate intracerebral bone chips solely by digital palpation of the brain in 16 out of 42 cases of civilian gunshot wounds to the brain.

Even more important, intracranial trajectories gain a new quality by the rigid skull functioning as a non-yielding wall. Because brain tissue is almost incompressible, intracranial temporary cavitation and surrounding overpressure meet counter-pressure from the skull. The skull will, so to speak, try to overcome the principle of nonconfinement of the cavity by denying the free space necessary for a gradual decrease of radial tissue displacement and associated overpressure. The volume of the intracranial temporary cavity will consequently stay smaller than a cavity formed under identical conditions in tissue not confined in a casing. Intracranial overpressures around the expanding temporary cavity, however, clearly exceed the pressures found in nonconfined tissue [4, 10, 45, 46]. These high dynamic pressures, the asymmetric shape of the temporary cavity, and unilaterally fixed tissue structures lead to shear forces within brain tissue. The unyielding skull does not allow the brain to expand, so the brain will transfer the overpressures to the skull. In other words, the brain's surface gets pushed with great force against the inner table of the neurocranium and the brain stem gets forced down into the foramen magnum. Consequently, the layer of cerebral tissue

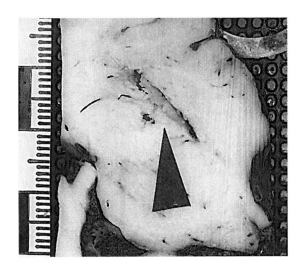

Fig. 9.7 Intracerebral bone fragment (*arrow*) at a distance of several cm from the tract and surrounded by petechial haemorrhages. The 3rd and 4th ventricles left of the arrow are filled with blood

Fig. 9.8 Subarachnoid
haemorrhage and cortical
contusion zone in the form
of ball haemorrhages
(Hematoxylin & Eosin)

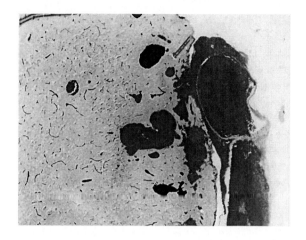

between temporary cavity and skull is compressed much more strongly than
tissue not confined in a rigid casing and shearing of brain tissue is increased by
bone structures projecting into the skull cavity.

Analogous to blunt trauma, enhanced compression can result in contusion
of brain tissue discernible as (cortical) contusion zones in superficial layers of
the brain remote from the trajectory [28, 44, 47, 48, 49] (Fig. 9.8). The stretching
and especially shearing of tissue is responsible for intracerebral petechial
hemorrhages remote from the tract in the form of classical perivascular ring
hemorrhages or spherical hemorrhages [28, 41, 43] (Fig. 9.9). They are simply
the result of an enlarged zone of extravasation due to the enhanced effect of
temporary cavitation. Preferential neuroanatomical sites are more central parts
of the brain such as the basal ganglia, midbrain, pons, and cerebellum (Fig. 9.9).

Fig. 9.9 Numerous
intracerebral haemorrhages
in the left thalamus
remote from the tract. The
macroscopical appearance is
similar to the haemorrhages
depicted in Fig. 9.7
(Hematoxylin & Eosin)

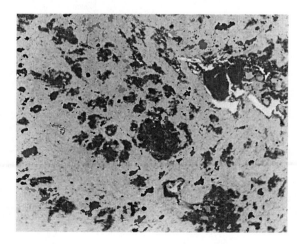

Fig. 9.10 Indirect fracture
(*arrow*) in the right anterior
cranial fossa after a suicidal
gunshot with a .45 ACP
FMJ bullet with the wound
tract above the middle and
posterior cranial fossa.
There was immediate
incapacitation in this case

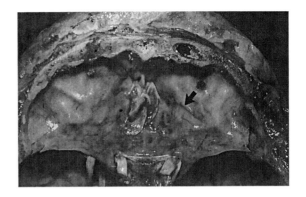

The skull will at first be slightly stretched by intracranial overpressures. If the skull's capacity to elastically stretch is surpassed, there will be indirect skull fractures, i.e., fracture lines without contact to the primary bony entrance and exit defects. Because the base of the skull is inhomogenous and less resistant to stretching than the vault, preferential locations are the roofs of the orbitae (Fig. 9.10) and the ethmoidal plates in the anterior cranial fossa [50]. While secondary radial fractures originating from the gunshot defects are induced by the bullet's impact, tertiary concentric fractures connecting the radial fracture lines (Fig. 9.11) are indirect heaving fractures [51, 52, 53] functioning as additional stress relief for internal overpressures. If the internal pressures are high enough, indirect skull fractures will combine to an "explosive" type of head injury [54] with comminuted fractures of the skull and laceration of the brain (Fig. 9.12).

So the rigid skull which protects the brain from most blunt trauma also makes the brain by far the most susceptible organ in the body to penetrating ballistic injury. Intracranial pressure peaks and its effects vary greatly, depending on

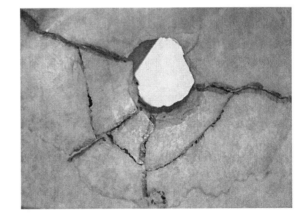

Fig. 9.11 Indirect (con-
centric) heaving fractures
around an exit wound in the
left temple after gunshot
with a .44 lead projectile.
The concentric fracture lines
are produced indirectly by
intracranial overpressure
while the radial fracture
lines are caused directly by
impact of the projectile

Fig. 9.12 Partial exenteration of the brain after a close-range gunshot with a 12/70 shotgun using a Brennecke shotgun slug (lead projectile, mass approx. 30 g, velocity approx. 450 m/s). This clearly demonstrates that no "high-velocity" missile is required for such an "explosive" type of head injury

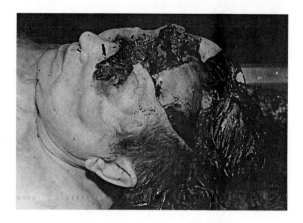

ballistic and anatomical parameters. Mathematically, the peak pressures recorded vary in direct proportion to the projected cross-sectional area of the missile and the square of its velocity but in inverse proportion to the distance from the point of origin [4, 10, 45, 46]. In more practical terms, bullet wounds from handguns and rifles differ considerably with regard to their effect in penetrating gunshots to the head. Bullets from conventional handguns can produce indirect skull fractures and pronounced cerebral tissue disruption [28]. Centerfire rifles, whether military or hunting, almost invariably cause a strong "explosive" effect with comminution of bone and laceration of at least part of the brain [42, 55, 56, 57]. Hits from shotguns differ substantially depending on the range of fire. Close range shots have a tremendous effect similar to centerfire rifles by literally riddling brain tissue and blasting the skull [58, 59] (Fig. 9.12).

9.3 Incapacitation

Determining a person's capability to act following a gunshot wound can be of major importance in crime scene reconstruction and in differentiation between homicide and suicide. If a person who has been shot is not able to shoot back, attack or escape, certain events can be ruled out. This can assist the identification of the person who fired the gun and the reconstruction of the sequence of shots and activities. Therefore, questions concerning the possibility of physical activity following a given gunshot wound are repeatedly raised in court.

Stopping power is a term very similar to incapacitation, although the point of view has changed to one from behind the trigger. The use of firearms by police officers is frequently intended to stop the momentary activity of a suspect by rapid incapacitation. Because stopping power and incapacitation both address the same phenomenon, this issue is also relevant to law enforcement agencies.

9.3.1 Definition and Mechanisms of Incapacitation

There are a variety of definitions mostly concentrating on the inability to act in a conscious and purposeful manner such as escaping or attacking [60, 61]. Others have used complex definitions primarily based on the degree of consciousness and on underlying neurophysiological processes [62]. In this context, a functional definition of capability to act independent of the state of consciousness or intention will be used: capability to act is the ability to participate in the interaction between victim and perpetrator or victim and environment, resulting in discernible events or stains. Thus, incapacitation is an early and necessarily occurring inability to perform complex and longer lasting movements. The activity does not have to be appropriate in the situation at hand. For example, pocketing or storing the firearm following a suicidal gunshot is not always achieved intentionally or purposefully. Incapacitation is based on physiological effects independent of psychological mechanisms such as pain or fright because it has to be independent of the victim's "cooperation".

Reliable incapacitation based on physiological effects according to the above definition is closely connected to death and can only be produced by decreasing the functioning capability of the central nervous system (CNS) [12, 63, 64]. The two sole mechanisms to accomplish this are direct disruption of brain tissue or indirect elimination of the CNS by cerebral hypoxemia from bleeding, both causing unconsciousness [12, 63, 64, 65].

There is no other way to prevent a determined person from further action. Many victims will collapse immediately when hit by a bullet as will some who were missed but think they were hit. They do so on a psychological basis but this is inconsistent and erratic [65]. The only thing to count on is that it will not work in the case of determined and highly motivated persons or in the case of those under the influence of drugs or adrenalin. Excessive pain, for example, must first be perceived and then this perception of pain must cause an emotional reaction. So reliable incapacitation is solely based on physiological effects independent of any unpredictable psychological factors.

Another alleged mechanism of incapacitation is high energy-transfer [31] or high energy deposit [66]. Energy deposit is an abstract value, considering neither the way (crush/stretch) or location energy is transferred nor the type of tissue involved (compare Sect. 2.2). Therefore, the amount of energy is of limited value in predicting effects in an actual shooting. The momentum transferred to the target does not knock the human body down or drive it significantly backwards [65, 67], even if shown so a thousand times on television. The impulse transferred to an adult from a .45 ACP round results in a negligible backwards motion of approximately 5 cm/s [67]. Injury or even incapacitation from shock waves [68] or a mysterious "nerve shock" postulated especially in hunting are not supported by a single experiment or by theoretical considerations [20, 33, 69].

Hampered physical activity but not incapacitation may be produced by injuries to sensory or optic brain areas, the spinal cord and large peripheral nerves, static structures such as long bones or joints and by pneumothorax [33].

9.3.2 Immediate Incapacitation

Instantaneous incapacitation can only be produced by direct disruption of brain tissue [64, 65]. In the case of gunshot injuries causing acute bleeding, the speed of blood loss is too slow and compensation mechanisms are too effective for immediate loss of consciousness and incapacitation [64]. So the only way to stop immediately the activity of another person are penetrating gunshots to the head.

Because of the enhanced intracranial tissue disruption and the functional significance of the CNS, craniocerebral gunshot wounds result in a high early mortality rate of 90% and more [70, 71] and commonly in immediate incapacitation. However, in the last century, numerous publications reported sustained capability to act following penetrating gunshot wounds of the head. Since these were case reports or small case series, no systematic correlations between wounding and capability to act could be detected. Therefore, all accessible cases have been reviewed [72]. A large number of case reports had to be excluded from this reexamination because of doubtful capability to act or lacking morphological or ballistic documentation; there remained 53 case reports from 42 sources for systematical analysis.

Favourable conditions for sustained capability to act are present in cases where the additional wounding resulting from the special wound ballistic qualities of the head are minimized. Thus, more than 70% of the guns used fired slow and light-weight bullets: 6.35-mm Browning, .22 rimfire or extremely ineffective projectiles such as ancient, improper, or self-made missiles (Table 9.1). Only two large handguns resulting in intracerebral wounding were used: A .38 spec. bullet which solely wounded the base of the right temporal lobe [73] and a .45 lead bullet which seriously injured the left frontal lobe but whose trajectory was limited to the anterior fossa of the skull [74]. A centerfire rifle or a shotgun from close-range were never employed in cases of intracerebral tracts. A coincidence of several lucky circumstances made sustained capability to act possible in two cases of military centerfire rifle bullets passing longitudinally between the frontal lobes without direct contact with brain tissue [75, 76].

Of the trajectories, 28% were outside the neurocranium. At least 70% of the craniocerebral tracts passed above the anterior fossa of the skull (Table 9.2), wounding the frontal parts of the brain. Apart from a neurophysiological approach, this preference can additionally be explained by the base of the anterior cranial fossa and the sella turcica area which serve as a bony barrier protecting those parts of the brain located in its "shadow" relative to the trajectory against cavitational tissue displacement and associated overpressures. This is particularly true for the brain stem. Intracerebral trajectories not located above the anterior

Table 9.1 Summary of the firearms used

Firearms used	$N = 53$
Pocket-revolvers and old, low-energy handguns	$n = 10$ (19%)
Modified blank handguns or selfmade/improper ammunition	$n = 5$ (9%)
.22 pistol	$n = 2$ (4%)
5.6-mm rimfire rifle	$n = 4$ (7%)
6.35-mm pistol	$n = 13$ (25%)
7.65-mm pistol	$n = 8$ (15%)
.45 Colt revolver	$n = 1$ (2%)
.38 special revolver	$n = 1$ (2%)
Centerfire rifle	$n = 3$ (6%)
Shotgun (contact shot)	$n = 1$ (2%)
Not exactly known	$n = 5$ (9%)

fossa were caused by slow and light-weight bullets preferring one temporal lobe. Additionally, one parietal and one occipital lobe were each injured once by a very ineffective projectile [77] and by a 7.65-mm bullet reduced in velocity [78]. Morphological signs of high intracranial pressure peaks (cortical contusion zones, indirect skull fractures, perivascular hemorrhages) and secondary missiles were poorly documented but appear to be very rare.

Therefore, sustained capability to act following craniocerebral gunshots is very unlikely if one of the following two conditions are fulfilled:

1. Use of a firearm from about 9-mm Parabellum upwards in terms of penetration power and wounding potential (large handguns, centerfire rifles). To increase further the probability of incapacitation, intracerebral trajectories above the anterior cranial fossa or very short ones can be excluded.
2. Definite occurrence of signs of high intracranial overpressures: indirect skull fractures, intracerebral petechial hemorrhages remote from the tract and cortical contusion zones.

Incapacitation can be determined beyond any doubt if central nervous centers essential for physical activity are wounded directly. In the literature reviewed [72], not a single case of injury to the brain stem, the diencephalon, the cerebellum, or major paths of motor conduction has been described. The

Table 9.2 Summary of brain areas injured or wound tracts

Wounded brain areas or trajectories	$N = 53$
One or both frontal lobes	$n = 17$ (32%)
Transtemporal (no autopsy or no precise cerebral morphological findings)	$n = 11$ (21%)
One temporal lobe	$n = 6$ (11%)
Right parietal lobe	$n = 1$ (2%)
Extraneurocranial	$n = 15$ (28%)
Intraneurocranial but extracerebral	$n = 3$ (6%)

Table 9.3 Targets of immediate incapacitation

Upper cervical spinal cord, brain stem including the mid-brain, diencephalon incl. central grey
  matter, cerebellum, major paths of motor conduction, motor cortex

central grey matter can also be included, for there was only one "grazing" shot
of the most ventral parts of the caput of the caudate nucleus [79]. The motor
cortex was injured once by a slow projectile probably restricting wounding to
the permanent tract and resulting in acute hemiplegia [77]. Immediate incapacitation, therefore, can only be produced reliably by injury to the brain regions
listed in Table 9.3.

9.3.3 Commotio Cerebri and Cerebral Pressure

Theoretically, incapacitation from gunshots to the CNS can result from
primary or from secondary effects of the bullet. The major primary effect is
disruption of brain tissue resulting in focal disturbances or loss of consciousness
and has been discussed above. Commotio cerebri where the major symptoms
are immediate unconsciousness and loss of muscle tone may be another
primary effect. The generation of commotio cerebri has been discussed in
cases of penetrating ballistic head injury for a long time [77, 80, 81] and was
thought to originate from the momentum transferred from the impacting
projectile to the skull. However, the mechanogenesis of commotio cerebri is a
matter of sudden acceleration of the skull, which by means of inertia results in
wounding of the brain. The crucial physical parameter in this is the change of
impulse per unit time or in other words the product of mass and acceleration of
the head. A maximum acceleration of the skull will be achieved when the mass
of the impacting object is equivalent to that of the head and when the velocity of
the object is relatively high.

A projectile has a very small mass but a very high velocity resulting in an ultra-
short time span during which the projectile is acting upon the skull. Because of
inertia, the skull as a whole will not really move during transfer of the impulse.
Instead, during impact there will be a high transfer of momentum and energy
locally but no direct load on the entire skull. The result is the perforation of
the skull without marked acceleration of the head. The penetrating character of
gunshots to the head thus does not allow a substantial transfer of impulse to
the head as a whole. In accordance with these theoretical considerations are
observations from battlefields reporting lack of commotio cerebri in penetrating
gunshots to the head [49, 82].

Cerebral pressure is the major secondary effect of ballistic brain injury.
However, the latent period in the range of minutes until the intracranial pressure
rises substantially in animal experiments [83, 84, 85, 86] is too long to produce
immediate or very rapid incapacitation following a head shot, although during

the further course elevated intracranial pressure can of course become sympto-
matic. So immediate incapacitation can only be the result of disruption of brain
tissue by the bullet.

9.3.4 Rapid Incapacitation

Acute cerebral hypoxemia can be caused by massive blood loss (or a double-sided
pneumothorax). Injuries associated with acute and massive bleeding will
cause circulatory depression and reduced perfusion of the CNS with subsequent
unconsciousness. However, immediate circulatory arrest is very rare in cardiac or
vascular gunshot wounds and even if this occurs, the oxygen stored in the CNS
ensures a potential for physical activity for about 10s [64, 65]. This is illustrated by
numerous case-reports. Marsh et al. [87] described two six-shot suicides, one of
which involved three .22 bullets striking the heart. A young man had been
conscious for several minutes after receiving two perforating and one grazing
gunshot wound of the heart from .22 bullets [88]. The highest number of suicidal
gunshots recorded is nine including a complete disruption of the apex of the heart
from seven .25 FMJ bullets [89]. Other cases of physical activity following
penetrating gunshot wounds to the heart have been published by Spitz et al.
[60] and Levy and Rao [90]. In a "worst-case" scenario described by DiMaio [91],
a man was able to walk 20 m after sustaining a hit from a 12-gauge shotgun from
a range of 3–4 m which destroyed his entire heart. Missliwetz [92] reported a
similar close range shotgun case with laceration of the posterior wall of the heart
and complete transection of the thoracic aorta where the young man still walked
a distance of 6 m. These very rare examples of immediate circulatory arrest from
gunshot wounds demonstrate without any doubt that a potential for physical
activity is present in such cases.

Therefore, trajectories involving the heart, the aorta (especially the thoracic
part) or the truncus of the pulmonary artery can cause rapid incapacitation
(Table 9.4) but they cannot be relied upon to terminate the physical activity of
the victim immediately [64, 65].

9.3.5 Delayed Incapacitation

The latent period until incapacitation in cases of considerable ballistic injury
to the lungs, liver, kidneys, spleen, and large vessels originating from the
aorta or central veins will be substantially longer [64, 65]. The slower rate of

Table 9.4 Targets of rapid incapacitation

Heart, aorta, truncus pulmonalis

Table 9.5 Targets of delayed incapacitation

Large arteries and veins, lungs, liver, spleen, kidneys

bleeding and the circulatory compensation mechanisms [64] usually offer the potential for sustained physical activity in the range of one or several minutes depending on the injury present (Table 9.5) and a considerable number of such case reports have been published (e.g., [60, 63, 90, 91]). So just about every person sustaining one or more gunshot wounds to the thorax including the heart possesses the potential for physical activity for at least a short period of time. But this potential for physical activity is not always exhausted: 80% of 62 gunshot fatalities collapsed following the assault [60], although it is not clearly stated how promptly they collapsed. Obviously, the mental or emotional condition of the victim, especially the expectancy of or being prepared for a hit, play an important role. Some may be stunned by surprise, fright or pain and some may instinctively choose not to act. But this psychological aspect can be neither predicted nor reconstructed. The only thing to rely on is that it will have no effect in the cases of trained, motivated, excited or stimulated individuals. Determination, adrenaline, or chemicals even enable persons to discharge aimed gunshots after sustaining a penetrating heart injury: A victim of a .32 caliber gunshot wound penetrating his heart, lung, and liver managed to fire back and wounded the assailant in the chest [60].

9.4 Backspatter

In most perforating gunshot wounds, blood and tissue is ejected from the exit wound. In many gunshot wounds, biological material is also propelled retrogradely out of the entrance wound towards the firearm. This phenomenon has been recognized for a long time as "Rückschleuderspuren" [94, 95, 96] and was later named backspatter [97, 98].

The stains resulting from backspatter can be very important in crime scene reconstruction because of the direction against the line of fire. There can be a transfer of stains from the victim to the interior of the barrel, the outside of the weapon, the person shooting, and persons or objects in the vicinity. Unlike gunshot residues, these stains can be individualized so that the transfer of stains can be demonstrated to be specific for the production of a clearly defined gunshot injury. Determination of the weapon used and the person firing, the shooting distance or the posture of the victim can be accomplished by analysis of backspatter stains, which should therefore form an integral part of all reconstructions of shooting incidents.

9.4.1 Mechanisms of Production

In terminal ballistics, backward hurling of gelatine [11, 99] and isolated muscle [100] and backward fragmentation of glass [101, 102] and bone [30] are well documented. The occurrence and the quantity of backspatter depend on a variety of ballistic and anatomical parameters. The kinetic energy necessary for the acceleration of blood and tissue particles can come from three different sources:

1. *Subcutaneous gas effect*: The rapid expansion of hot muzzle gases trapped below the elastic skin and especially between the skin and a bony abutment causes the temporary development of a pocket-like subcutaneous space. When this space collapses immediately, the biological particles are expelled together with the resulting backwards stream of escaping gases [94, 96, 98, 103, 104, 105].
2. *Temporary cavity*: Temporary cavitation produces overpressures inside the wound which also escape retrogradely to the line of fire [102, 103, 105]. Anatomical structures similar to liquid-filled cavities such as the head, the heart, or the eye provide the best conditions for violent temporary cavitation and backward hurling of particles.
3. *Tail splashing*: If a projectile penetrates tissue, there is always backward streaming of fluid and tissue particles along the lateral surface of the bullet in the direction of the entrance wound [11, 99, 103].

In most cases, these three driving forces act combined. The hot muzzle gases can only be effective in contact and close-to-contact gunshots, especially in the presence of a bony abutment. The presence of backspattered brain particles [106, 107] can only be explained by intracranial temporary cavitation, which is clearly enhanced by the confined space of the neurocranium (see Sect. 2.4). Therefore, backspatter mainly occurs in close-range gunshots to the head but is not limited to such cases, as is demonstrated by a gunshot to the heart (liquid-filled cavity) from a distance of 4 m resulting in massive backspatter travelling up to 2.5 m [105]. The spin of the bullet [108] or a momentary suction effect of the barrel aspiring material into the muzzle [106, 109] clearly do not contribute to backspatter [102, 103].

9.4.2 Experiments

While case reports (e.g., [94, 105, 110]) only shed some light on the topic, experimental investigations are difficult for obvious reasons. Mock experiments using primitive "head-models" constructed from blood-soaked sponges wrapped in plastic, rubber or tape [98, 104] resulted in small droplets from contact or almost contact shots only travelling a maximum distance of 30–60 cm. However, these findings are not reliable because there is neither a confined subcutaneous space for the hot gases to expand, nor is there a rigid skull to give rise to the high intracranial pressures during the formation of the temporary cavity. This applies even more to gunshots into soft pine covered with polyurethane foam saturated with blood [97].

Only controlled animal experiments interpreted by comparison with man can produce reliable results. Wagner [108] fired gunshots to rabbits using a 7.65-mm pistol but lacerated the small animals rather than creating backspatter. MacDonnell [97] performed shooting experiments on dogs but did not give detailed results or the experimental set-up. Burnett [111] has used pigs for the investigation of microscopic bone and bone-plus-bullet particles in backspatter and found tiny bone chips by SEM/EDX-analysis (scanning electron microscopy and energy dispersive X ray analysis) up to a distance of 37 cm from the entrance wound.

In experimental gunshots to the heads of calves [103, 112, 113] using 9-mm Parabellum ammunition from shooting distances of 0–10 cm, backspatter was documented after every gunshot. The number of macrostains (stains with a diameter >0.5 mm) varied from 31 to 324 per gunshot and appeared to be independent of the short shooting distances. The maximum distance macrodroplets travelled varied from 72 to 119 cm but the majority of droplets accumulated between 0 and 50 cm. The number of microbackspatter stains (diameter <0.5 mm) per gunshot varied between 39 and 262 and the maximum travelling distance was 69 cm while the vast majority of microdroplets accumulated between 0 and 40 cm. Microstains exclusively were circular to slightly oval due to the high surface tension of the tiny droplets. The morphology of macrobackspatter stains varied from round to elongated with circular, drop-like stains in the form of exclamation marks predominating (Fig. 9.13). Small macrostains (0.5–4 mm) made up more than 90% of the macrostains and no systematic relationship between distance travelled and size of the stains could be established. The direction a single droplet can take is every possible angle between the most tangential ones to the skin surface. This resulted in a semicircle of 180° (or a semisphere) covered with stains

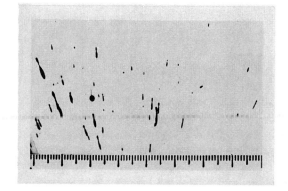

Fig. 9.13 Morphology of macrobackspatter stains on a horizontal surface in front of and 60 cm below the entrance wound after a near contact gunshot to the temple using a 9-mm Parabellum FMJ bullet. The entrance wound was roughly located where the long axis of the elongated stains converge

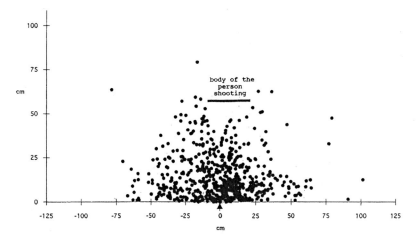

Fig. 9.14 Superimposed stain distribution of six close-range gunshots to the temple in front of and 60 cm below the entrance wound. The *small arrow* (0 cm) marks the location of the entrance wound

and not a triangle as assumed by MacDonnell [97]. The superimposed distribution of the stains from six gunshots is depicted in Fig. 9.14. The occurrence of skin ruptures of the entrance wound is not necessary for backspatter. Backspatter of tiny fragments of bone, fat, muscle and skin was recovered in most cases.

The succession of events was documented on high speed film and started with the recoil of the firearm, immediately followed by a blow-out effect of the skin. Large droplets exited approximately 0.7–4 ms after the bullet impacted the skin. The calculated minimum initial velocity of these droplets was in the range of 10 m/s.

In the same investigation [113], the firearms, the surgical gloves and the right sleeve worn by the person shooting were examined with a stereomicroscope. Backspatter of blood was found on the firearms and sleeves in half and on the gloves in two thirds of the cases. Most droplets were 1–3 mm in size and circular or elongated in shape but there was also a fine spray of tiny blood deposits. The distribution of the droplets on the firearms varied including regions shielded by prominent parts while the droplets on the person shooting were predominantly located on the extensor side of the fingers and the radial aspect of the hands and sleeves (Fig. 9.15).

9.4.3 Empirical Observations

In addition to blood, backspatter of brain tissue, fat, muscle, bone fragments, skin, hair, and even ocular tissue has been recovered from the shooting hand and/or the firearm in case-work following gunshots to the head [94, 96, 105, 106, 107]. Maximum travelling distances of 2 and 4 m have been documented

Fig. 9.15 Bloodstains on the
right glove predominantly
located at the extensor side
of the fingers after firing a
contact gunshot to the head

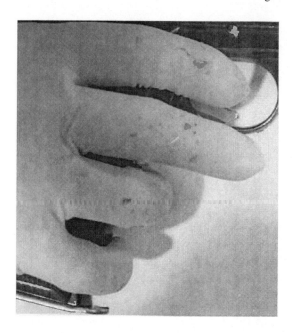

[103, 110]. After suicidal gunshots to the head, bloodspatter on the hands was
found with the naked eye at the time of autopsy in 14–35% [107, 114]. In a large
series of 1200 suicides, the exterior surface of the barrel reacted positive for
blood in 75% and the interior surface in 55% [115]. However, the morphology
of the blood deposits was not evaluated and blood can also be transferred by
contact or other mechanisms.

So in close-range gunshots to the head, backspatter is produced in all cases
and is deposited frequently on the firearm and person shooting. The presence of
backspatter stains establishes a clear link between a person or object and a
clearly defined gunshot, especially if the stains are individualized by DNA-analysis. Characteristic for backspatter are small or tiny droplet or splashing stains;
elongated shapes are roughly aimed at the entrance wound while the distribution
can vary greatly. The number and size of the stains can be very small. Thus, the
detection or exclusion of backspatter stains in practical case-work necessitates
magnification and appropriate lighting or chemical analysis, especially if the tiny
stains do not contrast with the background, e.g., a dark-coloured firearm (Fig.
9.16) or clothing. However, no rash conclusions should be drawn from the absence
of backspatter stains on the firearm and hands because the number of droplets in a
single gunshot can be so small that these structures may not be hit by a single
droplet. In these instances, special attention should be directed to the shoes and
pants of a suspect because these objects are likely to be in the downwards para-
bolic flight path of the droplets. In our case-work experience, the number of
positive findings also depends on the delay until the examination is carried out

Fig. 9.16 A tiny bloodstain (*below*) and a tiny bone chip (*above*) on the barrel of a firearm after a near-contact gunshot to the head. The *black bar to the right* marks a distance of 1 mm

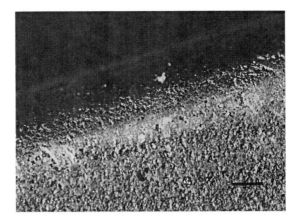

\because the small droplets can detach from the metal, skin or textiles during manipulations or transportation. Early inspection is therefore recommended.

9.5 Trajectory Reconstruction from Trace Evidence on Spent Bullets

Contact between two objects commonly results in bidirectional transfer of material. This principle forms the basis of modern trace evidence analysis. Trace evidence may be the decisive factor in reconstruction of the scene of crime and in identifying the persons and objects involved. Due to the substantial impact forces involved, bullets striking an object appear to represent favourable conditions for such a transfer of material but air friction and subsequent impacts may also cause loss of deposits. In principle, biologic and non-biologic deposits can be present on a spent bullet and both forms of trace evidence can be relevant depending on the case constellation.

9.5.1 Intermediate Targets

Contact of a fired bullet with an intermediate target of sufficient resistance is a very important factor: the bullet will ricochet, fragment or perforate, the trajectory will show a deviation and the stability of the bullet will be affected. The latter will cause the bullet to tumble and a tumbling bullet will produce an atypical gunshot entrance wound. The verification of a ricochet by analysis of trace evidence can have considerable legal implications because the intention to kill will commonly not be assumed. In addition, valuable information concerning the trajectory of the bullet can be gained.

In a few case reports dedicated to this field, the bullet deposits were only investigated on deformed lead bullets [116, 117], which represent very favourable conditions for the deposition of trace evidence.

In an experimental investigation [118], 9-mm Parabellum FMJ bullets were fired at various intermediate targets and at combinations of intermediate targets and tissue located in line. After recovery from a bullet collector, the bullets were examined using a scanning electron microscope and an energy-dispersive X-ray spectrometer (SEM/EDS). Elements of preexisting environmental deposits, mostly in the form of small spheres (Fig. 9.17), were already present on unfired bullets and elements from the bullet collector, the jacket, the charge and primer could be consistently detected as a "background".

In impact dynamics, ductile and fragile target media are distinguished [119]. Ductile material is elastic and can be stretched before perforation whereas fragile material is brittle and will break before a noticeable stretching occurs. Abundant deposits of the fragile materials concrete (Fig. 9.18), flat glass, asphalt and gypsum-board (Fig. 9.19) could be visualised on every bullet by SEM. The transfer dynamics involved a direct imprint of target material on the bullet surface and thus preferential locations at the tip but also indirect deposition over the entire surface ("powder effect") when the bullet travels through a cloud of shattered target particles. X-ray microanalysis demonstrated matching spectra of the elemental composition of these fragile deposits and of the targets contacted (Fig. 9.20A,B). After perforation of the ductile materials wood and car body parts, the scarce deposits on the bullets did not show characteristic spectra. This was due to the complex perforation dynamics of ductile materials involving elastic radial displacement or punching out of a plug. If multi-layered car metal targets were hit, few and variable fragments were scattered on the bullet surface and titanium indicative of paintwork could be determined on only a minority of bullets. The elemental composition of wood itself was heterogeneous but the fibrous morphology of the deposits was typical.

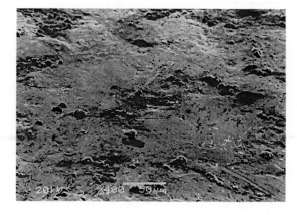

Fig. 9.17 Scanning electron microscopy image: preexisting deposits on the surface of a brand-new and unfired 9-mm FMJ bullet. Most contaminations presented in the form of small spherical Al-Si-combinations

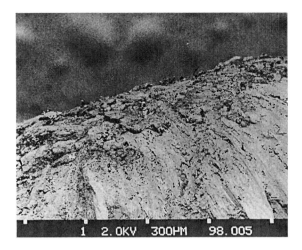

Fig. 9.18 Scanning electron microscopy image: concrete deposits on the tip of a 9-mm FMJ bullet after perforation of concrete

The SEM/EDS findings in gunshots including subsequent perforation of tissue were similar. In particular, the trace evidence primarily transferred to the bullets was not eliminated by secondary contact and the determination of the fragile target materials was not affected.

So when a person is killed or injured by a gunshot, the presence of a ricochet and the target material can be determined. It appears clear from these results and also from own case-work experience that a complete loss of fragile trace evidence in subsequent impacts or penetration of a human body does not occur. The determination of fragile target materials is therefore possible by the combined evidence of morphological and analytical findings. This possibility needs to be considered before an evidential bullet is mishandled: Blood, tissue, and nonbiological material may be washed from the bullet and loss or contamination may occur during transportation or storage. A directed search of the scene should then be conducted. The intermediate target will show a bullet impact mark/perforation defect, which additionally represents an ideal reference point

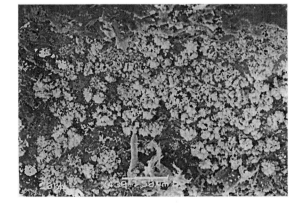

Fig. 9.19 Scanning electron microscopy image: gypsum-board deposits on a 9-mm FMJ bullet after perforation of gypsum-board

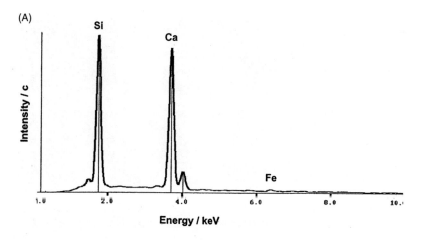

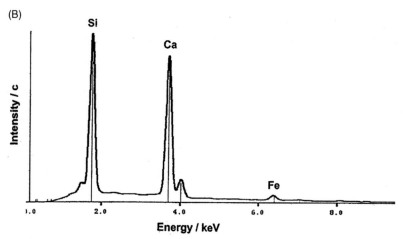

Fig. 9.20 Energy-dispersive X-ray spectrometer (EDS)-spectra: Comparison of the EDS-spectrum of: **A** the concrete perforated; **B** the bullet deposits shown in Fig. 9.18

for trajectory reconstruction. Investigation of the scene is also necessary because contact with an intermediate target may occur before or after a human body is perforated but the sequence of events can usually not be derived from trace evidence on FMJ bullets.

9.5.2 Biological Deposits

In cases of gunfights involving several persons, it can be crucial to know who killed or injured whom. A perforating bullet found at the scene can commonly be linked to one of the firearms involved via comparison of rifling marks but in addition, the bullet must be linked to the person through whom it has passed. A technique capable of demonstrating and simultaneously individualizing biological material is therefore necessary to reliably determine who killed or injured whom using which bullet.

Human trace evidence on bullets has been investigated by routine cytological methods but individualisation is commonly not possible, and cells or even cell layers can be found in the cavities of hollow point bullets but are rarely found on the smooth surfaces of FMJ bullets [120, 121, 122].

Individualisation of tissue deposits on FMJ bullets was successfully carried out by polymerase chain reaction (PCR)-typing of short tandem repeats (STRs) in both experiments [123] and case-work [124]. It could also be shown that the amplification of mitochondrial DNA on spent bullets is a useful additional method and that subsequent impacts on intermediate targets do not eliminate enough biological deposits to render DNA analysis impossible [125]. Neither visualisation by SEM nor separate swabbing was successful in establishing preferential locations of cells on bullets [125].

So DNA analysis of tissue deposits on spent bullets represents a sensitive method capable of demonstrating and at the same time individualising minute tissue fragments transferred during perforation of a human body. This makes it possible to determine who was killed or injured by which bullet. Additional comparison of the bullet with the firearms involved can possibly identify the person shooting this particular bullet. The decision whether DNA typing is to be performed should be made as soon as possible because the bullets must be protected from contamination and loss of material. The recovery of cellular material by swabbing the bullet can be easily and rapidly performed at the scene so that further examinations will not be delayed.

References

1. Fackler ML (1988) Wound ballistics. A review of common misconceptions. JAMA 259:2730–2736
2. Fackler ML, Malinowski JA (1985) The wound profile: a visual method for quantifying gunshot wound components. J Trauma 25:522–529
3. Harvey EN, Butler EG, McMillan JH, Puckett WO (1945) Mechanism of wounding. War Med 8:91–104
4. Harvey EN, Korr IM, Oster G, McMillan JH (1947) Secondary damage in wounding due to pressure changes accompanying the passage of high velocity missiles. Surgery 21:218–239
5. Bowen TE, Bellamy RF (1988) Emergency war surgery, Second United States Revision of the Emergency War Surgery Handbook. United States Department Of Defence, Washington, DC, pp 13–33
6. Callender GR, French RW (1935) Wound ballistics. Studies in the mechanism of wound production by rifle bullets. Mil Surg 77:177–201
7. Scott R (1983) Pathology of injuries caused by high-velocity missiles. Clin Lab Med 3:273–294

8. Krauss M (1957) Studies in wound ballistics: temporary cavity effects in soft tissues. Mil Med 121:221–231
9. Sellier K, Kneubuehl BP (1994) Wound ballistics and the scientific background. Elsevier, Amsterdam London New York Tokyo, pp 144–149, 245
10. Zhang J, Yoganandan N, Pintar FA, Gennarelli TA (2005) Temporary cavity and pressure distribution in a brain simulant following ballistic penetration. J Neurotrauma 22:1335–1347
11. Black AN, Burns BD, Zuckerman S (1941) An experimental study of the wounding mechanism of high-velocity missiles. Br Med J 2:872–874
12. Karger B (1995) Penetrating gunshots to the head and lack of immediate incapacitation. I. Wound ballistics and mechanisms of incapacitation. Int J Legal Med 108:53–61
13. Lindsey D (1980) The idolatry of velocity, or lies, damn lies, and ballistics. J Trauma 20:1068–1069
14. Beyer JC (1962) Wound ballistics. Office of the Surgeon General, Department of the Army, Washington, DC, p 135
15. Boyer CN, Holland GE, Seely JF (2005) Flash X-ray observations of cavitation in cadaver thighs caused by high-velocity bullets. J Trauma 59:1463–1468
16. Fackler ML, Surinchak JS, Malinowski JA, Bowen RE (1984) Bullet fragmentation: a major cause of tissue disruption. J Trauma 24:35–39
17. Dzieman AJ, Mendelson JA, Lindsey D (1961) Comparison of the wounding characteristics of some commonly encountered bullets. J Trauma 1:341–353
18. Hopkinson DAW, Watts JC (1963) Studies in experimental missile injuries of skeletal muscle. Proc R Soc Med 56:461–468
19. Kocher T (1895) Zur Lehre von den Schußwunden durch die Kleinkalibergeschosse. G. Fischer & Co, Cassel
20. Fackler ML, Peters CE (1991) The "shock wave" myth (and comment). Wound Ballistics Rev 1:38–40
21. Fackler ML, Bellamy RF, Malinowski JA (1988) The wound profile: illustration of the missile-tissue interaction. J Trauma 28(Suppl):S21–S29
22. Fackler ML, Surinchak JS, Malinowski JA, Bowen RE (1984) Wounding potential of the russian AK-74 assault rifle. J Trauma 24:263–266
23. Cooper GJ, Ryan JM (1990) Interaction of penetrating missiles with tissues: some common misapprehensions and implications for wound management. Br J Surg 77:606–610
24. Metter D, Schulz E (1983) Morphologische Merkmale der Schußwunden in Leber und Milz. Z Rechtsmed 90:167–172
25. Fackler ML (1989) Wounding patterns of military rifle bullets. Int Defense Review 1:59–64
26. Ragsdale BD, Josselson A (1988) Experimental gunshot fractures. J Trauma 28(Suppl): S109–S115
27. Sellier K (1971) Über Geschossablenkung und Geschossdeformation. Z Rechtsmed 69:217–251
28. Karger B, Puskas Z, Ruwald B, Teige K, Schuirer G (1998) Morphological findings in the brain after experimental gunshots using radiology, pathology and histology. Int J Legal Med 111:314–319
29. Robens W, Küsswetter W (1982) Fracture typing to human bone by assault missile trauma. Acta Chir Scand, Suppl 508:223–227
30. Lorenz R (1948) Der Schußkanal im Röntgenbilde. Dtsch Z Gerichtl Med 39:435–448
31. Sturdivan L (1969) Terminal behavior of the 5.56 mm ball in soft targets. Rep 1447. Ballistic Research Laboratory, Aberdeen Proving Grounds
32. Ragsdale BD (1984) Gunshot wounds: historical perspective. Mil Med 149:301–315

33. Karger B (2003) Schussverletzungen. In: Brinkmann B, Madea B (eds) Handbuch der Rechtsmedizin I. Springer, Berlin Heidelberg New York, pp 593–682

34. Albreht M, Scepanovic D, Ceramilac A, Milivojevic V, Berger S, Tasic G, Tatic V, Todoric M, Popovic D, Nanusevic N (1979) Experimental soft tissue wounds caused by standard military rifles. Acta Chir Scand Suppl 489:185–198

35. Berlin R, Gelin LE, Janzon B, Lewis DH, Rybeck B, Sandegard J, Seeman T (1976) Local effects of assault rifle bullets in live tissues. Acta Chir Scand Suppl 459:1–84

36. Berlin R, Janzon B, Rybeck B, Sandegard J, Seeman T (1977) Local effects of assault rifle bullets in live tissues: Part II: Further studies in live tissues and relations to some simulant media. Acta Chir Scand Suppl 477:5–57

37. Berlin R, Janzon B, Nordström G, Schantz B (1978) The extent of tissue damage in missile wounds one and six hours after the infliction of trauma studied by the current method of debridement. Acta Chir Scand 144:213–217

38. Jussila J, Kjellstrom BT, Leppaniemi A (2005) Ballistic variables and tissue devitalisation in penetrating injury – establishing relationship through meta-analysis of a number of pig tests. Injury 36:282–292

39. Scepanovic D, Albrecht M, Erdeljan D (1982) A method for predicting effects of military rifles. Acta Chir Scand Suppl 508:29–37

40. Tikka S, Seeman T (1988) Local tissue destruction in high-energy missile trauma and its dependence on energy transfer. Ann Med Milit Fenn 62:17–20

41. Allen IV, Scott R, Tanner JA (1982) Experimental high-velocity missile head injury. Injury 14:183–193

42. Clemedson CJ, Falconer B, Frankenberg L, Jönsson A, Wennerstrand J (1973) Head injuries caused by small-calibre, high-velocity bullets. Z Rechtsmed 73:103–114

43. Finnie JW (1993) Pathology of experimental traumatic craniocerebral missile injury. J Comp Pathol 108:93–101

44. Kirkpatrick JB, DiMaio VJM (1978) Civilian gunshot wounds of the brain. J Neurosurg 48:185–198

45. Dittmann W (1986) Wundballistische Untersuchungen zur Klinik der Schädel-Hirn-Schußverletzungen. Wehrmed Monatsschr 33:3–14

46. Watkins FP, Pearce BP, Stainer MC (1988) Physical effects of the penetration of head simulants by steel spheres. J Trauma 28(1)(Suppl):S40–S54

47. Freytag E (1963) Autopsy findings in head injuries from firearms. Statistical evaluation of 254 cases. Arch Pathol 76:215–225

48. Henn R, Liebhardt E (1969) Zur Topik außerhalb des Schußkanals gelegener Hirnrindenblutungen. Arch Kriminol 143:188–191

49. Spatz H (1941) Gehirnpathologie im Kriege. Von den Gehirnwunden. Zentralbl Neurochir 6:162–212

50. Klaue R (1949) Die indirekten Frakturen der vorderen Schädelgrube beim Schädeldachschuß. Dtsch Z Nervenheilkd 161:167–193

51. Kolsky H (1980) The role of stress waves in penetration processes. In: Labile RC (ed) Ballistic materials and penetration mechanics. Elsevier, New York, pp 185–223

52. König HG, Schmidt V (1989) Beobachtungen zur Ausbreitungsgeschwindigkeit und Entstehungsursache von Berstungsfrakturen beim Schuß. Beitr Gerichtl Med 47:247–255

53. Smith OC, Berryman HE, Lahren CH (1987) Cranial fracture patterns and estimate of direction from low velocity gunshot wounds. J Forensic Sci 32:1416–1421

54. Butler FG, Puckett WO, Harvey EN, McMillan JH (1945) Experiments on head wounding by high velocity missiles. J Neurosurg 2:358–363

55. DiMaio VJM, Zumwalt RE (1977) Rifle wounds from high velocity, center-fire hunting ammunition. J Forensic Sci 22:132–140

56. Knudsen PJT, Theilade P (1993) Terminal ballistics of the 7.62 mm NATO bullet. Autopsy findings. Int J Legal Med 106:61–67

57. Peng L, Cheng Z, Guangji Z, Yinqiou L, Reifeng G (1990) An experimental study of craniocerebral injury caused by 7.62 mm bullets in dogs. J Trauma (China) 6(Suppl): 187–191
58. Karger B, Banaschak S (1997) Two cases of exenteration of the brain from Brenneke shotgun slugs. Int J Legal Med 110:323–325
59. Sight WP (1969) Ballistic analysis of shotgun injuries to the central nervous system. J Neurosurg 31:25–33
60. Spitz WU, Petty CS, Fisher RS (1961) Physical activity until collapse following fatal injury by firearms and sharp pointed weapons. J Forensic Sci 6:290–300
61. Walcher K (1929) Über Bewußtlosigkeit und Handlungsunfähigkeit. Dtsch Z Gerichtl Med 13:313–322
62. Petersohn F (1967) Über die Aktions- und Handlungsfähigkeit bei schweren Schädeltraumen. Dtsch Z Gerichtl Med 59:259–270
63. Karger B, Brinkmann B (1997) Multiple gunshot suicides: potential for physical activity and medico-legal aspects. Int J Legal Med 110:188–192
64. Newgard K (1992) The physiological effects of handgun bullets. Wound Ballistics Rev 1:12–17
65. Fackler ML (1992) Police handgun ammunition selection. Wound Ballistics 1:32–37
66. DiMaio VJM, Jones JA, Caruth WW III, Anderson LL, Petty CS (1974) A comparison of the wounding effects of commercially available handgun ammunition suitable for police use. FBI Law Enf Bull 43:3–8
67. Karger B, Kneubuehl BP (1997) On the physics of momentum in ballistics: can the human body be displaced or knocked down by small arms projectiles? Int J Legal Med 109:147–149
68. Suneson A, Hansson H-A, Seeman T (1988) Central and peripheral nervous damage following high-energy missile wounds in the thigh. J Trauma 28(Suppl):S197–S203
69. Jason A (1991) The "twilight zone" of wound ballistics. Wound Ballistics Rev 1(1):8–9
70. Kaufman HH, Loyola WP, Makela ME, Frankowsky RF, Wagner KA, Bustein DP, Gildenberg PC (1986) Gunshot wounds to the head: a perspective. Neurosurg 18:689–695
71. Siccardi D, Cavaliere R, Pau A, Lubinu F, Turtas S, Viale GL (1991) Penetrating craniocerebral missile injuries in civilians: a retrospective analysis of 314 cases. Surg Neurol 35:455–460
72. Karger B (1995) Penetrating gunshots to the head and lack of immediate incapacitation. II. Review of case reports. Int J Legal Med 108:117–126
73. Bratzke H, Pöll W, Kaden B (1985) Ungewöhnliche Handlungsfähigkeit nach Kopfsteckschuß. Arch Kriminol 175:31–39
74. Smith S (1943) Voluntary acts after a gunshot wound of the brain. Police J 16:108–110
75. Fryc O, Krompecher T (1979) Überlebenszeit und Handlungsfähigkeit bei tödlichen Verletzungen. Beitr Gerichtl Med 37:389–392
76. Krauland W (1952) Zur Handlungsfähigkeit Kopfschußverletzter. Acta Neurochir 2:233–239
77. Klages U, Weithoener D, Frössler H, Terwort H (1975) Überlebenszeit, Handlungsfähigkeit und röntgenologische Diagnostik bei Schußverletzungen des Schädels. Z Rechtsmed 76:307–319
78. Maxeiner H, Schneider V, Betsch J, Piefke K (1986) Suizid mit drei Kopfsteckschüssen. In: Eisenmenger W, Liebhardt E, Schuck M (eds) Medizin und Recht. Springer, Berlin Heidelberg New York, pp 317–325
79. Herbich J (1955) Neun Jahre überlebte Gehirn- und Herzschußverletzung mit Einheilung beider Geschosse, nach Selbstmordversuch. Beitr Gerichtl Med 20:22–34
80. Goroncy C (1924) Handlungsfähigkeit Kopfschußverletzter. Dtsch Z Gerichtl Med 4:145–164
81. Naegeli O (1884) Zwei perforierende Hirnschüsse. Mord oder Selbstmord? Vjschr Gerichtl Medicin 40:231–264

82. Payr E (1922) Der frische Schädelschuß. In: Schjerning O von (ed) Handbuch der ärztlichen Erfahrungen im Weltkrieg 1914/1918, Bd 1. Barth, Leipzig, pp 285–410
83. Carey ME, Sarna GS, Farrel JB, Happel LT (1989) Experimental missile wound to the brain. J Neurosurg 71:754–764
84. Crockard HA, Brown FD, Johns LM, Mullan S (1977) An experimental cerebral missile injury model in primates. J Neurosurg 46:776–783
85. Crockard HA, Brown FD, Calica AB, Johns LM, Mullan S (1977) Physiological consequences of experimental cerebral missile injury and use of data analysis to predict survival. J Neurosurg 46:784–794
86. Gerber AM, Moody RA (1972) Craniocerebral missile injuries in the monkey: an experimental physiological model. J Neurosurg 36:43–49
87. Marsh TO, Brown ER, Burkhardt RP, Davis JH (1989) Two six-shot suicides in close geographic and temporal proximity. J Forensic Sci 34:491–494
88. Hudson P (1981) Multishot firearm suicide. Examination of 58 cases. Am J Forensic Med Pathol 2:239–242
89. Habbe D, Thomas GE, Gould J (1989) Nine-gunshot suicide. Am J Forensic Med Pathol 10:335–337
90. Levy V, Rao VJ (1988) Survival time in gunshot and stab wound victims. Am J Forensic Med Pathol 9:215–217
91. DiMaio VJM (1985) Gunshot wounds. Practical aspects of firearms, ballistics and forensic techniques. Elsevier, New York Amsterdam Oxford
92. Missliwetz J (1990) Ungewöhnliche Handlungsfähigkeit bei Herzdurchschuß durch Schrotgarbe. Arch Kriminol 185:129–135
93. Introna F, Smialek JE (1989) Suicide from multiple gunshot wounds. Am J Forensic Med Pathol 10:275–284
94. Fraenckel P, Straßmann G (1924) Zur Entfernungsbestimmung bei Nahschüssen. Arch Kriminol 76:314–316
95. Hofmann v ER (1898) Lehrbuch der Gerichtlichen Medizin, 8. ed. Wien, Leipzig, p 389
96. Werkgartner A (1924) Eigenartige Hautverletzungen durch Schüsse aus angesetzten Selbstladepistolen. Beitr Gerichtl Med 6:148–161
97. MacDonell HL (1982) Bloodstain pattern interpretation. Laboratory of Forensic Science Publishers, New York, pp 16–21
98. Stephens BG, Allen TB (1983) Back spatter of blood from gunshot wounds – observations and experimental simulation. J Forensic Sci 28:437–439
99. Amato JJ, Billy LJ, Lawson NS, Rich NM (1974) High velocity missile injury. An experimental study of the retentive forces of tissue. Am J Surg 127:454–458
101. Lamprecht K (1959) Schuß durch Fensterglas. Arch Kriminol 97:128–132
102. Sellier K (1982) Schusswaffen und Schusswirkungen I. Schmidt-Römhild, Lübeck
103. Karger B, Nüsse R, Schroeder G, Wüstenbecker S, Brinkmann B (1996) Backspatter from experimental close-range shots to the head. I. Macrobackspatter. Int J Legal Med 109:66–74
104. Pex JO, Vaughan CH (1987) Observations of high velocity bloodspatter on adjacent objects. J Forensic Sci 32:1587–1594
105. Weimann W (1931) Über das Verspritzen von Gewebeteilen aus Einschußöffnungen und seine kriminalistische Bedeutung. Dtsch Z Gerichtl Med 17:92–105
106. 106. Brüning A, Wiethold F (1934) Die Untersuchung von Selbstmörderschußwaffen. *Deutsche* Zeitschrift Gerichtliche Med 23:71–82
107. Zwingli M (1941) Über Spuren an der Schießhand nach Schuß mit Faustfeuerwaffen. Arch Kriminol 108:1–26
108. Wagner HJ (1963) Experimentelle Untersuchungen über Art und Ausmaß der Rückschleuderung von Blut und Gewebeteilen beim absoluten und relativen Nahschuß. Dtsch Z Gerichtl Med 54:258–266

109. Knight B (1977) Firearm injuries. In: Tedeschi CG, Eckert WG, Tedeschi LG (eds) Forensic medicine. Saunders, Philadelphia London Toronto, pp 510–526
110. Verhoff MA, Karger B (2003) Atypical gunshot entrance wound and extensive backspatter. Int J Legal Med 117:229–231
111. Burnett BR (1991) Detection of bone and bone-plus-bullet particles in backspatter from close-range shots to heads. J Forensic Sci 36:1745–1752
112. Karger B, Nüsse R, Tröger HD, Brinkmann B (1997) Backspatter from experimental close-range shots to the head. II. Microbackspatter and the morphology of bloodstains. Int J Legal Med 110:27–30
113. Karger B, Nüsse R, Bajanowski T (2002) Backspatter on the firearm and hand in experimental close-range gunshots to the head. Am J Forensic Med Pathol 23:211–213
114. Betz P, Peschel O, Stiefel D, Eisenmenger W (1995) Frequency of blood spatters on the shooting hand and of conjunctival petechiae following suicidal gunshot wounds to the head. Forensic Sci Int 76:47–53
115. Stone IC (1992) Characteristics of firearms and gunshot wounds as markers of suicide. Am J Forensic Med Pathol 13:275–280
116. DiMaio VJM, Dana SE, Taylor WE, Ondrusek J (1987) Use of scanning electron microscopy and energy dispersive X-ray analysis (SEM/EDX) in identification of foreign material on bullets. J Forensic Sci 32:38–47
117. Petraco N, DeForest PR (1990) Trajectory reconstructions I: trace evidence in flight. J Forensic Sci 35:1284–1296
118. Karger B, Hoekstra A, Schmidt PF (2001) Trajectory reconstruction from trace evidence on spent bullets. I. Deposits from intermediate targets. Int J Legal Med 115:16–22
119. Goldsmith W (1999) Non-ideal projectile impact on targets. Int J Impact Eng 22:95–395
120. Knudsen PJT (1993) Cytology in ballistics. An experimental investigation of tissue fragments on full metal jacketed bullets using routine cytological techniques. Int J Legal Med 106:15–18
121. Nichols CA, Sens MA (1990) Recovery and evaluation by cytologic techniques of trace material retained on bullets. Am J Forensic Med Pathol 11:17–34
122. Nichols CA, Sens MA (1991) Cytologic manifestations of ballistic injury. Am J Clin Pathol 95:660–669
123. Karger B, Meyer E, Knudsen PJT, Brinkmann B (1996) DNA typing of cellular material on perforating bullets. Int J Legal Med 108:177–179
124. Karger B, Meyer E, DuChesne A (1997) STR analysis on perforating FMJ bullets and a new VWA variant allele. Int J Legal Med 110:101–103
125. Karger B, Stehmann B, Hohoff C, Brinkmann B (2001) Trajectory reconstruction from trace evidence on spent bullets. II. Are tissue deposits eliminated by subsequent impacts? Int J Legal Med 114:343–345

Part VI
Identification

Chapter 10
Unique Characteristics at Autopsy that may be Useful in Identifying Human Remains

Ellie K. Simpson and Roger W. Byard

Contents

R.W. Byard
University of Adelaide, Adelaide, South Australia, Australia
e-mail: byard.roger@saugov.sa.gov.au

M. Tsokos (ed.), *Forensic Pathology Reviews, Volume 5*,
doi: 10.1007/978-1-59745-110-9_10, © Humana Press, Totowa, NJ 2008

Abstract When a person dies, it is a legal requirement in most countries for the body to be formally identified. In Australia, it is the responsibility of the State Coroners to accept the identification and to release the body for burial. Usually, identification can be carried out by friends or relatives viewing the body and confirming the identity to a member of the police force (visual identification). In some cases, however, postmortem changes such as decomposition, or facial trauma or disfigurement, incineration or skeletonisation make visual identification unacceptable. In this instance other methods of identification are attempted. These include dental, fingerprints, DNA or, as a last resort, circumstantial identification. On a national and global scale, the issue of identification becomes a particular challenge in situations of multiple fatalities, for example in circumstances of natural disaster or tragic events such as aeroplane crashes, genocide, war or terrorist attacks. In these situations, identification of victims becomes one of the primary aims of the disaster relief teams. During the postmortem examination, the pathologist facilitates identification by examining the body and documenting any unique characteristics that may be useful in identifying the person. This information can then be used to corroborate any other information on the identification, and becomes especially useful when visual identification is not possible.

Keywords Mass disaster · Identification · Fingerprints · Birthmarks · Frontal sinus comparison · Tattoo · Postmortem changes

10.1 Introduction

The identification of a person in situations of mass disaster differs from methods commonly used in conventional coronial/medical examiner investigations. For most coronial cases, members of the deceased's family or their friends are available to conduct a visual identification, locate treating dentists or medical practitioners, provide DNA samples for comparison and also inform the Coroner and police about any identifying property, features and relevant medical history that may be used in corroborating identification. The body is usually located relatively recently after death, which increases the likelihood of a visual identification being acceptable. In situations of multiple fatalities, family and friends may have perished along with the victim, thus sometimes precluding visual identification. Similarly, the death of close family members may prevent DNA samples from being taken for comparison with the victim. Further complicating visual identification is the probability that the body has undergone trauma or postmortem changes such as decomposition, thus making visual identification unacceptable. Finally, as was seen in the Asian Tsunami disaster of 26th December 2004, the death of people in a country they were visiting also complicates identification, since so many nations may be involved in searching for their citizens under less than optimal conditions (Fig. 10.1).

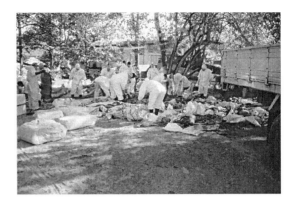

Fig. 10.1 Initial processing of unidentified individuals at a site in Thailand following the December 26, 2004 tsunami disaster

10.2 Methods of Identification

The following methods of identification are listed alphabetically to prevent any perceived order of importance. However, the most commonly used, or primary, methods of identification are visual, dental, fingerprints and DNA. This is due to a number of factors such as reduced cost and time constraints for visual identification; the individuality of dental, fingerprint and DNA characteristics; the persistence of teeth, fingerprints and DNA after death (property can be lost or removed from a body which makes it difficult to link back to the deceased); and the increased reliability of identification when based on scientific methods.

10.2.1 Age Assessment

Age assessment can be separated into categories of biological and chronological age. The biological age is an estimate of the physical age of the person using dental and skeletal characteristics, whereas the chronological age is an estimation of the length of time that the person has been alive. Chronological age assessment cannot be accurately determined, but relies on verbal reporting, whereas biological age assessment requires examination of the teeth, body, or skeleton by an expert. Under normal conditions of growth and development, estimations of biological age should correspond with the chronological age of the individual. If an individual has been exposed to serious illness, malnutrition or general poor health, estimates of biological age may differ from the chronological age, making the individual appear either older or younger than their chronological age. Generally, markers of these conditions are present in the skeleton and can be incorporated into the skeletal age assessment as possible factors of variation. The condition of the body will often limit the type of assessment – a person looking at a recently deceased person will usually be able to provide an estimation of age, whereas a decomposed, skeletonised or traumatised deceased will need to be examined by a person experienced with these methods of identification. Broad age categories such as infant, juvenile, adolescent and early/middle/late adulthood are easier to determine. Generally speaking, the younger a person is, the more accurate age estimation can be, with fetal material usually being the most accurate. This is because there is increasing individual variation in biological characteristics with advancing age, especially after the first three decades.

10.2.2 Birthmarks

Birthmarks can be temporary or permanent, and can often be recognised by family and friends on visual inspection. The commonly seen birthmarks include salmon pink patch, strawberry naevus, port wine stain and cavernous hemangioma. "Moles" (pigmented skin lesions) are also very common and can also be described and recognised by family members. Both birthmarks and pigmented lesions can be shown to relatives in photographic form, which may be a preferred alternative to viewing the body.

10.2.3 Body Piercing

Body piercing is commonly seen in many cultures, and in both sexes. Some piercing may be temporary, and jewellery may be attached to the body using clips, screws or adhesive. Typical areas of the body for piercing are the ear, face, nipples, navel and genitals. These and other body adornments (see Sect. 2.11) may be torn off from the body due to trauma or may be looted.

10.2.4 Clothing

Clothing may be lost or damaged by the time a body is found. As with other types of property, distinctions must be made between clothing on the body and clothing associated with or next to the body. Even small remnants of material in the axilla or groin can be examined for an indication of fabric and colour (Fig. 10.2). Labels can be examined for the location of manufacture or purchase. Uniforms can provide information on the rank of an individual. The size of clothing can give an estimation of stature and body build; however differences in clothing sizes in different countries should be accounted for. Homemade clothing on a body may be able to be matched with material found at their home. If footwear is present it might give indications of unusual wear patterns resulting from differences in gait. Occupational residues such as oil and paint may also be present and may assist with identification. Possible complications

Fig. 10.2 Remnants of clothing from a burnt body that could be checked for place of manufacture, size, and other individual features

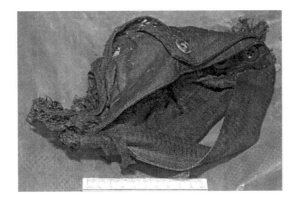

with identification using clothing are that it can be torn from the body in circumstances of strong winds (including free-fall), high-speed impact or in strong flood-waters. It can also be burnt in fires, although remnants can often be found in the axilla and groin regions. It must also be remembered that clothing on a body may be new, second-hand or borrowed, and therefore may not be recognised by relatives as belonging to that person.

10.2.5 Currency

Currency, if found associated with a body, can provide information on the person's country of origin or their holiday destination (Fig. 10.3). Similarly, postage stamps may also indicate nationality. Coins may survive fires. Unfortunately currency may be looted from bodies and therefore may not be present by the time identification teams arrive.

Fig. 10.3 Example of currency, a cigarette butt, and jewellery found on a body. The currency may give an indication of the country of origin; the cigarette butt could be tested for DNA while the jewellery is quite individual and should be recognisable to relatives

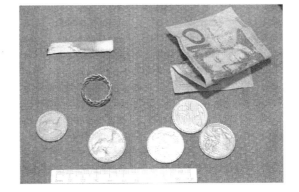

10.2.6 Dental Identification

Dental identification is usually performed by forensic odontologists. The dentition often remains in circumstances when other identifying information has been lost, for example in circumstances of intense heat. The teeth, along with bones, can be used for age estimation. This is performed by examining the stage of eruption and the patterns of wear on individual teeth. Evidence of dental treatment is recorded and compared to dental records collected from families. However, with numerous countries supplementing their water supplies with fluoride, and with generally better oral hygiene, the number of children requiring fillings is declining. In addition, records kept by dentists may be incomplete and unless an individual has had complex work done on their teeth, identification purely on dentition may be difficult. Antemortem and postmortem radiographs can be very useful in dental comparisons. The type of work performed on the teeth can give an indication of the country where the reconstruction was done. Destruction of medical and dental records after certain periods of time is current practice in certain jurisdictions, which means that information that could be used to identify an individual may be lost. An additional point here is that placing a name, serial number or some other unique marking on prostheses such as dentures would greatly assist the identification process. These markings would provide an initial point of inquiry to the practitioner or manufacturer that could then lead to identification of the deceased. Many cases where dental identifications are required possess dentures, which often cannot be reliably matched to an individual due to the loose fit of the dentures to the edentulous mandible and maxilla. Thus, if the dentures contained a person's name or the name of a dental practitioner, it would be much easier to identify the individual.

10.2.7 DNA

DNA has become a crucial factor in many postmortem identifications over the last 20 years. If first-degree relatives (father, mother, and child) are available to provide a reference sample for comparison, and a suitable postmortem sample is obtained, the chances of obtaining a match are quite high. Somatic muscle has been found to be a good sample for postmortem DNA testing. This is because it is less likely to be contaminated than other samples such as blood, and because deep muscle often survives impact and fire. Furthermore, small samples of tissue can be used for polymerase chain reaction (PCR) amplification. Frozen samples of muscle can be stored indefinitely, so that bodies can then be stored awaiting identification. However, DNA testing is both costly and time consuming. Also, in some disasters whole families may be victims and therefore no first-degree relatives are available to provide comparison samples. If first-degree relatives are not available to provide comparison samples, it may be necessary to locate personal items of the deceased and to obtain a DNA sample from them. Possible items that may contain DNA of the individual include toothbrushes, hairbrushes, shavers, clothes, towels, used dishes, and toys [1].

10.2.8 Documents

Documents, when found with a body, can provide personal information about the bearer, or at least some information linking them with a particular country or government. Such documents may include passports, driver's licences, credit or bank cards, receipts, cheque books, business cards, or any other piece of paper (Fig. 10.4). Documents containing photographs of the bearer are particularly valuable. Some other document-related personal information that may assist with the identification of a person includes keys (domestic or vehicular), metal identification tags or military dog tags. As with currency and jewellery, it must also be remembered that information found associated with the body may not belong to that person, but may have been held for some other reason. Therefore, such information should generally be only used as a guide for other more reliable and individual methods of identification.

10.2.9 Fingerprint Identification

Fingerprint identification is considered to be one of the most reliable methods of identification. This is due to the fact that all fingerprints are unique and standard methods of identification have been developed that are globally accepted. Some methods differ in the number of comparisons acceptable for

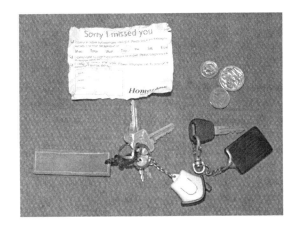

Fig. 10.4 Documents, currency, and keys (vehicle and residential) found on a body that could be traced back to the individual and assist with identification

identification, for example in criminal cases a 16 point match is needed, while a coroner/medical examiner may accept a 10 point match as positive identification. Many countries have large databases of fingerprints that can be matched to those of unidentified persons. Furthermore, when searching for comparison prints they are often found in locations that can be reliably matched to the individual, for example on their vehicle or on personal items. In some circumstances hands have been removed from bodies and retained as evidence. More frequently prints are taken from a body and filed for future comparisons pending the arrival of known prints. In some cases where fingerprints are not possible, palm, foot, ear and lip prints can be examined and compared in a similar manner, since, like fingerprints, these are also unique among individuals. It should be remembered that these methods have been less commonly used than fingerprint identification and methods of comparison such as the minimum number of acceptable matching points have not been standardised to the same level as fingerprints.

10.2.10 Frontal Sinus Comparison

Frontal sinus comparison is based on the anatomy of the frontal sinus, a convoluted cavity found in the midline of the frontal bone that is thought to be unique between individuals. If a person has had a radiograph taken of this part of the skull during life, a postmortem radiograph of the same area can be compared for anatomical similarity. The frontal sinus develops after the first year of life, but sometimes is not visible on radiographs until after about seven years. Until a person is 15 years old, the sinus can grow at a rate of 1.5 mm per year. From 18 years onwards, the frontal sinus is largely stable and any changes after this age are due to trauma, infections or other disease. Due to a later puberty and a consequently longer growth period, the frontal sinus is on average larger in males than females. In recent years it has been suggested that the comparison of antemortem and postmortem radiographs for identification is not valid, since the uniqueness of these anatomical structures has not been stringently tested [2, 3, 4].

10.2.11 Jewellery

Jewellery can often be traced to an individual as many people wear numerous pieces that are highly individualistic. Jewellery is mainly worn for decoration and can be found on fingers, toes, wrists, ankles, neck, around the waist and in the hair, as piercings, or on clothing. In general, females tend to have more jewellery than males. Due to its construction many items resist fires and damage and, depending on its location, may not be torn from the body in situations of trauma. On occasion, it may also indicate that the wearer is subject to a particular medical condition. Relatives will often recognise a sentimental piece of jewellery on a deceased person or in a photograph. In the case of expensive items, the jewellery may be insured and there will be records of the description of the piece, as well as photographs and valuations. Engravings may also be present that can be linked to an individual. However, it must be realised that for some jewellery that has been handed down through generations, the names on the engravings may differ from that of the bearer. The same can be said for engravings where a person's name has changed due to a change in marital status. If initials are engraved they may also match the initials of numerous people on the missing persons list. If an item is common, for example a plain gold wedding band without engraving (Fig. 10.5), it will be harder to link to an individual. Other information obtained from jewellery may include club insignias, zodiac signs or birthstones signifying the date of birth or religious persuasion of the victim. Jewellery can be constructed from precious metals, such as gold, silver or platinum. In this case the items may have a hallmark punched into the metal, providing information on the manufacturer, standard mark (type of metal), assay office and date letter.

10.2.12 Laundry Marks

Laundry marks are no longer as common as they have been in the past. These are marks that were used in laundries in the past, and are classified into two types – NATMAR in the USA and POLYMARK in the UK. POLYMARK is made of adhesive cloth tape that is fixed to the garment. It can be in one of six colours and either striped or plain, resulting in 12 possible variations. A five-digit code is also printed on the label; however there is no standard code usage,

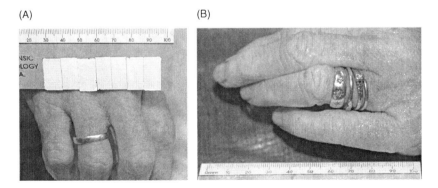

(A)   (B)

Fig. 10.5 Examples of common (**A**) and uncommon (**B**) jewellery that could be used for identification purposes. The uncommon jewellery would be much more useful as an identifier than the common piece (a traditional gold coloured wedding band)

and no central records, reducing their value as a possible identifier, unless an individual laundry is searched for paper records of the mark.

10.2.13 Lottery Tickets

Lottery tickets can often be traced to the country of purchase and also to the location of sale, as most national lottery tickets contain a retailer code. Since it can be deduced that the bearer probably bought the ticket close to their home or work, the list of possible missing people can be narrowed accordingly. In some countries the majority of the eligible population may purchase a weekly lottery ticket, which may be found amongst documents on their person. This may be useful for local disasters, but may not contribute much to the identification of foreign tourists, for example, who would be unlikely to purchase lottery tickets on their holiday.

10.2.14 Medical Records

Medical records may be collected once a person has been reported as missing. Examination of the body and the medical records can reveal evidence of medical intervention in the deceased that matches descriptions in the medical records. These records can take the form of notes, photographs, radiographs or other medical images, or simply a report from relatives about previous medical history. In cases of multiple fatalities, the evidence of medical intervention may help to establish or exclude identity. Occasionally at autopsy unique features may become apparent that may have been incidentally noted at the time of other medical treatment, but can greatly enhance the probability of identification. This includes the morphology of the frontal sinuses [2, 3, 4], cranial suture patterns [5], morphology and trabecular architecture of the bones of the hand [6], comparisons of chest radiographs [7], and trabecular morphology of the distal femur and proximal tibia [8]. Other examples are the comparison of bony markings [9], orthopedic devices or implants [10], evidence of medical intervention [11], phleboliths [12], and even the presence of an intraocular lens [13]. Similar issues exist with the comparison of antemortem and postmortem radiographs regarding the level of detail or certainty that should be reached in order for an identification to be made. A common assumption made when comparing radiographs of antemortem and postmortem features is that the characters compared in a radiograph are unique, and the absence of any inexplicable differences has been considered sufficient for an identification to be made. However, as for frontal sinuses (above) it has been found that such comparisons relied on in the past for identification purposes have not been stringently tested for uniqueness, and as a result, such forms of identification are now being tested for scientific validity, reliability and relevance. The level of detail for comparisons of anatomical features is also being examined [5, 8, 14]. For example, is it enough to state overall similarities between radiographs or should there be a minimum number of corresponding features in order for a positive identification to be made? The primary consideration is the absence of any inexplicable inconsistencies between antemortem and postmortem records [15].

10.2.15 Mobile Phones

Mobile phones have increased greatly in numbers over recent years and in most countries are carried by a large percentage of the population. They are carried by adults as well as an increasing number of children, and are often registered to a single user, with name and address details held by the service provider. However, there are a large number of pre-paid or "pay as you go" mobile phones on the market and these are not generally registered to a particular user. Mobile phones can be used as a guide to identification since the mobile number is (theoretically) unique. Some phones also have code numbers on the body or other identifying features. The chip inside the phone can withstand some trauma, apart from fire, and the information on it may be retrieved to assist identification, such as the last number dialled and stored numbers of relatives and friends. Occasionally fingerprints may also be present on the body of the phone. The network provider of the phone can also be displayed by the phone, which may assist in determining the country of origin of the owner.

10.2.16 Physical Characteristics

Physical characteristics are often used to describe missing people, and the documentation of these is the first step towards visual identification of a body (Fig. 10.6). The most common physical characteristics cited include height, weight, sex, race, eye colour, hair colour, skin colour, body build and any distinguishing marks such as scars, tattoos, or birthmarks. Some of these are less distinguishable in decomposed or damaged remains, such as eye colour, which deteriorates rapidly, and skin colour, which may be affected by decomposition. While hair colour can be easily changed and may be unreliable, the pattern of baldness or hair distribution is generally persistent and similarities between antemortem and postmortem appearances can be described. Another point to remember is the distinction between gender and anatomical sex, where the physical description of a body or body part given by forensic pathologists or anthropologists will be based on the anatomical sexual characteristics of the body (male, female, transsexual, hermaphrodite, pseudohermaphrodite, gynaecomastic), while the description given by relatives may reflect the social gender

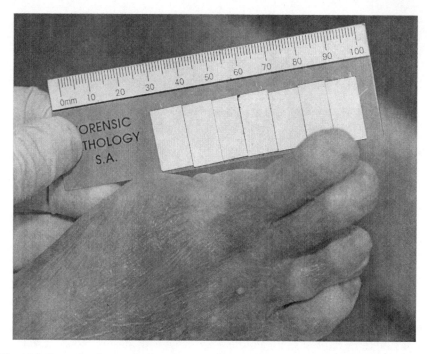

Fig. 10.6 Example of a physical characteristic showing a foot with an amputated right toe. For identification purposes this finding would be matched with a physical description provided by relatives

of the person. Estimates of stature can also become less reliable after death. Estimates of stature can be shortened by flexure of muscles due to rigor mortis or exposure to heat, and lengthened due to flaccidity or with decomposition. Incomplete bodies or body parts can also lead to an increased error in stature estimates. Similarly, a simple error in measuring postmortem stature from toe to crown instead of from heel to crown may result in estimates of stature differing significantly from antemortem reports. Other descriptions of physical appearance can be made based on body build, such as classification into endomorph, mesomorph and ectomorph body shapes. Racial classifications may be in broad categories of appearance such as caucasoid, mongoloid or negroid. However, the biological variability of physical characteristics must also be considered. Classification into racial types can be relatively straightforward in a non-decomposed body, but becomes more difficult when standard categories such as skin pigmentation are no longer reliably determined. Other indications of racial or population origin could be determined from property such as clothing and ornaments, or particular physical characteristics such as body piercing or tattoos; however these should not be substantially relied upon. In cases of mass fatalities of numerous nationalities, there is a temptation to classify and sort bodies initially according to their apparent population of origin based on physical characteristics. This may be done for socio-political reasons, and with considerable migration and interbreeding among populations, this may lead to more problems, rather than simplifying the identification process.

10.2.17 Scars

Scars are an invariable consequence of damage to the dermis and remain for the duration of a person's life. Scars can be accidentally or intentionally inflicted, and are often easily remembered by friends and relatives as identifying features (Fig. 10.7). People with darker skin pigmentation tend to develop keloid scars. Surgical scars can provide information on medical history. Self-inflicted scars may indicate previous suicide attempts or self-mutilation, while other scars may provide information on cultural or social persuasions.

10.2.18 Serology

Serology of an individual's blood type can help narrow down the search for a missing person. Global population studies of serology have revealed 300 blood grouping systems, resulting in 500 million possible blood groups. The blood group does not change during life, apart from possible transient changes after receipt of a universal type blood transfusion. If the blood type of both biological parents is known, determination of a victim's serology can help exclude them from a match. The most commonly known blood groupings are the ABO and

(A)   (B)

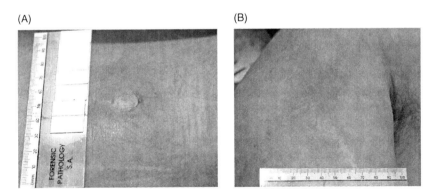

Fig. 10.7 Different forms of scars that could be used to identify an individual based on descriptions provided by relatives. A Distinctive scar to the cubital fossa region. B Fairly non-descript area of scarring to the upper arm

Rhesus grouping systems, the frequencies of which vary between populations. Globally, the O blood type ranges between 50% to 80% frequency, while the A blood type ranges between 10% and 35% and the B blood type is the rarest allele, present in less than 10% of the global population. These frequencies vary among geographic regions and social groups and some alleles are therefore more common in localised areas than others. For example, while the O blood type is the most common type in the world, in Sweden, Norway and among Australian Aborigines, the A blood type predominates. The lowest frequencies of O alleles are seen in Eastern Europe and Central Asia. Frequencies of the B blood type are most common in Central Asia, while they are lowest in the Americas and Australia [16]. The Rhesus factor, which provides the '+' or '−' sign to the ABO alleles, also varies between geographic regions. For example, RhD is present in 15–17% of Europeans, 3–5% of Africans and < 0.1% in Asian populations [17].

10.2.19 Spectacles or Corrective Lenses

Spectacles or corrective lenses are worn by an increasing proportion of the population. In Australia, 52% of the adult population have eyesight problems, with about 8% of children and 9% pf people aged between 15 and 24 years [18]. In addition to common visual problems such as myopia, hyperopia or presbyopia, most people also have some degree of astigmatism-axis value. These two factors can be measured in corrective lenses and the results compared to antemortem records made by their optician or optometrist. Spectacles, like jewellery, clothing and documents, may be lost from a body in the event of a disaster, or may be looted after death. In addition, spectacles found on a person's face are much more likely to belong to that person than those found next to or near a body, in which case they may have originated from a different person.

10.2.20 Tattoos

Tattoos are an indelible mark or pattern on the skin (See chapter 11). They may be accidentally or intentionally obtained. Some are amateur, such as prison or gang tattoos, while others are professionally applied. Some tattoos may also be applied for medical reasons, for example as markers for radiotherapy. Other people may have names, dates, blood types, or records of army service as tattoos. Tattoos can be visible in decomposed cases and can also persist after considerable time immersed in water. If there is superficial burning from fire, tattoos can also be obtained from the dermis of a person's skin. Some tattoo designs are common, such as roses, hearts and devils, while others are rare (Fig. 10.8). People frequently have multiple tattoos, which greatly assists identification. As with scars, tattoos are often remembered by friends or relatives.

Fig. 10.8 An example of a distinctive tattoo that would assist in identification

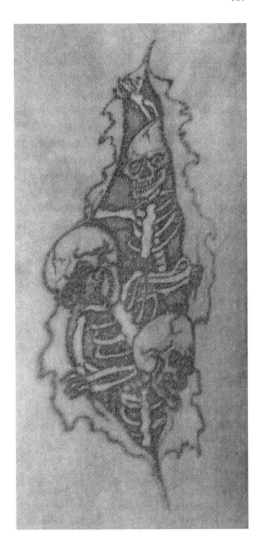

10.2.21 Vehicles

Vehicles can also be used as a guide to identification, since the registration records of vehicle licence plates, engine/chassis numbers and details of ownership are usually held in central government departments. Following a disaster, vehicles may be found abandoned in car parks or involved in the disaster itself, and can lead to a missing person. Vehicle licence plates may give an indication of the region where the vehicle is registered. Car keys found on a body can also be used to search for a vehicle or type of vehicle.

10.2.22 Visual Identification

Visual identification is the most frequently used method of identification. This involves a person who is familiar with the deceased stating that the victim is a particular person. In some circumstances, it can be less reliable than other methods, for example if there are multiple fatalities or there is significant trauma or disfigurement. Ante- or postmortem animal depredation may be responsible for removing identifying features such as the face [19, 20, 21]. Families can often be extremely distressed about the death of a relative and may find it hard to identify a body positively. Visual identification may be made unreliable by the facial features being affected by death and not appearing as they did in life. Often, if numerous people from the same family are involved in the disaster, there may be nobody to view the body and conduct a visual identification. On occasion, photographs of the body can be shown to relatives to avoid them having to view the body; however this can have problems similar to those with visual identification in the mortuary. Visual identification can be substantiated by viewing of property, such as jewellery, clothing and documents found on the body, as long as this property can be reliably concluded as having belonged to that individual.

10.3 Practical Aspects of Identification Procedures

While this is not an exhaustive list of identification methods, it is believed that it represents the methods most commonly used, especially in incidents of mass fatalities. Finally, it must also be remembered that identification by exclusion may also be useful.

The primary methods of identification of the deceased are visual, dental, fingerprints, and DNA. These methods are preferred due to reduced cost and time constraints for visual identification, the individuality of dental, fingerprint, and DNA characteristics, the persistence of teeth, fingerprints, and DNA after death, and the increased reliability of identification when based on scientific methods. In situations of multiple fatalities, it is common practice to request at least two identifiers in order to prevent possible errors. Many reports of identification of mass disasters, however, report the significant contribution of dental identification, and this has been recognised by the *Interpol Disaster Victim Identification Guide*, which states that if a positive match is found using dental identification it can be relied on as a stand-alone identifier. A recent overview of the identification effort following the Asian Tsunami disaster of 26th December 2004 found that 79% of the identifications from January to May 2005 had been provided by dental comparison. Of the remaining 21%, 9% were identified using fingerprints as the sole identifier, and 15% were identified by combinations of various methods, such as dental + fingerprints, physical characteristics + fingerprints, dental + physical characteristics and dental + fingerprints + physical characteristics. During this time identification using DNA accounted for 0.5% of the total; however this number may increase, along with the contributions of fingerprints, as the identification process continues [22].

The identification of human remains is an area that is constantly being reevaluated in the light of new developments. Situations of mass fatalities under various conditions often lead to new techniques being developed. For example, following the September 11, 2001 terrorist attacks on the New York World Trade Center towers, the team of experts in charge of identification using DNA developed new technologies to analyse the 20,000 victim samples. This included the examination of mitochondrial DNA instead of nuclear DNA, and the implementation of complex software analysis to search for matches among the 10,000 family reference samples [23, 24]. However, in February 2005 it was reported that the examination of DNA from remains recovered from the World Trade Center attacks has been halted due to the fact that the investigators had reached the limits of the technology to obtain profiles from the remaining pieces of tissue [25]. The extraction of DNA from the remaining samples will only continue once the technology has been improved. A recent case in South Australia involving innovative DNA analysis involved human remains recovered from the sea in the Great Australian Bight. A fishing trawler operating in the Great Australian Bight along the southern coastline of Australia dredged up two rubber boots containing the remains of lower limbs and feet, possibly from an adult male (Fig. 10.9). DNA was extracted from wedges of left and right tibiae using the laboratory protocol of incubation in 20% Chelex, proteinase K (10 mg/mL) and 0.1 M DTT for 4 h with intermittent vortexing. This resulted in a complete DNA profile being obtained from the bone. Police records were obtained of fishermen who had disappeared in the area, believed to have drowned, over the past 20 years. Reference samples from the wife and son of a fisherman who had disappeared 11 years earlier were compared with the profile obtained from the bone samples, and were found to correspond [26]. In other cases, extraction of DNA and genomic STR profiling from buried bones have been unsuccessful due to degradation of the DNA and inhibition of the PCR process, needing use of either mtDNA analysis or mini-STRs or SNPs. The reasons for successful extraction of DNA in this case are not yet clear. It is possible that the combination of cold water, darkness and the fact that the bones were contained in socks and rubber boots preserved the DNA in this case [26, 27].

In situations of multiple fatalities physical characteristics or individual features may be used for separating people into broad population groups or other possible categories. However, there is a danger here in relying on untested and unvalidated methods, and any new procedures or characteristics suggested during the identification stage should not be relied on to separate people into groups or to be used as a basis for a positive identification. Instead, these suggested new methods should be noted and then tested under controlled conditions before being applied on new data in the field.

Fig. 10.9 One of two boots
containing foot bones that
was recovered from the sea
and enabled identification of
the deceased using DNA
evidence. The individual had
been missing for over 10
years

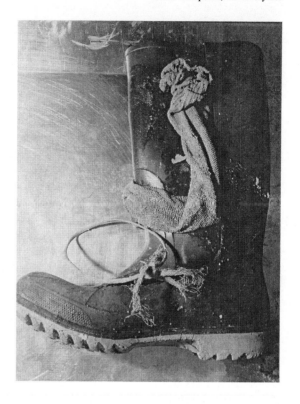

The potential for identification based on individual characteristics of a medical or orthopedic device using antemortem and postmortem comparison of radiographs has been well established, although recent questions regarding the evidential validity of these comparisons raise pertinent issues [4]. Another area that has not been investigated to the same extent is the use of a unique coding number on medical implants or orthopedic devices, which could then be traced back to clinicians and ultimately to patients [28]. At present, there are no formal requirements for coding of medical devices in Australia, while in the USA the requirements are for life-sustaining or life-supporting implants only to be marked [29, 30]. Many orthopedic devices are also used for fixation in both humans and non-humans, which can also complicate potential identification if fragmentary remains are located. Current record-keeping requirements are insufficient and are unlikely to lead to a positive identification unless the identity of the remains is already suspected.

One of the most important factors in the identification of human remains is the timely collection of data. Since a number of methods of identification rely on the comparison of antemortem and postmortem material it becomes imperative that this material is collected as soon as practicable once a person is reported as missing. Timely collection of records of suspected missing persons should be routine in order to prevent destruction of records before identification is complete. With regard to other types of identification using postmortem records, the collection of samples for fingerprints and DNA should also occur in a timely manner to prevent decay or loss of comparative material. While DNA samples can also be collected from relatives and compared to the DNA profile of the deceased, this is only achievable if the relatives are available to provide a reference sample. If several members of the same family are killed in the same incident, it may be difficult to locate a first-degree relative to provide reference samples. For this reason, collection of DNA from personal items such as toothbrushes, hairbrushes, shavers, clothes and toys of suspected missing people should also be done as soon as possible.

10.4 Conclusions

When a person dies, and for whatever reason the body cannot be identified visually, there are a number of potentially unique characteristics that can be looked for at autopsy that can assist with the identification. While the primary identifiers such as dental, DNA, and fingerprints remain the most reliable methods, there are many other less scientific identifiers that may assist with the identification. These become especially useful in cases of multiple fatalities, when any individual feature may be the one that establishes the identification of an individual or excludes them from the list of possible matches. The methods of identification listed here are not exhaustive but represent the more commonly used primary and secondary methods of identification. It is imagined that, with time and technological advances, this list will evolve to include new developments in the field; however, it is unlikely that any methods would ever be removed from the list. Identification of the deceased is a vital part of the repatriation and burial system, and errors or uncertainties act to delay this process, often causing considerable distress to families. A coordinated, systemic approach to the collection and recording of identification information will greatly reduce the likelihood of errors, such as false matches or false exclusions. Past situations of mass fatalities have proven that different investigators have various approaches to the issue of postmortem identification. This is especially so when victims originate from countries or regions distant to the event, as investigators then have to deal with additional factors such as communication difficulties, differing legal systems, problems with collection of records from the victims home, and any perceived or actual media pressure to speed up the identification process. While problems like these can result in a less organised and professional approach to the identification, it may also be said that each situation of multiple fatalities is an opportunity to learn from previous problems and to not repeat them. In the past, it has been unusual for the same identification teams to be sent to subsequent disasters; however, the benefit of past experience for situations such as these is increasingly evident. Unfortunately, the current global situation of terrorist attacks makes the probability of more multiple fatalities high. It is hoped that, out of these tragedies, increasingly better management of disasters and disaster victim identification will lessen the burden on societies and the families of the victims.

References

1. Meyer HJ (2003) The Kaprun cable car fire disaster – aspects of forensic organisation following a mass fatality with 155 victims. Forensic Sci Int 138:1–7
2. Haglund WD (1992) Remains identification by frontal sinus radiographs. J Forensic Sci 37:1207
3. Kirk NJ, Wood RE, Goldstein M (2002) Skeletal identification using the frontal sinus region: a retrospective study of 39 cases. J Forensic Sci 47:318–323
4. Christensen AM (2004) The impact of *Daubert*: Implications of testimony and research in forensic anthropology (and the use of frontal sinuses in personal identification). J Forensic Sci 49:427–430
5. Kuehn CM, Taylor KM, Mann FA, Wilson AJ, Harruff RC (2002) Validation of chest X-ray comparisons for unknown decedent identification. J Forensic Sci 47:725–729
6. Koot MG, Sauer NJ, Fenton TW (2005) Radiographic human identification using bones of the hand: a validation study. J Forensic Sci 50:263–268
7. Rogers TL, Allard TT (2004) Expert testimony and positive identification of human remains through cranial suture patterns. J Forensic Sci 49:203–237
8. Mann RW (1998) Use of bone trabeculae to establish positive identification. Forensic Sci Int 98:91–99
9. Angyal M, Dérczy K (1998) Personal identification on the basis of ante-mortem and post-mortem radiographs. J Forensic Sci 43:1089–1093
10. Bennett JL, Benedix DC (1999) Positive identification of cremains recovered from an automobile based on the presence of an internal fixation device. J Forensic Sci 44:1296–1298
11. Hogge JP, Messmer JM, Fierro MF (1995) Positive identification by post-surgical defects from unilateral lambdoid synostectomy: A case report. J Forensic Sci 40:688–691
12. Kahana T, Hiss J (2002) Suprapelvic and pelvic phleboliths – a reliable radiographic marker for positive identification. J Clin Forensic Med 9:115–118
13. Isaacs TW, Margolius KA, Chester GH (1997) Post-mortem identification by means of a recovered intraocular lens. Am J Forensic Med Pathol 18:404–405
14. Skinner M (1988) Method and theory in deciding identity of skeletonized human remains. Can Soc Forensic Sci 21:114–134
15. Kieser JA, Firth NA, Buckley H (2001) Dental misidentification on the basis of presumed unique features. J Forensic Odontostomatol 19:36–39
16. O'Neill D (2005) Distribution of blood types. *http://anthro.palomar.edu/vary_3.htm*
17. Westhoff CM (2004) The Rh blood group system in review: a new face for the next decade. Transfusion 44:1663–1673
18. Australian Bureau of Statistics (2006) National Health survey: summary of results. 4364.0 *www.abs.gov.au*
19. Byard RW, James RA, Gilbert JD (2002) Diagnostic problems associated with cadaveric trauma from animal activity. Am J Forensic Med Pathol 23:238–244
20. Tsokos M, Schulz F (1999) Indoor postmortem animal interference by carnivores and rodents: report of two cases and review of the literature. Int J Leg Med 112:115–119

21. Tsokos M, Byard RW, Püschel K (2007) Extensive and mutilating craniofacial trauma involving defleshing and decapitation: unusual features of fatal dog attack in the young. Am J Forens Med Pathol 28:131–136

22. James H (editor) (2005) Thai tsunami victim identification – overview to date. J Forensic Odontostomatol 23:1–18

23. Vastag B (2002) Out of tragedy, identification innovation. J Am Med Assoc 10:1221–1223

24. Gill JR (2006) 9/11 and the New York City Office of Chief Medical Examiner. Forensic Sci Med Pathol 2:29–32

25. Powell M (2005) Identification of 9/11 remains comes to an end. *http://www.washington-post.com/ac2/wp-dyn/A47866-2005Feb23*

26. Both K, Simpson E, Byard RW (2008) The identification of submerged skeletonised remains. J Clin Forensic Med 29:69–71

27. Ludes B, Keyser-Tracqui C (2005) Anthropology: role of DNA. In: Payne-James J, Byard RW, Corey T, Henderson C (eds) Encyclopedia of forensic and legal medicine, vol 1. Elsevier/Academic Press, Amsterdam, pp 127–132

28. Ubelaker DH, Jacobs CH (1995) Identification of orthopedic device manufacturer. J Forensic Sci 40:168–170

29. TGA (2004) Medical Device Evaluation Committee meeting 2004/2: Summary of key resolutions. *http://www.tga.gov.au/docs/html/mdec/mdec_2004res.htm*

30. FDA. Device Advice. *http://www.fda.gov/cdrh/devadvice/353.htm*

Chapter 11
The Forensic and Cultural Implications of Tattooing

Glenda E. Cains and Roger W. Byard

Contents

Abstract Tattooing for decorative purposes has occurred in most communities for many thousands of years. Tattoos have been used as an indicator of high status, or have been used to mark slaves and prisoners indelibly. In tribal communities, elaborate tattooing rituals have been associated with rites of passage into adulthood. Tattooing may be inadvertent, associated with

R.W. Byard
University of Adelaide, Adelaide, South Australia, Australia
e-mail: byard.roger@saugov.sa.gov.au

M. Tsokos (ed.), *Forensic Pathology Reviews, Volume 5*,
doi: 10.1007/978-1-59745-110-9_11, © Humana Press, Totowa, NJ 2008

occupations such as welding or coal mining, and has been used in medicine to mark anatomical locations to assist with radiotherapy, or to identify an area that requires careful re-examination at follow-up. Clubs, street gangs and criminal organisations, such as the *Yakuza* in Japan, have all used tattoos as markers of membership. In the forensic environment, tattoos can be extremely useful in assisting with body identification, and in giving an indication of possible life styles and history. For example, commemorative military tattoos are most often found in war veterans, rudimentary line tattoos with antisocial and anti-police messages often indicate previous imprisonment, and marihuana leaves, mushrooms or "ecstasy" suggest drug usage. In recent years there has been a resurgence of interest in tattoos in Western countries, particularly among the young, and so there will be more cases seen in mortuaries in the future where particular tattoos may be found to assist with identification.

Keywords Tattoos · Identification · Gangs · Tribal marking

11.1 Introduction

The term "tattoo" refers to the act or practice of marking the skin with indelible patterns, pictures, legends, etc., by making punctures in it and inserting pigments (earlier *tattow*, from Polynesian *tatau*) [1, 2] (Fig. 11.1). As tattoos are routinely encountered within the mortuary environment, it is important to understand the history, development and culture of tattooing practices, particularly as there has been somewhat of a renaissance in Western countries over the past 15 years. It is estimated that 10–16% of adolescents now have tattoos, compared to 3–9% of the general population [3]. Tattoos may now be found on any type of person, not just in "lower-class men, notably sailors and soldiers" and "prostitutes of the lowest class" as was previously asserted [4], and so assumptions about the lifestyle of the tattooed individual have to be guarded. Tattoos can, however, be used to help with the identification of unknown deceased persons, and may give some indication of social and cultural background [5] (Fig. 11.2). Due to changing trends and styles, tattoos can no longer be used to identify specific cultural groups

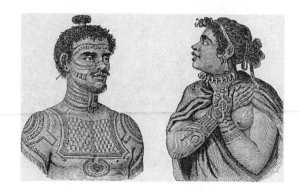

Fig. 11.1 Traditional tattooing of both sexes from the Marquesas Islands of the South Pacific. (Taken from *The Races of Mankind being a Popular Description of the Characteristics, Manners and Customs of the Principal Varieties of The Human Family*, 1868 [2].)

Fig. 11.2 Complex tattoos
in a man from Cambodia

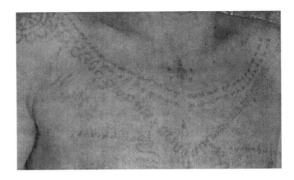

precisely, as "traditional tribal" style, or calligraphy; tattoos can now be found on persons with no connection to the culture where the style originated.

11.2 Historical and Cultural Background

The practice of tattooing human skin has been around for millennia and has been described in almost every culture, from the highlands of Peru, to Inuit communities, to the Pacific Islands where it is still practiced today. The earliest evidence of tattooing comes from the upper Paleolithic era (38,000–10,000 BC) and archeological artefacts recovered in Europe have included skin puncturing tools and pigment reserves. These items have been found together with small, decorated figurines, engraved with what appear to be tattoos [6]. Mummies of court dancing girls or concubines from the 11th dynasty of ancient Egypt in the second millennium BC have revealed tattoos, and there is both archaeological and written evidence to indicate that tattooing was widespread across early Europe, practiced by many different peoples including the Scythians, Celts, Picts and Germanic tribes [7]. Special techniques, including infra-red examination of the skin, have been used to enhance designs from early remains for examination [8].

The Bronze Age has provided many mummified and preserved remains bearing a multitude of tattoos that have added much to our understanding of the historical significance of the practice. For example, a Bronze Age warrior, named *Ötzi* (or *Oetzae*) for the Alpine region in which he was discovered, was found to have several tattoos marked with dark blue ink. A series of parallel lines over the lumbar spine and ankle and a cross on the inside of one knee seemed to correspond to underlying arthritic disease, and so it has been suggested that the tattoos may have been related to therapeutic activities [4, 9, 10].

The practice of tattooing evolved further in the Iron Age, with many examples being found across Europe and into Asia. One of the most spectacular examples of Iron Age tattooing can be found on the remains of a chieftain of the nomadic Siberian warrior tribe, the *Pazyryk*, who resided on the Russian steppes in the sixth to the second century BC. The unearthing of an undisturbed grave, filled with elaborate grave goods and the well-preserved body of this chieftain, was an important archaeological find, added to by the presence of extensive and complex tattoos. Along with many stylised animal designs, there were also parallel lines similar to those discovered on "Ötzi", again suggesting a possible therapeutic or magical use for these markings [6]. In 1994, in Ukok on the Siberian plateau, the frozen Iron Age body of a young woman from the same culture was discovered. Similar grave goods were found and the body was extensively tattooed with comparable designs to those of the male warrior [6]. Both of these finds, with the richness of the grave goods, suggests that tattoos were used to denote a high and honourable status among these people.

In Classical Greece, tattoos first began to be regarded as the mark of an "outsider" and in an effort to clearly distinguish between civilised peoples (Greeks) and barbarians (Celts, Scythians and Germanic tribes) any person with tattoos was poorly regarded [4]. Tattoos began to be used to identify slaves and criminals. For example, the Romans used both tattoos and branding to clearly stigmatise and identify slaves and criminals, and later they were also utilised by military personnel and tradesmen to identify their occupations. It was at this time that the first examples of Christian tattoos appeared. As Christianity was both an unofficial and outlawed religion, followers used tattoos as a covert method of recognition. This practice flourished until an edict from Pope Hadrian in the year 787 AD forbad any Christian to be tattooed [7]. In Britain in 1717, tattooing replaced branding as a method of marking deserters from the army and continued until 1879 with deserters being tattooed with a "D". In 1832 tattoos were used to identify French convicts who had been sentenced to forced labour [4, 7].

However, the acceptability of tattoos has always been subject to the whims of fashion and in medieval Europe crusaders and pilgrims to the Holy Land often tattooed their bodies with Christian symbols, such as the Cross of Jerusalem, and a shrine in Loreto offered tattoos to its pilgrims [4]. In the nineteenth century, tattoos were considered fashionable among female members of European and English aristocracy, with Lady Randolph Churchill sporting a tattoo of a snake around her wrist [11].

The Japanese have a long history of tattooing dating back to the fifth century BC and, as with many other cultures, those most likely to be tattooed were traditionally considered to be outside "normal" society. This persists today with the *Yakuza*, or "Japanese mafia", perpetuating the practice of a full body, or "suit", of highly coloured and intricate tattoos [7] (Fig. 11.3A).

Perhaps the most enduring and well-known examples of traditional tattoos are those adorning peoples of the South Pacific islands. Each group has its own designs and, as with the Scythians and other early cultures, tattoos were mostly reserved for the upper classes of warriors and chieftains. Known as Moko among the Maori for facial tattoos, and Pe'a among the Samoans for tattoos from the waist to the knees [12], these types of tattoos are unique in that they have sometimes survived in their traditional form to this day (Fig. 11.3B). It was not until Captain James Cook and others journeyed to the Pacific region that tattooing, as we know it in the West today, developed. Early explorers such as Dampier and Bougainville brought back tattooed individuals from

(A)   (B)

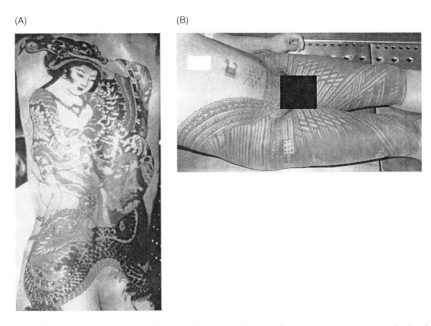

Fig. 11.3 **A** A complex and multicolored oriental design of a Japanese woman on the back. **B** A complicated monochromatic traditional design on the legs and buttocks of an adult Polynesian male

Mindanao and Tahiti for exhibition in Europe and Cook first published detailed observations of tattooing, as witnessed in Tahiti and New Zealand. Many of his and subsequent sailors had themselves tattooed and also took the practice back to Europe with them, practicing their art on each other during the long voyages home [4, 7]. Not all groups in this part of the world used tattooing for body modification, with the Tasmanians for example, relying instead on quite elaborate scarification [13]. Elaborate scarification is still found among certain African tribal groups (Fig. 11.4). The interest in tattoos continued to develop into the nineteenth century with sideshow exhibits often featuring a "Tattooed Lady" [4].

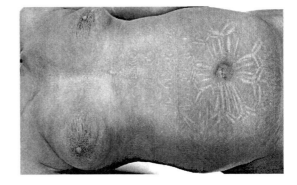

Fig. 11.4 Elaborate decorative scarification of the abdomen and upper chest in a Dinka woman from Southern Sudan

11.3 Techniques of Tattooing

Traditional tribal tattoos were often produced by cutting the skin and rubbing in soot or other pigments. The Inuit used relatively crude instruments such as a bone needle coated in soot that was drawn through the skin [7]. Other cultures used sticks, bones, shells and animal teeth to make instruments with sharpened ends that were capable of quite fine work. Today, most tattoos are produced using an electric machine with multiple needles that cycle between 50 to 300 times per minute, little changed from the machine that Edison designed in 1877 for making embroidery patterns [7, 10]. Ink is picked up by the needles from wells and injected into the papillary and reticular dermis to a level of 1–2 mm, creating a permanent design. The components of various dyes have remained relatively unchanged for many years and include India ink, mercuric sulfide (cinnabar), cadmium, chromium and cobalt salts [7].

The techniques and complexity of tattoos in Western cultures have changed significantly over the last 10 years. Prior to this most tattoos had relatively thick black outlines filled in with solid blocks of colour. The designs were usually simple and bold with a lack of fine detail and are known as "traditional western" (Fig. 11.5). The introduction of the "fine line" style has allowed for more complex and intricate designs such as those based on photographic images shown in Fig. 11.6. As most people acquire their first tattoos in their late teens to early

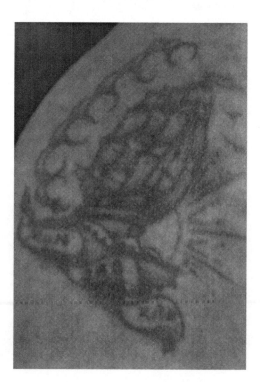

Fig. 11.5 A "traditional Western" tattoo with a ship, setting sun and scroll

Fig. 11.6 A fine line
contemporary Western style
tattoo depicting a woman

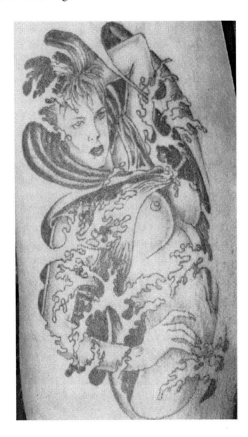

20s, the differentiation between new, fine line tattoos and those of the older thick outline style may help to establish the approximate age of a tattooed individual.

Contemporary amateur tattoos created with sharp instruments and ink are often found in individuals who have acquired them in institutions such as prisons and often have a "humorous" or an antisocial message (Fig. 11.7). As they are often created using unsanitary practices they are of more concern in the mortuary

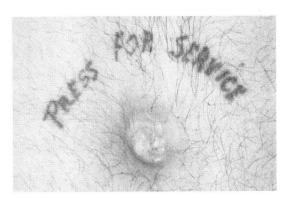

Fig. 11.7 A crude tattoo of
the navel with 'press for
service'

environment as the possibility of infectious diseases such as hepatitis C or AIDS being present is much higher than in individuals with professionally produced tattoos.

11.4 Non-intentional Tattoos

These are tattoos that are produced as a result of the occupation or lifestyle of the individual. For example, coal miners are often easily recognised by the carbon dust that becomes trapped in the skin of their face and hands (Fig. 11.8). Amalgam tattoos can be produced on the gingival surfaces after dental treatment and this can be used as an identifying feature [10]. Probably the most common example of non-intentional tattooing encountered in the mortuary is that of gun shot residue. The distribution and pattern of such tattooing can be used to estimate the distance of the discharge of the firearm from the body, and also to identify entry wounds [10, 14].

11.5 Specific Tattoo Styles

Despite considerable changes in styles tattoos generally fall into several easily defined categories.

11.5.1 Traditional Western

This is the older style of tattoo, often found among sailors or ex-navy personnel. Designs include hearts, roses, daggers, animals, sailing ships and scrolls with the names of family members (Fig. 11.5). The designs sometimes had specific meanings; for example a swallow on the chest indicated that a sailor had travelled 5000 miles [6], and a cobweb that the wearer had killed someone [12]. Most people nowadays who have these types of tattoos are unaware of the symbolism associated with them, and have usually chosen the design for esthetic reasons. The designs tend to be bold and colourful and are often

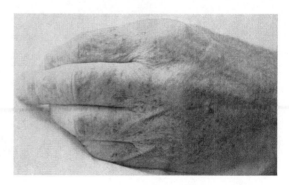

Fig. 11.8 Occupational tattooing of the hand with coal dust in a miner

displayed on the walls of tattoo studios. They are commonly referred to as "flash" [7].

11.5.2 Traditional Tribal

These include designs such as those used in Polynesia, Africa and in South East Asia (Figs. 11.1–11.3). The designs have specific meanings and usually represent a transition in status. They are customarily produced by expert tribesmen using traditional tools. The designs are monochromatic produced in black ink only and are usually geometric.

11.5.3 Traditional Eastern

These designs are usually intricate and colourful, depicting complex scenes that often tell a story. The style is said to have originated when peasants, who were forbidden to wear colourful clothing, tattooed a "suit" of vibrant designs onto their bodies.

11.5.4 Contemporary Western

This encompasses new fine line styles and detailed photorealistic work that is produced in either greyscale (where the designs are produced using shades of grey) or colour, with new shades such as vibrant purples, and advances in shading techniques.

11.5.5 Contemporary Tribal

This, more than any other style, was responsible for the resurgence of interest in tattoos in the West. The tattoos are usually monochromatic, although occasionally some colour is used. The style is defined by sweeping solid curves and sharp points, with un-tattooed spaces left in between to form intricate designs (Fig. 11.9). Celtic designs are also included in this category.

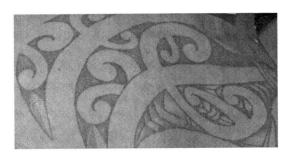

Fig. 11.9 A contemporary Western tribal style tattoo

(A)   (B)

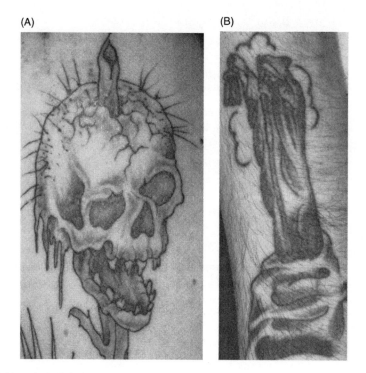

Fig. 11.10 **A** A skull design. **B** A Grim Reaper design

11.5.6 Gang and Prison

Designs are often crude, with an emphasis on death and violence, and include
the grim reaper, skulls, serpents and tombstones (Fig. 11.10A,B).

11.6 Reasons for Tattooing

11.6.1 Decorative

Most tattoos in the West are acquired for purely decorative purposes, with
little or no symbolic significance, and have been chosen off the wall, or from
catalogues at tattoo parlours. Customised tattoos, often designed by the
wearer to reflect personal taste and content, are becoming more popular,
and may be used to celebrate a special occasion, such as the birth of a child,
the beginning, or end, of a relationship, or other significant life achievements.
Alternatively they may also be used as a permanent memorial for loved ones
who have died.

11.6.2 Voluntary Group Membership

Some individuals are tattooed to reflect membership of a group or gang, most commonly paramilitary, street or motorcycle groups. For example the Californian Pachuco street gang signify membership with a cross between the thumb and first finger [15]. The Yakuza in Japan have been previously mentioned. Military personnel are another group who use tattoos to denote membership of specific platoons or involvement in specific fields of combat (Fig. 11.11). Illicit drug users are also commonly tattooed, both to advertise their drug of choice (Fig. 11.12) and to disguise scars from repeated venipunctures. Tattoos designed to reflect sexual orientation are not common but a bluebird adjacent to the thumb on the left hand (Fig. 11.13A), was said to have been a recognition sign for male homosexuals [16]. Other designs such as the rainbow flag pictured in Fig. 11.13B may also reflect a gay lifestyle.

11.6.3 Involuntary Group Membership

Inmates of Nazi concentration camps in World War II had identification numbers tattooed on their arms, a practice reminiscent of Roman methods of identifying slaves and criminals (Fig. 11.14). Nowadays, grandchildren of inmates sometimes have the number tattooed on their forearms as a commemorative.

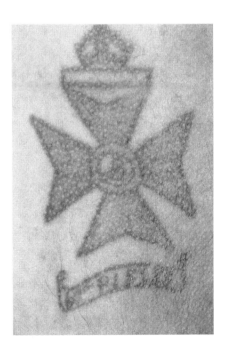

Fig. 11.11 A crude services tattoo in a World War II veteran

Fig. 11.12 A design in a drug user with mushrooms, a marihuana leaf and "Life be out of it"

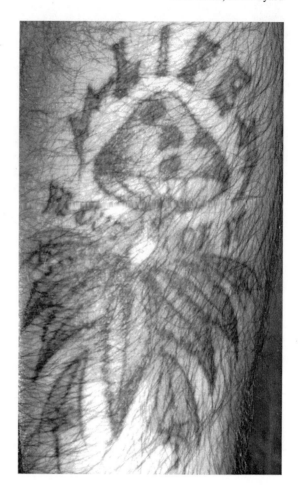

11.6.4 Religious and Political

Tattoos depicting religious themes are a method for people to advertise their religion, despite both the Bible and the Koran forbidding this practice [7] (Fig. 11.15) – "Ye shall not make any cuttings in your flesh for the dead, nor imprint any marks upon you; I am the Lord": *Leviticus* 19:28.

In contrast, in other religions such as Hinduism, tattoos are used to ensure fertility and to ward off the evil eye, and are seen as a normal expression of faith. Tattoos may also be used to exhibit political or ideological values, the most common of these being fascist or racist symbols and images adopted by neo-nazis and white supremacists (Fig. 11.16 A,B). Many tattoo artists refuse to apply racist images or messages, or designs that may be deemed offensive. Patriotic symbols such as flags and emblems are also common.

(A)   (B)

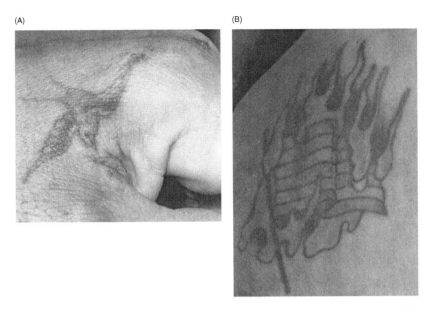

Fig. 11.13 **A** A swallow in the web space at the base of the thumb of the left hand. **B** A rainbow flag indicating support for gay rights

11.6.5 Cosmetic and Medical

Tattoos have been used cosmetically for centuries. The most common kinds of cosmetic tattoos are those of "permanent makeup", such as eyeliner and lip liner. Tattoos are also used cosmetically to cover birthmarks or scars. Probably the most common form of cosmetic, medically-administered tattoo involves reconstruction of the areola following mastectomy procedures. This method

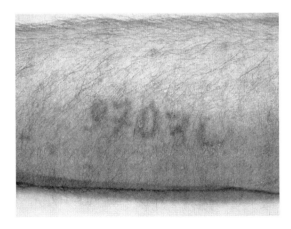

Fig. 11.14 Tattooing of the arm of a Nazi ex-concentration camp inmate (*Kindly provided By Dr T Lyons, Newcastle*)

Fig. 11.15 An Orthodox
cross

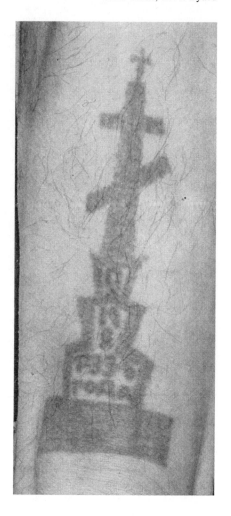

has been used successfully for many years with little to no adverse reactions reported in the literature [17]. Similar techniques have been used to disguise areas of facial scarring, to camouflage hemangiomas or areas of vitiligo, or to tattoo "hair follicles" into bald areas [18]. Of importance to pathologists are tattoos that may be used to hide or disguise areas of medical interest, such as skin lesions and surgical scars. Corneal tattooing to disguise opacities is an ancient practice thought to be first used by Galen (ca. 129–ca. 200). It resurfaced as a medical procedure in the early part of the last century and has recently been modified to include the use of excimer laser technology [19].

Small dots or crosses are sometimes used in radiotherapy as permanent points of orientation for continuing treatment (Fig. 11.17). "Internal" medical tattooing includes the injection of India ink at the site of colonic polyp removal,

(A)   (B)

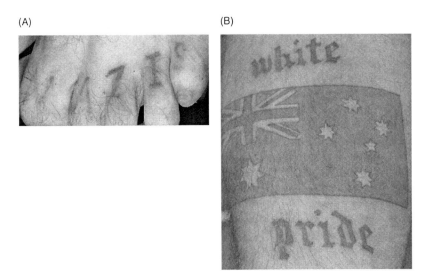

Fig. 11.16 A 'N' 'A' 'Z' 'I' 'S' across the toes. **B** 'White Pride' and the Australian flag

to allow for follow-up examinations of the area, in addition to similar procedures for follow-up of Barrett esophagus [20].

In certain cultural groups in West Africa, traditional healers utilise tattoos
and scarification as therapeutic tools. For example, a thin line on the forehead
may be drawn to treat epilepsy, and tattoos may be systematically drawn on the
hands and legs for cases of peripheral neuropathy [21]. Whilst these types of
tattoos are not commonly encountered in the West, their incidence may increase
with increasing immigration of West African people. In cases where there is
little information on the medical history, these types of tattoos may help to
identify possible underlying conditions.

11.6.6 Medical Information

In recent years, there have been instances where medical practitioners have
encountered tattooed messages of an instructional nature [22, 23]. These tattoos
may appear in older patients, or in those with a chronic medical condition who

Fig. 11.17 Three small blue dots across the upper chest in a woman with a past history of
thyroid cancer treated with radiotherapy

for metal allergy reasons are unable to wear medical alert bracelets [24] Such permanent markings are used for a number of reasons:

1. Some are specific condition-related instructions, directing the attention of treating physicians to a condition such as a drug allergy, or to previous treatments that are not to be repeated. These messages are advisory in nature, alerting but not specifically directing the physician to any particular course of action [22, 24].

2. Another form that these types of tattoos may take poses more complex issues for paramedics and physicians. These consist of instructions that direct health care workers either not to undertake cardiopulmonary resuscitation ("DND" = "Do not defibrillate or cardiovert"), or not to prolong life by using feeding gastrostomy (PEG) tubes [23] (Fig. 11.18). These are found on persons who have decided that they do not wish to have medical resuscitative procedures performed on them in the event of a serious accident or injury. This raises an ethical dilemma for treating health professionals: to follow the advice of the tattoo without a verbal instruction from the unconscious patient, or to follow normal resuscitation procedures [25].

3. A third type of medical information tattoo includes those that specify particular medications and treatments being used, or particular conditions that may quickly incapacitate an individual, such as insulin-dependent diabetes mellitus. Military personnel may also have their blood groups tattooed on their upper arms to assist medical personnel with resuscitative efforts.

11.6.7 Psychological Issues

Many studies have linked tattoos with mental illness and high-risk behaviour and it has been suggested that tattoos can be used as a diagnostic indicator for psychiatric problems such as anti-social personality disorder, schizophrenia, borderline personality disorders, fetishism and paraphilias, in addition to alcohol and drug abuse [15, 26, 27]. As a number of these studies have been

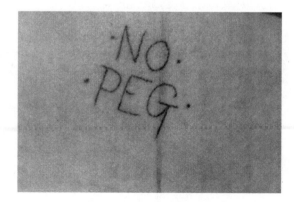

Fig. 11.18 "NO PEG" on the abdomen of a nurse indicting her desire not to have a feeding gastrostomy tube in the event of her incapacitation

Fig. 11.19 A highlighted scar of the neck from a self-inflicted injury with the word "damage" beneath in a suicide victim

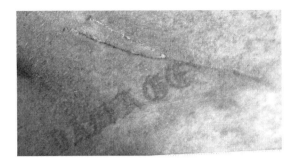

conducted within mental health facilities, bias is an obvious problem [14]. However, while the stereotype of the "outsider" being tattooed must be resisted, there are certain individuals whose tattoos do indicate antisocial behaviour or psychiatric illness [28]. For example, there are often strong links between adolescents who are tattooed or pierced at a young age (<13 years) and high-risk behaviours such as drug abuse, gang membership and violence [28, 29]. Other studies have shown that individuals tattooed and pierced after the age of 20 years do not appear to engage in these behaviours to the same degree as younger individuals [29].

Figure 11.19 shows a self-inflicted scar of the side of the neck that has been highlighted by tattooing over the top, with the word "Damage" beneath. The tattoo belonged to 29-year-old man with a history of self-mutilation and intravenous drug abuse who had committed suicide. A schizophrenic man in his 20s who also committed suicide was noted in our mortuary to have tattoos of female genitalia and antisocial messages over his cheeks and forehead (Fig. 11.20A–C). Lombroso had commented in the nineteenth century "that

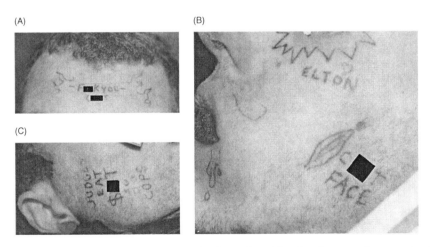

Fig. 11.20 A–C Antisocial messages on the face of a schizophrenic man who committed suicide by hanging

Fig. 11.21 Crude tattooing of the penis associated with plastic bead implants

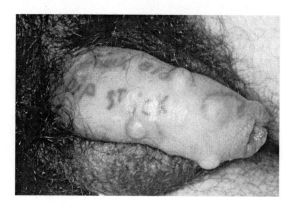

the convicts with numerous tattoos are natural and dangerous criminals, and that the worst and most bestial types are distinguished by their obscene and cynical designs" [4]. Such tattoos may be associated with other forms of body modification such as penile spherules (Fig. 11.21).

11.6.8 Veterinary

It has become standard practice in some areas of small animal veterinary practice to tattoo animals with identification numbers to prevent misidentification. Tattooing animals for identification purposes also occurs in animal laboratories [30].

11.7 Pathological Features and Complications of Tattoos

Tattoos undergo a sequence of changes due to tissue responses to injected pigments. The first reaction is erythema and swelling, followed by sloughing of the epidermis without blistering. After 5–7 days a tattoo will be indurated with crusting of the surface followed by healing after about 14 days [12]. In histological sections tattoos appear as aggregates of black material within the interstitium and macrophages within the dermis, usually without significant inflammatory reaction. Adjacent regional lymph nodes may also show aggregated pigment (Fig. 11.22 A,B), a feature described by Casper in the mid-nineteenth century [31]. The only diagnostic difficulty that might arise is misinterpretation of the significance of the pigment if the macroscopic details of the case were not known [32].

Complications of tattooing are rare if sterile equipment is used under aseptic conditions. The obvious concerns are when tattoos are produced by amateurs and in unsanitary conditions such as those found in prisons. As there is no method of sterilising equipment between clients, the potential for transmission

(A)   (B)

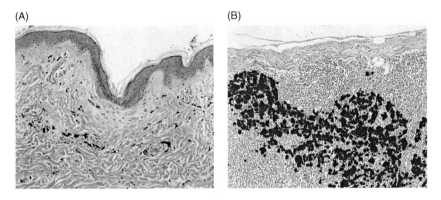

Fig. 11.22 A Black pigment in the upper dermis in a typical tattoo (Hematoxylin and Eosin x 120). **B** Further black pigment was present in an adjacent draining axillary lymph node (Hematoxylin and Eosin x 100)

of blood borne diseases such as hepatitis C is high, although confirmation of human immunodeficiency virus (HIV) transmission via tattooing is lacking. Less serious problems consist of localised tissue reactions and bacterial infections [33, 34, 35].

The incidence of the transfer of other diseases via professionally-produced tattoos is very low, although there have been reported cases of inoculation with leprosy, where affected individuals all presented with lepromatous lesions within tattooed areas. Subsequent inquiry in one series of cases, however, revealed that all of the affected individuals obtained their tattoos from roadside tattoo artists with no sterilisation facilities. In all of the patients reported, lesions appeared from 6 to 23 years after the tattoos had been obtained [36]. Syphilis represents another disease that has been associated historically with tattoos, again where artists did not sterilise or even clean equipment between customers. One theory suggests that syphilis may have been transmitted when an infected tattoo artist moistened a tattoo needle with saliva, during the tattooing process [7, 37].

Tattoo-associated dermatoses [38] may also be observed and have been classified into three major categories: allergic/granulomatous/lichenoid reactions, inoculation/infection and coincidental lesions [37].

Allergic reactions to red mercuric-based inks are common with swelling, erythema and pruritis, and in recent years alternatives to the mercuric-based red inks have been developed which include sienna/red ochre (ferric hydrate), cadmium red (cadmium selenide) and organic vegetable dyes such as Sandalwood and Brazilwood. These alternatives seem to have reduced, but not completely solved, the problem of red dye sensitivity and reactions [39]. Granulomatous reactions due to chronic inflammatory reactions to tattoo pigment granules may occur [37, 40], as may lichenoid reactions due to delayed hypersensitivity simulating a graft vs host response [39]. Cutaneous sarcoidosis has been reported in tattoos [40]. Rarely the diagnosis of a skin tumor such as a mela-noma may be delayed if it has developed within a tattoo [41]. The theoretical possibility of arachnoiditis or neuropathy secondary to an inflammatory reac-tion following an epidural injection through tattoo pigment has also been raised, although this has not been reported to date [42].

11.8 Removal

Occasionally, there may be evidence that a tattoo has been removed. This may be though such methods as dermabrasion followed by the application of caustic chemicals such as tannic acid and silver nitrate (*Variot's* method) or trichlor-oacetic acid, salabrasion (with salt), cryosurgery, surgical resection or laser ablation. Most of these methods result in scarring. Alternatively, a larger tattoo may have been superimposed over another in an attempt to either disguise or obliterate the previous work [6].

11.9 Forensic Uses

While the increase in the popularity of tattoos in the West may have resulted in individuals from all socio-economic backgrounds presenting to autopsy with tattoos, there are still a number of useful pieces of information that may be gleaned from particular designs. Tattoos may provide information on the possible occupation and club/gang affiliations of the deceased, drug taking habits, previous military service, prison history, names of family members, medical conditions, previous travel destinations, and religious and cultural background. Certain tattoos critical of police are very characteristic of indivi-duals with prison records and when found usually indicate that the deceased will in all likelihood have police record with fingerprints on file (Fig. 11.23).

Tattoos may be extremely useful in identifying individuals, as dermal pig-ments remain remarkably intact even after there has been considerable putre-faction and loss of superficial skin layers. Tattoos were one of the features that were specifically looked for in badly decomposed bodies in Thailand during the recent Disaster Victim Identification operation following the 2004 Tsunami.

A well-known case in Australian forensic history occurred in 1935 and involved the identification of a murder victim, James Smith, by a faded tattoo of two boxers on his right arm. The victim had been murdered and dismem-bered, and then dumped into the ocean off Sydney, where the arm was ingested by a passing tiger shark. The less-than-well shark subsequently disgorged the arm after its capture and is displayed at the Coogee Aquarium [43]. Figure 11.24 shows a putrefied hand from a murder victim in South Australia whose badly decomposed body was uncovered in sand dunes by a dog. He had been shot in

Fig. 11.23 A pig in a police
uniform with the letters
"ACAC"

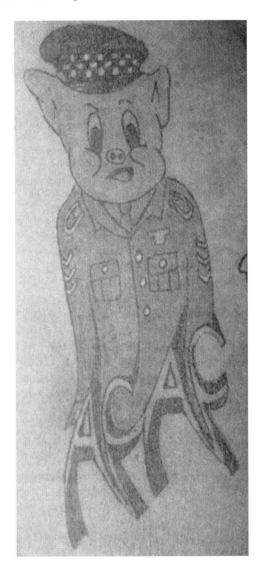

the head. The distinctive tattoo of a map of Australia with the word "love"
enabled presumptive identification to be made.

11.10 Conclusions

Encountering tattoos within the mortuary environment may be of more
value to the pathologist than just another interesting feature of the deceased.
Tattoos should be clearly described, with their location, type and major features

Fig. 11.24 A putrefied and
incomplete hand with a
clearly discernable tattoo
including a map of Australia

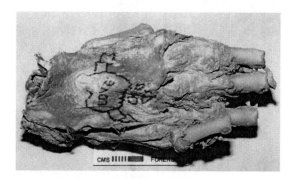

noted. Any text, names or dates should be recorded, and photographs taken of significant tattoos, particularly if there are issues with identification of the deceased. There is a wealth of information that can be gained by such investigations: the style and design may give an approximate age or cultural background; the design may be a custom piece that is able to be identified by an artist; easily identifiable designs such as military insignias or motor cycle club emblems may point to particular associations of the deceased and add background information to the case. Any designs in possible injection sites such as the cubital fossae should be closely investigated to exclude the disguising of venipuncture marks, and importantly, any persons exhibiting amateur tattoos should be treated with caution, as their infectious status may be questionable.

References

1. Macquarie Library (1985) The Macquarie Dictionary, 2 nd rev edn. The Macquarie Library, Sydney
2. Brown R (1868) The races of mankind being a popular description of the characteristics, manners and customs of the principal varieties of the human family, vol II. Cassell Petter amp; Galpin, London, p 53
3. Roberts TA, Ryan SA (2002) Tattooing and high risk behaviours in adolescents. Pediatrics 110:1058–1063
4. Caplan J (1997) 'Speaking scars': the tattoo in popular practice and medico-legal debate in nineteenth-century Europe. Hist Workshop J 44:107–142
5. Kuczkowski KM (2003) Diagnostic tattoo in a parturient with ecstasy use. Anaesthesia 58:1251–1252
6. Green T (2003) The tattoo encyclopedia, a guide to choosing your tattoo. Simon amp; Schuster, New York
7. Sperry K (1991) Tattoos and tattooing. Part 1. History and methodology. Am J Forensic Med Path 12:313–319
8. Hansen JPH, Melgaard J, Nordqvist J (1985) The mummies of Qilakitsoq. National Geographic 167:191–207
9. Murphy WA, Nedden D, Gostner P, Knapp R, Recheis W, Seidler H (2003) The iceman: discovery and imaging. Radiology 226:614–629
10. Swift B (2004) Body art and modification. In: Rutty GN (ed.) Essentials of autopsy practice: recent advances, topics and developments. Springer, London, pp 159–186

11. Armstrong ML, Gabriel DC (1993) Tattoos on women: marks of distinction or abomination? Dermatol Nurs 5:107–113
12. Langlois NEI, Little D (2005) Tattoos, medico-legal significance. In: Payne-James J, Byard RW, Corey TS, Henderson C (eds) The encyclopedia of forensic and legal medicine, vol 4. Elsevier, Amsterdam, pp 263–268
13. Plomley NJB (1983) The Baudin expedition and the Tasmanian aborigines 1802. Blubber Head Press, Hobart
14. Pozgain I, Barkic J, Filakovic P, Koic O (2004) Tattoo and personality traits in Croatian veterans. Yons Med J 45:300–305
15. Raspa RF, Cusak J (1990) Psychiatric implications of tattoos. Am Fam Physician 41:1481–1486
16. Picton B (1971) Murder, suicide or accident. The forensic pathologist at work. Robert Hale and Company, London
17. Spear SL, Arias J (1995) Long-term experience with nipple – areola tattooing. Ann Plast Surg 35:232–236
18. Tsur H, Kaplan HY (1993) Camouflaging hairless areas on the male face by artistic tattoo. Plast Reconstr Surg 92:357–360
19. Anastas CN, McGhee CN, Webber SK, Bryce IG (1995) Corneal tattooing revisited: excimer laser in the treatment of unsightly leukomata. Aust NZ J Opthalmol 23:227–230
20. Shatz BA, Thavorides V (1991) Colonic tattoo for follow-up of endoscopic sessile polypectomy. Gastrointest Endosc 37:59–60
21. Balogou AA, Dodzro KC, Grunitzky EK (2000) Traditional tattoos with neurological diseases in Togo. Bull Soc Path Exot 93:361–364
22. Barclay P, King H (2002) Tattoo medi-alert. Anaesthesia 57:625
23. Juhl MH (1997) A tattoo in time: I want my last wish to be clearly visible so it will be honoured by the doctor who treats me. Newsweek 130:19
24. O'Neil M, Dubrey SW, Grocott-Mason R (2003) An unusual tattoo. Heart 89:474
25. Iverson KV (1992) The 'no-code' tattoo – an ethical dilemma. West J Med 156:309–312
26. Kim JJ (1991) A cultural psychiatric study on tattoos of young Korean males. Yons Med J 32:255–262
27. ApplebyJJ (1991) Implications of tattoos. Am Fam Physic 43:1162–1163
28. Stephens MB (2003) Behavioral risks associated with tattooing. Fam Med 35:52–54
29. Carroll ST, Riffenburgh RH, Roberts TA, Myhre EB (2002) Tattoos and body piercings as indicators of adolescent risk-taking behaviours. Pediatrics 109:1021–1027
30. Avery DL, Spyker JM (1977) Foot tattoo of neonatal mice. Lab Anim Sci 27:110–112
31. Casper JL (1861) A handbook of the practice of forensic medicine, vol.1. New Sydenham Society, London, p 109
32. Friedman T, Westreich M, Mozes SN, Dorenbaum A, Herman O (2003) Tattoo pigment in lymph nodes mimicking metastatic malignant melanoma. Plast Reconstr Surg 111:2120–2122
33. Long GE, Rickman LS (1994) Infectious complications of tattoos. Clin Infect Dis 18:610–619
34. Nishioka S de A, Gyorkos TW, MacLean JD (2002) Tattoos and transfusion transmitted disease risk: implications for the screening of blood donors in Brazil. Braz J Infect Dis 6:172–180
35. Makkai T, McAllister I (2001) Prevalence of tattooing and body piercing in the Australian community. Commun Dis Intell 25:67–72
36. Ghorpade A (2002) Inoculation (tattoo) leprosy: a report of 31 cases. J Eur Dermatol Venereol 16:494–499
37. Jacob CI (2002) Tattoo-associated dermatoses: a case report and review of the literature. Dermatol Surg 28:962–965
38. Leggiadro RJ, Boscamp JR, Sapadin AN (2003) Temporary tattoo dermatitis. J Pediatrics 142:586

39. Mortimer NJ, Chave TA, Johnston GA (2003) Red tattoo reactions Clin Exper Dermatol 28:508–510
40. Papageorgiou PP, Hongcharu W, Chu AC (1999) Systemic sarcoidosis presenting with multiple tattoo granulomas and an extra-tattoo cutaneous granuloma. J Eur Acad Dermatol Venereol 12:51–53
41. Khan IU, Moiemen NS, Firth J, Frame JD (1999) Malignant melanoma disguised by a tattoo. Br J Plast Surg 52:598
42. Douglas MJ, Swenerton JE (2002) Epidural anaesthesia in three patients with lumbar tattoos: a review of possible implications. Can J Anaes 49:1057–1060
43. Coppleston VM (1968) Shark attack. Pacific Books, Melbourne, pp 14–22

Part VII
Serial Murder

Chapter 12
The Interaction, Roles, and Responsibilities of the FBI Profiler and the Forensic Pathologist in the Investigation of Serial Murder

Tracey S. Corey, David T. Resch and Mark A. Hilts

Contents

Abstract Of the many challenges facing the law enforcement community, one of the most difficult is the investigation of serial murder cases since these are high-profile, resource intensive investigations that provide unique challenges to the investigators. In addition, it is not uncommon for serial murder cases to extend across multiple jurisdictions, creating communication, investigation, and prosecution problems. The motivations of serial killers can be complex, and are more likely to be related to internal fantasies or desires, than to more traditional motivations such as financial gain. FBI Special Agents assigned to the *Behavioral Analysis Units of the National Center for Analysis of Violent Crime* are regularly called upon for assistance in the investigation of serial murder. A close working relationship between the medical examiner and forensic pathologist, respectively, with the primary investigator is essential to overcome challenges associated with investigating serial murder. In many serial homicide cases, the last activities and

T.S. Corey
University of Louisville, School of Medicine and Office of the Kentucky Medical Examiner, Louisville, KY
e-mail: traceyscorey@aol.com

M. Tsokos (ed.), *Forensic Pathology Reviews, Volume 5*,
doi: 10.1007/978-1-59745-110-9_12, © Humana Press, Totowa, NJ 2008

whereabouts of the victim are not known. In such cases, when a body is discovered, the forensic pathologist may be able to assist in determining final activities or events. In certain instances, the forensic pathologist may shed light on activities during the interval between disappearance and body discovery by analysis of findings such as stomach contents, and comparison of these findings with verifiable known accounts of the decedent's activities in the period immediately preceding the disappearance. Investigatively and behaviourally, these findings will provide essential information regarding the window of opportunity that the offender had to commit the murder, as well as other important information, such as whether the offender kept the victim alive for a period of time before killing her/him.

Keywords Serial murder · Criminal investigative analysis · Serial homicide · Criminal profiling · Behavioral analysis unit · Forensic pathology

12.1 Introduction

Of the many challenges facing the law enforcement community, one of the most difficult is the investigation of serial murder cases. These are high-profile, resource intensive, time-sensitive investigations that, while relatively rare compared to the total number of murders, provide many unique challenges to the investigators charged with their resolution.

From a case management perspective, multiple homicide cases committed by a common offender will drain resources more quickly than the same number of cases committed by different offenders. For example, in addition to the usual duties of investigators, medical examiners, crime scene personnel, and laboratory resources in a murder case, in a serial murder investigation, all information and evidence must be intercompared. Victims must be studied to determine where their lives may have intersected with the offender. Forensic evidence must be compared between crime scenes. Injury patterns must be determined and analyzed by the medical examiner. The sheer volume of information and leads that develop in a serial murder case often overwhelm traditional case management techniques. It is not uncommon for serial murder cases to extend across multiple jurisdictions, creating communication, investigation, and prosecution problems. Dealing with the intense media and public attention that accompanies serial murder cases can drain additional time and resources. The pressure to resolve the cases before another victim is killed places tremendous strain on the members of the investigative team [1].

In addition to issues related to the sheer volume of work created by multiple cases, serial murders are generally different from most murder cases in other ways that can serve to frustrate traditional investigative methods. The motivations of serial killers can be complex, and are more likely to be related to internal fantasies or desires, than to more traditional motivations such as financial gain. Serial murder cases are predatory and premeditated in nature, and lack the interpersonal conflict and provocation common in many non-serial offenses. In most serial murder cases there is no prior relationship between the killer and his victims [2].

Even more unique challenges are presented when the serial murder investigation encompasses medical/extended care professionals, infanticide, and poisoners. The reality may indeed exist that law enforcement will lack recognition of the series until identified by other professionals, such as medical examiners.

FBI special agents assigned to the *Behavioral Analysis Units of the National Center for Analysis of Violent Crime* (NCAVC), commonly referred to as FBI profilers, are regularly called upon for assistance in the investigation of violent crimes, including serial murder. Additionally, some state agencies and some local agencies, have personnel trained through the *International Criminal Investigative Analysis Fellowship*, which evolved from the FBI *Police Fellowship Training Program*. A close working relationship between the medical examiner, the primary investigator, and profiler is essential to overcome the aforementioned challenges associated with investigating serial murder. The profiler and the medical examiner, when faced with a series of murders, must each have a good working knowledge of the strengths and limitations of the other's field of study, to understand how to maximize the investigative tools available. Further, ideally, the medical examiner and profiler work hand-in-hand through the development of a case – such "real-time" cooperative efforts allow the fullest utilization of investigative possibilities as the case develops. Unfortunately, time constraints, geographic and jurisdictional limitations, and delayed identification of the serial nature of a string of homicides often result in the process being undertaken in a more retrospective and disjointed fashion. Even if a case or series has not been worked jointly from the outset, a collaborative review by the profiler and medical examiner may result in a fresh approach to a particular series which often leads to the development of new investigative strategies or thought processes – this may result in the recognition of previously overlooked evidence or patterns which may aid in the resolution of a particular case or series.

12.2 Criminal Investigative Analysis

The FBI defines *Criminal Investigative Analysis* (CIA) as the process of reviewing and assessing the facts of a criminal act, and interpreting offender behavior and interaction with the victim and the environment, as exhibited during the commission of the crime [1]. The premise of CIA is that the method and manner in which a crime is committed relates directly to the personality of the offender. CIA is not a substitute for a thorough, well-executed investigation. Good fundamental police work solves crimes. Rather, CIA is one of many tools available to the investigator faced with an unsolved homicide, or a series of unsolved homicides. The exchange of information regarding autopsy and crime scene findings, and the communication between the medical examiner and the profiler facilitates the CIA process [3].

The responsible profiler will take into account the totality of the known circumstances prior to rendering an opinion. This should include a review of all available case information, to include autopsy reports, police reports, crime scene sketches, media releases, maps, photographs (crime scene, autopsy, aerial, etc.), demographic data, and any other relevant information. The medical examiner's evaluation and autopsy protocol provide valuable insight into victimology and offender behavior. A consultation involving the profiler, the forensic pathologist, and the lead investigator is the best method to ensure complete understanding and integration of all information available. This consultation should be undertaken after each has had the opportunity to review all available reports. Situations and time constraints often prevent face to face meetings. In these instances, a thorough and complete review of all reports is essential.

CIA in a serial murder investigation often provides a better understanding of the offense, including the motivation of the offender, the victim selection process, and the crime scene dynamics. Additionally, in serial murder cases where there is no physical evidence linking a common offender, CIA may provide a behavioral linkage. Another function of CIA, in support of serial murder investigations, is the development of an unknown offender profile. The development of this profile is based upon the premise that the criminal's behavior exhibited at a crime scene will also be present in other areas of the criminal's life. The offender's personality characteristics will be reflected in the interaction of the offender with the victim and the environment [4]. If behavior at the crime scene is a reflection of the offender, then through the process of reviewing and assessing the facts of a criminal act and interpreting the interactions, the profiler may project a composite of an unknown offender through the description of certain traits and characteristics, which may include:

- Gender
- Age/maturity
- Criminal sophistication/criminal history
- Race/ethnicity
- Intelligence/education
- Employment status and skills
- Living circumstances
- Interpersonal relationships
- Personal fantasy

The CIA process is most useful for identifying a behavioral composite in an unknown offender when the crime involves a significant amount of interaction between the offender and the victim, as well as the offender and the crime scene. Crimes that involve fantasy-based, need-driven behavior such as postmortem manipulation, sadism, ritual behavior, exploration, sexual assault, staging, overkill, and evisceration are examples of behaviorally rich crimes. This unknown offender profile may assist in focusing the investigation in the direction of the most likely offender [5].

The responsible profiler only renders opinions when he has the necessary information, ideally taking into account the totality of circumstances surrounding the crime. Presenting a "threshold assessment," to the investigator or the media, is irresponsible and can be extremely detrimental to the investigation. The information obtained from the medical examiner is extremely useful to the thorough criminal investigative analysis.

12.3 Forensic Pathology in Serial Murder Investigation

12.3.1 Interaction of Law Enforcement and Pathologists

The forensic pathologist may assist investigators and profilers in the analysis of serial homicide by determining and/or defining:

- Cause, manner, and mechanism of death
- Pattern injuries
- Postmortem interval estimation
- Sequence of events and decedent activities
- Trace evidence collection and interpretation
- Identification of similarities and linkages in wound patterns and/or patterns of infliction of injury

Behaviorally, the profiler looks to the medical examiner for assistance in determining the nature, timing, and relative significance of injuries and trace evidence found on and about the corpus delicti. For example, is there evidence of a sexual assault? If so, how is that evidence manifested in the physical findings and biological samples collected? Is there evidence of vaginal, anal, or oral sexual assault? Is it possible to determine the temporal sequence of events of the attack? Is there physical evidence of the use of ligatures, even if ligatures are not present when the body is found? Are there superficial injuries consistent with torture and control? Is it possible to establish the order of injury infliction? Were some injuries inflicted postmortem? Is there evidence of removal of tissues, e.g., as souvenirs? Regarding the cause of death – would death have been quick? Is there evidence of postinjury survival? What actions would have been possible after the victim sustained various wounds? [6]. Knowledge of such details may be helpful in a number of investigative areas, including construction of a composite of the offender, development of media releases, and identification of link cases. Further, such information may be of use to identify themes when designing an interview strategy for the detective. For example, in 1994, a serial killer was operating in Miami, killing prostitutes and then dumping their bodies in nearby neighborhoods. The cause of death was identified as manual strangulation, with very little associated trauma, and almost no other injuries on most victims. In order to understand exactly how the offender was controlling and killing his victims, investigators and the local

FBI NCAVC coordinator met personally with the medical examiner. The medical examiner discussed his opinions, and demonstrated how he thought the killer was attacking. The medical examiner's opinion, that the offender was attacking from behind, was key to a better understanding of the killer and his actions, and was integrated in to the eventual profile prepared by the FBI.

12.3.2 Determination of Cause, Manner and Mechanism of Death

The determination of cause and manner of death in persons dying suddenly and unexpectedly represents the core of the practice of forensic pathology. The cause of death may be defined as the event, circumstance and/or disease process setting in motion the chain of events which ultimately culminates in the demise of the individual. In cases of known homicide, the forensic pathologist conducts a complete postmortem investigation in order to ascertain necessary facts and document physical findings to determine the cause of death. The causes of death in serial homicides are often linked to class characteristics of the victims. For instance, infant victims may be suffocated, and may be initially mistaken for sudden infant death syndrome (SIDS). A series of hospitalized murder victims may succumb to the purposeful administration of lethal injections of drugs or chemicals such as potassium. In both of these scenarios, it may be months or years before the serial nature of the deaths is recognized, and the homicidal manner of the deaths is properly identified.

Older children and adults succumbing to a serial killer in an average community setting may die from causes more easily recognized as violent; examples may include strangulation, beating, stabbing, and gunshot wounds. It is recognized that there is no "typical" serial murder, and serial murders may involve injuries ranging from subtle to disfiguring. The causes of death in serial homicide are myriad as well, ranging from minimal physical findings to immediately obvious trauma, including suffocation, sharp force injury, blunt force trauma, gunshot wounds and even electrocution. It is the role of the forensic pathologist to interpret the physical findings, in light of the historical information known and provided by investigators, to arrive at a logical and defensible opinion regarding the cause of death. Causes of death in serial murder are many, but in examining trends in large numbers of series, some generalizations emerge. First, many serial killers utilize a relatively consistent method of killing, which may evolve over time. The method used by the killer may be developed based on factors including:

- Motivation of the offender in the commission of the crime
- Experience, confidence, and criminal sophistication of the offender
- Physical characteristics of the offender and the victim
- Interaction between the offender and the victim
- Unexpected factors not anticipated by the offender [7]

The interplay of these various factors results in various causes of death and physical findings. This interplay is illustrated in two contrasting examples of serial killers: a mother who serially suffocates her young infants in their cribs over a period of years vs a man who serially abducts, rapes, and strangles prostitutes. Each is a serial killer, but the interaction of the perpetrator's characteristics, victim characteristics, and the perpetrator's motives result in a series with different physical findings and causes of death. Additionally, the identification and recognition of these cases as homicides will differ based in part on the nature of the physical findings (subtle vs blatant trauma), and the presentation of the victim (presenting at first as a suspected natural death vs immediate recognition of homicide by investigators).

The manner of death may be defined as the context or milieu in which the death occurs. For manner of death, there are five options:

- Natural
- Accident
- Homicide
- Suicide
- Undetermined

In medicolegal terms, the term "homicide" may be defined as *the intentional act of one leading to the death of another*. Note that the definition does not include any reference as to whether or not a criminal act occurred. This is not within the purview of the forensic pathologist, but rather should be determined independently by those within the criminal justice system – the investigators, the prosecutor, and the courts. Obviously, in cases of serial killings, the manner of death is homicide. However, in certain cases this may not be immediately apparent, especially in deaths involving suffocation of weak or debilitated individuals, or homicides caused by toxins. With some types of serial homicides, including serial infanticide and serial poisonings, the manner of death as homicide may not be apparent until several deaths are identified as related and suspicious.

The mechanism of death refers to the physiologic derangement, or pathophysiologic process that occurs within the body during the process of the death. Examples of mechanisms of death include cardiac arrhythmias, cardiovascular collapse and exsanguination. Understanding the mechanism of death may allow the pathologist to assess more accurately the case for possible causes of death, especially in cases of poisoning. Sometimes the signs and symptoms involved in the mechanism of death may be elucidated by review of medical records, and may suggest possible causes of death. In cases of serial killings in the hospital setting, the recognition of repeated patterns of mechanisms of death may precede recognition of the actual causes of death and the serial nature of the deaths. An example would be the recognition of signs and symptoms associated with hyperkalemia prior to the determination of an exogenous, injected source of potassium, and the retrospective identification of other deaths in the same institution due to the intentional injection of potassium chloride.

12.3.3 Pattern Injuries

A pattern injury may be defined as an injury in which the size and/or shape and/or contour correspond to a portion of the object which created it, a contour of the body, or a combination thereof. Recognition of pattern injuries by the forensic pathologist may be of crucial importance in the investigation of serial killings. An assailant may choose to use a certain type of instrument, or even the same instrument repeatedly. Recognition of patterns left by such instruments may allow the forensic pathologist to be the first investigator to link cases. This is especially true in areas in which many law enforcement jurisdictions feed into a single medical examiners office. If bodies are recovered from various areas, the medical examiner's office may represent the only common investigative agency.

Regarding pattern injuries, in general, impact with the same surface of a rigid object multiple times will leave relatively uniform patterns on the body. Assessment of these patterns may allow delineation of the instrument involved. It is important for the forensic pathologist to adequately document pattern injuries in multiple forms, including photographic, diagrammatic, and verbal form. As the professional tasked with the identification of the physical characteristics and evidence on the body, the forensic pathologist may be able to identify and recognize other patterns as well that may provide profilers with information necessary to behaviorally link cases. An example of a pattern of evidence placement is the placement of foreign bodies in orifices in multiple victims. Another example is the identification of similar ligatures and knots thereof in serial victims of bindings and/or strangulation. A third example is the linkage of multiple gunshot wound victims to a single weapon by recovery of the bullets at autopsy and examination by a firearms expert, as in the Washington DC sniper case.

In some cases, relatively superficial wounds may be more important from a forensic standpoint than the wound that actually caused the death. Examples of superficial wounds with greater forensic importance include patterns from torture prior to being killed by a gunshot wound. Evidence of torture and excessive bindings may lead the profiler to reach a conclusion regarding the presence of sexual sadism among the offender's motivations. Such a finding may lead to solid investigative suggestions, such as the inclusion of collateral material related to offender fantasy in search warrant applications, and the development of interview themes that take into account offender motivation.

12.3.4 Postmortem Interval Estimation

12.3.4.1 Early Postmortem Period

Factors to be assessed in the estimation of the time of death in the early postmortem period may include the following:

- Rigor mortis
- Livor mortis
- Vitreous potassium concentration
- Body temperature
- Early decomposition patterns
- Stomach contents
- Date and time last reliably known alive

With the exception of the last element listed above, these indicators for time of death in the early postmortem interval are highly variable, and depend on a number of factors which are not known, and cannot be controlled in an individual case. Most of these factors are essentially dependent on the conditions of the environment in which the body rests after death. The sooner the pathologist is notified of the case, and has an opportunity to examine the body, the more accurate the estimation may be. If time of death is of extreme importance in the investigation, this information should be immediately conveyed to the pathologist. If time, geographic constraints, and local procedures allow, a visit to the scene of death and/or body discovery will provide the pathologist with an opportunity for direct assessment of the postmortem factors such as rigor mortis, temperature, and lividity.

12.3.4.2 Later Postmortem Period

As decomposition continues, especially in outdoor scenes, the direct involvement of a forensic pathologist (with a forensic anthropologist as timing and availability allow) in the body recovery process becomes essential for proper and thorough evidence recovery. As decomposition with insect infestation and skeletonization proceed, the forensic pathologist may defer opinions regarding the postmortem interval to other forensic experts – specifically the forensic anthropologist and forensic entomologist. If insect activity is present and the determination of the postmortem interval is deemed a critical segment of the investigation, the forensic pathologist should contact a forensic entomologist as early as possible in the process, preferably before the scene is processed. Such early consultation will allow direct input and guidance by the entomologist regarding preferences of scene assessment and evidence documentation, recovery, and preservation.

12.4 Determination of Activities of Decedent

In many serial homicide cases, the last activities and whereabouts of the victim are not known – the victim is simply noted to be missing after failing to appear at a family, social, or occupational obligation. In such cases, when a body is discovered, the forensic pathologist may be able to assist in determining final activities or events. In certain instances, the forensic pathologist may shed light on activities during the interval between disappearance and body discovery by analysis of findings such as stomach contents, and comparison of these findings with verifiable known accounts of the decedent's activities in the period immediately preceding the disappearance. Investigatively and behaviorally, these findings will provide essential information regarding the window of opportunity that the offender had to commit the murder, as well as other important information, such as whether the offender kept the victim alive for a period of time before killing her/him.

Collection of a biological samples kit (often referred to as a "rape kit") may provide physical evidence linking the killer to the victim. Such physical evidence may also allow the identification of a serial crime, by linking the same perpetrator to multiple victims. Evidence collected during to biological samples examination and collection may include semen, hairs, and saliva. Even in cases in which the victim appears to be fully clothed, and without evidence of genital trauma, the biological samples kit should be collected. There are numerous cases in which the victim was redressed following the sexual assault, and in which there are no physical signs of genital trauma despite the recovery of biological evidence of sexual assault in the form of semen recovered from the vagina and/or rectum. Documentation of the state of the victim's clothing at the time of body discovery may allow identification of subtle clues. In the experience of one of the authors (T.S.C.), a young woman was abducted and murdered after developing engine trouble during an interstate trip. Her body was found several days after her abduction. When her body was discovered along the side of an interstate highway, she appeared to be fully dressed. But careful observation of the state of the clothing revealed subtle abnormalities, including twisting of the bra-strap. Despite the absence of physical injury to the genital region, the biological samples collection revealed the presence of semen, and it was this evidence that physically linked the perpetrator (an interstate commercial trucker) to the victim.

In some high profile cases, the state of digestion of stomach contents has played a prominent role in the investigation and courtroom presentation of the case. Gastric emptying times normally show average time intervals for small and large meals. But caution must be exercised when applying such general studies to a particular case. Stress may significantly alter the normal time course for such biological functions.

In victims displaying multiple wounds, the forensic pathologist may, in certain instances, be able to ascertain what activities or actions could be performed after sustaining the wounds, and further offer opinions regarding estimation of the post injury survival interval.

12.5 Collection of Trace Evidence

12.5.1 Cases in Which the Body is Discarded

In cases of serial homicide in which the victim bodies are discarded by the killer, collection of trace evidence may provide the necessary and essential link between cases. This link may come in the form of trace evidence such as carpet fibers, hairs, or even paint flecks. It is the responsibility of the forensic pathologist to insure that the body is handled and processed in a stepwise and thorough fashion to facilitate identification, collection, and maintenance of chain of custody of such evidence.

Ideally, the forensic pathologist will be able to attend the scene of body discovery and begin the search for, and maintenance of, trace evidence at that time. The manner in which this is conducted will vary greatly and is dictated by circumstances of the individual case. For example, a scene involving scattered skeletal elements will be processed in a different manner than a scene involving an intact body found in the early postmortem interval. Any items that are unlikely to survive the transport process should be collected at the scene. In general, clothing, ligatures, and other items are best left intact and in place on the body for examination at the autopsy suite. The hands and feet should be bagged in paper prior to the placement in the body bag. At the autopsy facility, the forensic pathologist will undertake a stepwise process of examining, documenting, removing, and cataloging all clothing and adherent trace evidence. Alternate light sources may be used to identify areas of dried secretions or fibers not easily detected with normal office lighting. Fingernail clippings and a standard biological sample kit (or rape kit) is collected when the state of preservation of the body permits. During the examination of the interior portion of the body, a DNA standard of the victim is collected and maintained. The use of a culposcope or other magnifying device may aid in the identification of trace evidence and small injuries.

12.5.2 In-hospital or In-home Deaths

In cases of suspected serial killings occurring in a home or hospital setting, the focus of trace evidence collection is different, as the suspected assailant will normally have interacted with the decedent in the environment. For instance, a mother suspected of serial suffocating her babies will of course have an innocent reasonable explanation for the presence of her hairs on the body or clothing of her baby. The focus of the type of trace evidence sought will therefore be different, and may include extensive testing of body fluids for the identification of possible exogenous substances such as electrolyte concentrations, and toxins.

12.6 Review of Wound Patterns

When a pattern of serial killing has been identified, the investigating law enforcement agency should gather all pertinent information regarding the death investigation and autopsy procedures of all known or suspected linked cases. Such cases may have been investigated by a number of different law enforcement agencies and forensic pathologists due to normal work schedule fluctuations, the passage of time, and the geographic location of the body at the time of discovery, and thus the jurisdiction of the investigating agency. The lead detective or task force members should collect and organize all death investigation documents and photographs, and submit these to a single forensic pathologist for a comprehensive review, along with the review by the profiler. Ideally these two reviews may be conducted simultaneously, with subsequent joint consultation by the profiler and the forensic pathologist with the lead investigator. The forensic pathologist working in concert with the profiler, may conduct a review of all cases, looking for similarities and patterns [8]. These pattern similarities may include:

- Physical attributes of the victims, specific pattern injuries linked to a particular instrument or type of instrument
- Patterns in the distribution of the wounds
- Body disposal methods
- Repetitive and/or consistent trace evidence (such as similarities in ligature materials or binding methods)

Other examples may include signature wound patterns or habits such as the placement of foreign bodies in orifices or unique pattern injuries such as paired electrical burns. A systematic comprehensive review of all cases by a single forensic pathologist, with review and consultation with the profiler may allow identification of previously undetected similarities in cases.

Quality death investigation is undertaken by a team of investigative professionals, each bringing their unique expertise and perspective to the investigative table. Such a cooperative endeavor maximizes the potential benefit of each specialty and promotes complete and comprehensive analysis of a particular series. The law enforcement investigator and the forensic pathologist each bring a unique set of investigative tools and perspectives to the case. Those rendering opinions without taking into account all available information and reasonable opportunities to consult with the medical examiner, run the risk of rendering a threshold assessment providing no positive input and possibly hindering efforts to apprehend the offender. The strengths of each investigative arm are maximized by an in depth "round table" discussion of each series. Using such a team approach, the attributes of each investigative perspective are potentiated by the input of the others.

References

1. Johns LG, Downes GF, Bible CD (2005) Resurrecting cold case serial homicide investigations. FBI Law Enforcement Bulletin 8/05. Federal Bureau of Investigation, Washington, D.C.
2. Brantley AC, Kosky RH (2005) Serial murder in the Netherlands: a look at motivation, behavior, and characteristics. FBI Law Enforcement Bulletin 1/05. Federal Bureau of Investigation, Washington, D.C.

3. Ankrom LG (2002) Criminal investigative analysis. Miscellaneous Publication of the FBI's National Center for the Analysis of Violent Crime, Department of Justice, Washington, D.C.
4. Hazelwood RR, Warren JI (2004) Linkage analysis: modus operandi, ritual, and signature in serial sexual crime, Aggression and violent behavior 9. Elsevier
5. Morton RJ, Lord WD (2005) Criminal profiling. In: Payne-James J, Byard RW, Corey TS, Henderson C (eds) Encyclopedia of forensic and legal medicine. Elsevier Academic Press, Amsterdam, pp 51–55
6. Safarik ME, Jarvis JP (2005) Examining attributes of homicides: toward quantifying qualitative values of injury severity. Homicide studies 9:183–203
7. Douglas JE, Munn C (1992) Violent crime scene analysis, modus operandi, signature, and staging. FBI Law Enforcement Bulletin 2/92. Federal Bureau of Investigation, Washington, D.C.
8. DiMaio VJ, DiMaio D (2001) Forensic pathology, 2nd edn. CRC Press, New York, N.Y.

Part VIII
Forensic Histopathology

Chapter 13
Forensic Histopathology

Gilbert Lau and Siang Hui Lai

Contents

Abstract   Forensic histopathology is the application of histological techniques and examination to forensic pathology practice. It is a unique and specialised aspect of pathology practice. This chapter highlights several differences in forensic histopathology practice compared to clinical and surgical histopathology practice. The various roles of microscopic tissue examination in forensic pathology practice are categorised and discussed. These are in relation to definitive pathological diagnosis, confirmation of equivocal and occult pathology, serving as a form of permanent record, and providing invaluable material for education and research. Case examples are included to illustrate the impact of routine histological examinations, special stain techniques, as well as

G. Lau
Centre for Forensic Medicine, Health Sciences Authority, Singapore
e-mail: gilbert_lau@hsa.gov.sg

M. Tsokos (ed.), *Forensic Pathology Reviews, Volume 5,*
doi: 10.1007/978-1-59745-110-9_13, © Humana Press, Totowa, NJ 2008

immunohistochemistry where appropriate, towards relevant pathological diagnoses, which may or may not be directly relevant to the establishment of the cause of death. Lastly, the chapter also aims to highlight some recent advances as well as the challenges ahead in this field.

Keywords Forensic histopathology · Surgical pathology · Immunohistochemistry · Sudden death · Iatrogenic death

13.1 Introduction

The application of histological techniques and examination in forensic pathology is an unique and specialised aspect of pathology practice. Compared to clinical histopathology practice, in which similar techniques are applied, there are several notable differences. First, the nature of specimens varies significantly between forensic pathology practice and clinical histopathology practice. In clinical histopathology practice, specimens and biopsies generally comprise parts, fragments, or segments of various organs, and diagnoses are made from histological sections of tissues obtained through targeted sampling of the specimens, usually after adequate fixation. In contrast, the forensic pathologist routinely examines organs in their entirety and, in the first instance, in their unfixed state. The organs are quite often already in varying stages of autolysis and putrefaction. The starting point of histological sampling and examination is different from the outset. Second, the spectrum of organ and tissue examination varies between clinical histopathology practice and forensic pathology practice. In histopathology practice, small biopsies of the breasts, the aerodigestive tract, the female genital tract, etc. form an integral part of the workload. Biopsies of the many organs such as the heart, lungs, liver, brain, and kidneys often fall into areas of sub-specialised histopathology practice. In contrast, the forensic pathologist routinely examines entire hearts, lungs, livers, brain, and kidneys albeit with slightly a different focus and emphasis. While the breasts, intestines, and lymph nodes are also examined, less attention would be given to those compared to the major organs that are more often associated with the cause of death. The ability to identify macroscopic pathology in unfixed whole organs is an essential prerequisite in forensic pathology practice. Having said that, it is, naturally and nevertheless, necessary for the forensic pathologist to be able to recognise pathology in all organs, properly examine and report on them. Third, the emphasis of histological examination of surgical and clinical specimens is on diagnosis and prognostication. Marginal clearance in surgical specimens for neoplastic lesions is of vital importance in planning further and subsequent management. Specific grading, refined typing and classification of various neoplasms are also of primary significance in treatment and prognosis. In contrast, the main aim in the forensic postmortem examination is to properly determine the cause of death. Often the cause of death is obvious after macroscopic examination without any histological input. In these cases, all other factors, including incidental pathologies, may be considered to be of secondary or academic significance.

Therefore, in forensic pathology practice, it is often unnecessary to undertake comprehensive tissue sampling of the major parenchymatous organs for histology in order to arrive at a precise cause of death. However, histological examination does have significant impact in several instances.

13.2 The Roles of Histology in Forensic Pathology Practice

The major roles of histology in forensic practice are as follows:

1. As a primary ancillary investigation in cases where macroscopic examinations fail to yield a specific or diagnostic pathology that accounts for death
2. To confirm and refine macroscopic diagnoses including incidental pathologies identified at autopsy
3. To confirm or refute antemortem diagnosis and clinical suspicions
4. To evaluate medical and surgical interventions as a means of medical audit
5. As a form of permanent documentation of pathologies identified at autopsy
6. As an essential source of material for medical undergraduate and postgraduate teaching
7. As a source of research

The authors recommend the practice of routine sampling of major parenchymatous organs such as the heart, lungs, liver, and kidneys for histological examination. At the very least, this could sharpen the forensic pathologist's approach in correlating macroscopic pathology, observed or suspected, with microscopic pathology.

In the following sections, the roles of histological analysis in routine forensic pathology practice are illustrated.

13.2.1 To Establish the Cause of Death

The determination of the definitive cause of death may depend on elucidating the histological features of inapparent or equivocal macroscopic lesions. In these cases, the lack of definitive pathology or the presence of borderline pathology requires ancillary confirmation for diagnosis. Examples include sudden deaths due to viral myocarditis, where the cellular response may be focal or patchy, rather than diffuse.

In cases of maternal deaths, amniotic fluid embolism is confirmed by the demonstration of the components of amniotic fluid within the pulmonary microvasculature and occasionally in other organs, such as the kidneys and liver. Epithelial squames, mucin, vernix caseosa (appearing as fat) and occasionally, lanugo hair can be most profitably identified by means of the Attwood's stain (for squames and mucin) or, if necessary, by immunohistochemical epithelial markers (e.g., AE1/3, Cam 5.2, LP34, CK 7, CK 20).

In disseminated intravascular coagulation, the detection of microscopic fibrin thrombi (aided by use of Martius Scarlet Blue or phosphotungstic acid hematoxylin [PTAH]), primarily within the pulmonary microvasculature and the renal glomeruli, is essential to establish the diagnosis.

In the recent epidemic of severe acute respiratory distress syndrome (SARS), histological examination contributed to the final diagnosis of a severe infectious disease caused by a novel coronavirus.

Histological examination of the lungs of SARS cases showed diffuse alveolar damage with varying degrees of organisation. There were associated cytopathological changes such as cytological atypia of pneumocytes, syncytial change, and giant cell formation. These were noted in deceased patients who had spent a longer period in intensive care units and there undergone mechanical ventilation (Fig. 13.1).

The SARS coronavirus was identified in the cytoplasm of alveolar lining cells by in-situ hybridisation using the oligonucleotide probe for the nuclear capsid region of the virus (Fig. 13.2).

Case #1: Sudden death due to acute viral myocarditis in a previously healthy 12-year-old girl A 12-year-old girl was brought to the emergency department in a state of collapse. Resuscitation was unsuccessful. The deceased's parents volunteered that she was previously healthy, but had apparently suffered from fever and headache for the past few days.

At autopsy, there were no obvious macroscopic pathological findings that could account for death. The main finding was non-specific acute pulmonary edema. The cause of death was left unascertained, pending further investigations. Histological examination of the heart, however, revealed a dense and florid inflammatory infiltrate comprising mainly lymphocytes within the myocardium. This was associated with necrosis of the myocardial fibres. The features were diagnostic of acute viral (lymphocytic) myocarditis (Fig. 13.3);

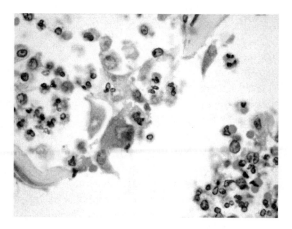

Fig. 13.1 Cytological atypia of the bronchial epithelium in the lungs of a SARS case (H&E ×1000). Reprinted with permission from Archives of Pathology & Laboratory Medicine. Copyright 2006. College of American Pathologists

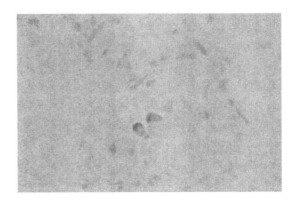

Fig. 13.2 Marking of coronavirus infected cells in the lungs by in-situ hybridisation using oligonucleotide probe for the nuclear capsid antigen of the virus. Reprinted with permission from Archives of Pathology & Laboratory Medicine. Copyright 2006. College of American Pathologists

histologically, the heart showed moderate and diffuse lymphocytic infiltration of the myocardium associated with myonecrolysis.

13.2.2 To Confirm and Refine the Diagnosis of Macroscopic Pathological Lesions

13.2.2.1 Confirmation of Macroscopic Pathological Lesions

At autopsy, pathology could present in several ways other than being quite occult as in the cases illustrated earlier. Lesions could be identified, suspected, or incidental. Not uncommonly, the macroscopic features of lesions such as bronchopneumonia, myocardial infarction, tuberculosis, pneumoconiosis (e.g., asbestosis, silicosis berylliosis, siderosis) or malignant tumours (e.g., mesothelioma, lymphoma) may be either equivocal or insufficiently specific for their comprehensive characterisation. In such instances, postmortem histopathology may contribute substantially to their evaluation.

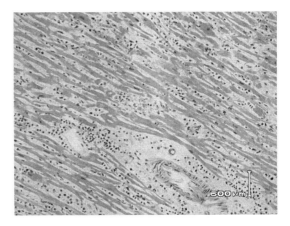

Fig. 13.3 Case #1: Viral myocarditis with marked lymphocytic infiltrate within the myocardium, accompanied by necrosis of the myocardial fibres (H&E ×400)

Fig. 13.4 Small, almost
innocuous, dry blister on
the finger

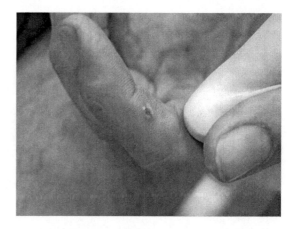

Figures 13.4 and 13.5 illustrate the macroscopic and microscopic features of
a suspicious electrical burn.

**Case #2: Sudden death due to acute pulmonary embolism by right atrial
myxoma** A 27-year-old female was admitted to hospital because of a three
week history of fever. Investigations revealed elevated erythrocyte sedimenta-
tion rate (ESR) of 93 mm/h. The level of C-reactive protein (CRP) was also
markedly elevated at 40.4 mg/L. However, there was no leukocytosis and
differential counts were within reference ranges. Microbiological and serol-
ogical investigations aiming at identifying a specific microorganism were
consistently negative. She was discharged after a few days with a diagnosis of
viral fever. Approximately one week later, she was found dead at home.

Autopsy revealed multiple jelly-like tumour fragments choked within the
main pulmonary artery, the right and left pulmonary arteries, as well as the
lobar pulmonary arterial tree of both lungs. The main tumour was a polypoid
jelly-like red fleshy mass that was attached to the right atrial wall, measuring
$4.0 \times 3.5 \times 3.0$ cm (Fig. 13.6).

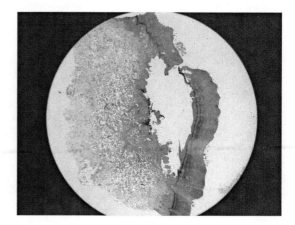

Fig. 13.5 The edges and
floor of the blister shown in
Fig. 13.4 expressed typical
features of electrothermal
damage (H&E × 40)

Fig. 13.6 Case #2: Friable, fleshy and jelly-like polypoid tumour attached to the medial wall of the right atrium

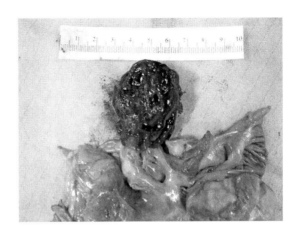

Fig. 13.6 Case #2: Friable, fleshy and jelly-like polypoid tumour attached to the medial wall of the right atrium

Microscopic examination of the tumour showed two components. The first was stellate or spindle myxoma cells containing moderate amounts of eosinophilic cytoplasm, occasionally forming perivascular aggregates. The second component was glandular elements lined by cuboidal epithelium containing cytoplasm that stained positive with mucicarmine, PAS-diastase and Alcian blue. The epithelial elements were surrounded by an expansive myxoid stroma showing large areas of hemorrhage. There were areas of fibrin and haemosiderin deposition within the stroma (Fig. 13.7).

The features were those of a right atrial myxoma that had fragmented and embolised into the pulmonary arterial tree, causing death from fatal acute pulmonary tumour embolism.

Case #3: Confirmation of Alzheimer's disease The deceased was a 77-year-old lady with a medical history of Alzheimer's disease. She was found collapsed at home in the bathroom and was conveyed to the emergency department in a state of collapse. Resuscitative attempts were unsuccessful.

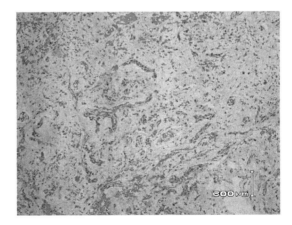

Fig. 13.7 Case #2: Microscopic examination of the tumour revealed scattered myxoma cells and glandular elements present within an expansive myxoid stroma. Areas of fibrin and hemosiderin deposition were noted in some areas (H&E ×100)

Fig. 13.8 Case #3: Numerous neuritic plaques are present in the brain (Bielchowski ×200)

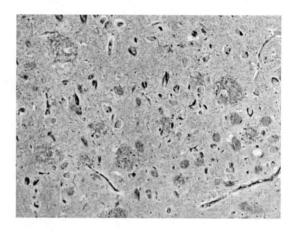

Autopsy revealed the cause of death to be due to bronchopneumonia. The brain weight was 1210 g. Microscopic examination showed neuronal loss and gliosis associated with many neuritic plaques and intraneuronal fibrillary tangles. These were noted using standard haematoxylin and eosin (H&E) staining, but were better demonstrated with the use of the Bielchowski technique (Figs. 13.8 and 13.9). The lesions were found in many areas of the brain including the hippocampi and cerebral cortices. The histological features supported the clinical antemortem diagnosis of Alzheimer's disease.

13.2.2.2 Histological Ageing of Lesions

The histological ageing of lesions permits the pathologist to ascertain whether a particular lesion or injury is consistent with been inflicted or sustained within an alleged time frame. Common examples include the following.

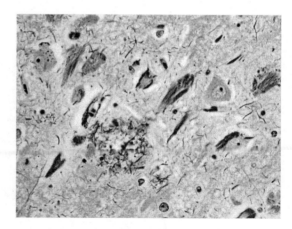

Fig. 13.9 Case #3: A neuritic plaque and intraneuronal fibrillary tangles at higher magnification (Bielchowski ×400)

Ageing of Wounds

The ageing of wounds (determination of wound age – e.g., incised wounds and lacerations) can be problematic as there may be much variation in the appearance of the inflammatory and histochemical changes which attend these injuries. Generally, polymorphonuclear and mononuclear infiltrates may be seen after 8 and 16 h, respectively. Earlier lesions may be aged by means of enzyme histochemistry on fresh frozen tissue specimens stained for histamine and serotonin (within the first hour of wounding), followed by adenosine triphosphatase and esterase (later than 1 h of wounding), aminopeptidase (2 h), acid phosphatase (4 h) and alkaline phosphatase (8 h) [1].

Subdural Hematoma

The wound age of recent and chronic subdural hemorrhage can be determined by a variety of histological criteria, namely those established by Munro and Merritt [2]. Much like the ageing of cerebral contusions, this is seldom a straightforward matter, but these criteria, although not absolute, may serve as useful guidelines particularly with respect to the temporal relation between the injury and alleged battery, homicide, or accident.

Pulmonary Thromboembolism

The forensic importance of estimating the age of pulmonary thromboembolism in relation to traumatic injury of the lower limbs, as well as significant or severe trauma to other parts of the body (as in the aftermath of a road accident), is evident. In this respect, it is essential that the residual or remaining deep venous thrombi, which are usually lodged within the deep veins of the lower limbs or the iliac veins, rather than the embolus per se, are examined as it is the evaluation of the thrombo-endothelial junction that provides useful chronological information (Fig. 13.10) [1].

Myocardial Infarction

Myocardial infarcts may supervene in instances of alleged battery or homicide, or may complicate injuries sustained in an accident. The ageing of myocardial infarction involves the use of routine histology with H&E, as well as special stains to render these lesions more prominent (e.g., Masson-Trichrome, acid fuchsin, PTAH). Early infarcts occurring within a few hours before death may be demonstrated by the use of histochemistry to detect the presence of the enzymes malate, succinic or lactic dehydrogenase; basement membrane components (e.g., fibronectin, laminin); cytoskeletal proteins (e.g., actin, desmin, α- and β-tubulin); cell-matrix adhesion molecules (e.g., vinculin, talin); fatty acid binding protein, and other molecules [1].

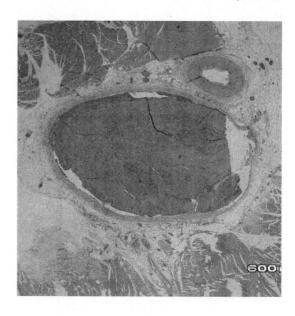

Fig. 13.10 Section through calf muscles revealing a deep vein thrombosis (H&E ×100)

13.2.3 Corroborating and Refuting Antemortem Diagnosis and Clinical Suspicions

13.2.3.1 Histological Evidence of Drug Dependency

Foreign body granuloma, formed around talc, starch, and other adulterants that are ingredients in various recreational and street drugs (e.g., heroin, cocaine, amphetamine derivatives, and their analogues), may be found at the sites of injection, or systemically, in the lungs and, occasionally, the liver and kidneys.

In addition, cocaine abuse may be associated with catecholamine-induced contraction band necrosis of the myocardium, eosinophilic myocarditis, or infective endocarditis. Heroin abuse may cause renal amyloidosis and focal segmental glomeruloslcerosis. These drugs of abuse may also result in potentially lethal rhabdomyolysis and subsequent renal failure.

Case #4: Drug abuse A 27-year-old man was found unconscious in the kitchen of a relative's house. He was pronounced dead on arrival at hospital. Police reported that the deceased had a past history of drug abuse.

Autopsy revealed nonspecific features of acute pulmonary edema. Microscopically, both lungs showed multiple foreign-body granuloma, highlighted under polarised light, scattered throughout the lung parenchyma. The granuloma were typically situated in perivascular locations. Occasional multinucleated giant cells were also present. Other common causes of granulomatous inflammation of the lungs were excluded. The features were typical of a "junkie's lung" that correlated with the history of intravenous drug abuse (Fig. 13.11).

Fig. 13.11 Case #4: Pulmonary granulomatous inflammation surrounding birefringent foreign bodies in the perivascular space of the lung parenchyma in a case of intravenous drug abuse (H&E ×400)

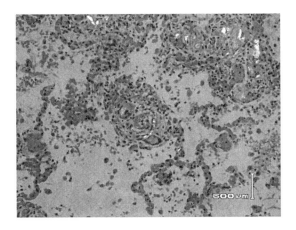

Toxicological analyses of postmortem blood samples revealed higher than therapeutic levels of midazolam, therapeutic levels of ephedrine and orphenadrine, as well as the presence of several other medications such as paracetamol, codeine, and promethazine. Notably buprenorphine was also detected in a postmortem blood sample. A similar profile was obtained from the postmortem urine sample.

The dangers of diversion buprenorphine abuse and its coabuse with benzodiazepines have seen several reports over the last decade [3]. Having excluded other causes of death in this case, the final cause of death was certified to be due to a mixed drug reaction.

13.2.3.2 Evaluation of Adverse Drug Reactions and Poisoning

Certain histological features may provide corroborative evidence in instances of suspected fatal adverse drug reaction, manifesting as mucocutaneous eruptions, hepatotoxicity, nephrotoxicity, cardiotoxicity , and neurotoxicity [4]. Some examples are as follows: centrilobular fatty change in the liver and hepatocellular necrosis in chloroform poisoning; perivenular, mid-zonal or massive hepatocellular necrosis in paracetamol poisoning; acute pulmonary hemorrhage followed by massive fibrosis and type II pneumocyte hyperplasia induced by paraquat poisoning, which may also result in toxic myocarditis as well as hepatic and renal tubular necrosis.

Chemical meningoencephalitis, renal tubular degeneration, myocardial degeneration with cardiac dilatation and bronchopneumonia, associated with the deposition of calcium oxalate crystals in the respective tissues, are characteristic of ethylene glycol poisoning (Fig. 13.12).

Case #5: Massive hepatocellular necrosis, possibly induced by orlistat A 62-year-old-man developed deepening jaundice after having consumed orlistat at a dosage of 120 mg tid over a period of 10 days, in an attempt to lose weight. His drug history included the occasional ingestion of paracetamol

Fig. 13.12 Oxalate crystals within the renal tubules of a victim of ethylene glycol poisoning (H&E ×400)

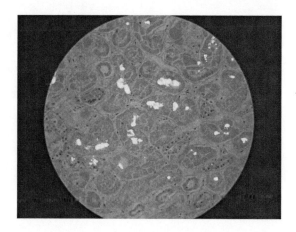

(apparently not exceeding two to four tablets on any one day). He also had no history of taking herbal preparations. There was also no record of any drug allergy or recent travel overseas. Apart from mild systemic hypertension and occasional alcohol ingestion, he had no other significant medical history.

The results of the initial post-admission liver function tests indicated severe deranged hepatic functions. Subsequent investigations for markers of a range of hepatitic viruses (anti-HAV IgM, anti-HBs, anti-HBc IgM, anti-HBe, HBsAg, anti-HCV, HCV RNA (Chiron), anti-HEV IgM, anti-EBV IgM, anti-CMV IgM and anti-leptospiral antibodies), HIV-1 and -2, and autoimmune disease (anti-mitochondrial and anti-nuclear antibodies) yielded largely negative results, with the exception of anti-smooth muscle antibodies, which were present at a low titre (1:100). Investigations for malarial parasites and *Clostridium difficile* toxin (stool sample) were also negative. A clinical drug screen, performed on a blood sample on the second post-admission day, yielded a non-toxic level of orlistat 33 mg/L (µg/mL). Concurrent clinical investigations excluded Wilson's disease, Budd-Chiari syndrome, and biliary disease.

A diagnosis of fulminant liver failure was made, presumably attributable to an adverse reaction to orlistat. Although the patient was considered as a candidate for liver transplantation, he died little more than three weeks after hospitalisation, having a nosocomial infection and developed renal failure in the process.

Postmortem histological examination of the liver showed complete loss of the normal hepatic architecture and massive hepatocellular necrosis, associated with marked portal and periportal cholestasis (Fig. 13.13), accompanied by collapse of the reticulin framework (Fig. 13.14). There was moderate, chronic portal inflammation, with occasional, relative preservation of a few periportal hepatocytes in some areas. Perivenular fibrosis was noted, but veno-occlusive disease and hepatic cirrhosis were absent. No Mallory bodies, giant mitochondria, or steatosis were observed in the residual hepatocytes. Toxicological analysis was negative.

Fig. 13.13 Case #5: Massive
hepatocellular necrosis
with marked periportal
cholestasis (PAS ×200)

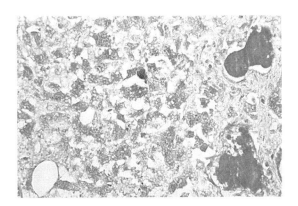

Comprehensive clinico-pathological correlation led to the almost inevitable
conclusion that this was likely to have been a case of drug-induced massive
hepatocellular necrosis, possibly related to the use of orlistat, which was implicated in a previously reported instance of non-fatal hepatitis [5].

Case #6: Adulteration of a slimming herbal combination by nitrosofenfluramine
A 42-year-old female succumbed to fulminant hepatic failure and eventual
multiple organ failure, after having ingested an undetermined quantity of a
herbal product over a period of approximately four months prior to the onset of
her illness. The product contained extracts of Herba Gynostemmae, Folium
Camelliae Sinensis, Succus Aloes Folii Siccatus, Semen Raphani, and Fructus
Crataegi and purportedly had slimming, "energising" and "cleansing" properties. She eventually underwent total hepatectomy, with porto-caval shunting, in
anticipation of an allogenic liver transplant. Unfortunately, her condition
deteriorated and she died within 48 h of the operation, approximately three
weeks post-admission.

Autopsy showed that the deceased had severe jaundice and was severely
obese (BMI: 47.1), with evidence of diffuse hemorrhage, including the presence
of 1350 mL of blood in the peritoneal cavity (which was likely to be iatrogenic in

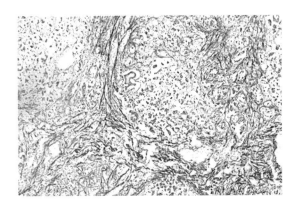

Fig. 13.14 Case #5: Collapse
of the hepatic reticulin
framework (Gordon &
Sweet's ×200)

nature). The liver had been removed and was later recovered as a formalin-fixed specimen. It was markedly contracted, comprising multiple micronodules interspersed with extensive areas of dense fibrotic tissue.

Microscopy showed the complete loss of the normal hepatic architecture, with massive parenchymal destruction and collapse of the reticulin framework (Fig. 13.15). The residual hepatocytes were disposed as nodules, displaying variable cellular regeneration and ballooning degeneration, within extensive areas of densely fibrous stroma (Fig. 13.16). There was florid ductal proliferation and mild to moderate, mixed inflammatory infiltrates, containing T-lymphocytes (CD3+, CD20−). Prominent focal cholestasis, mostly intracannalicular and intraductal in distribution, was present (Fig. 13.17). Excessive copper or iron deposition was not seen. These features were deemed to be consistent with repair and limited parenchymal regeneration following upon massive hepatocellular necrosis.

Analysis of a postmortem blood sample showed therapeutic and subtherapeutic concentrations of a variety of therapeutic agents administered to the patient during her last illness. Subsequent analysis of a sample of residual herbal capsules revealed that it was adulterated by fenfluramine, N-nitrosofenfluramine, nicotinamide, and thyroid extract. None of the herbal ingredients is currently known to be hepatotoxic (in contrast, Succus Aloes Folii Siccatus is apparently considered liver-protective) and much the same applies to fenfluramine, nicotinamide (except when taken in mega-doses), and thyroid extract. As nitrosamines are known to be variably hepatotoxic, and in the absence of a more plausible cause of liver damage, N-nitrosofenfluramine was deemed to be the likely cause of massive hepatocellular necrosis in this instance [6].

13.2.4 As an Audit Tool for Medical Treatment and Interventions

Last but not least, the authors wish to highlight the role of forensic histopathology as a tool for medical audit and forensic evaluation of iatrogenic

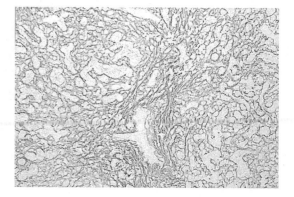

Fig. 13.15 Case #6: The liver microarchitecture showing collapse of the reticulin framework (Gordon & Sweet's ×100)

Fig. 13.16 Case 6: Massive hepatocellular necrosis with marked architectural distortion and dense stromal fibrosis (Masson Trichrome ×100)

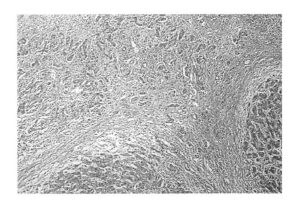

injuries. This is essential for proper clinico-pathological correlation, although the investigated pathological entity may or may not be related to the final cause of death.

This subject was discussed briefly by Lau recently [4]. Here, a more expansive consideration of the place of forensic histopathology in the evaluation of suspected or actual iatrogenic injuries is provided by means of a series of case studies.

Case #7: Clinically undiagnosed mediastinal large B-cell malignant lymphoma causing postanaesthetic respiratory distress in a patient with an ectopic pregnancy
A 32-year-old female was diagnosed as having an ectopic pregnancy at six weeks' amenorrhoea and underwent laparoscopic salpingectomy. During a preoperative anaesthetic review, she presented with a month-long history of a mild, persistent productive cough, which was attributed to an upper respiratory tract infection. She developed severe respiratory distress after extubation and died on the second postoperative day.

Autopsy revealed the presence of a large mediastinal tumour, the existence of which was apparently unsuspected preoperatively, but suggested by a

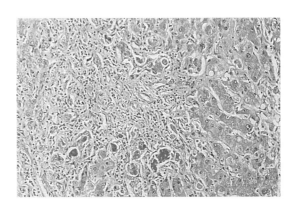

Fig. 13.17 Case #6: N-Nitrosofenfluramine-induced liver pathology: ductal proliferation, mixed inflammatory infiltrates and prominent cholestasis (PAS ×200)

Fig. 13.18 Case #7: A large
fleshy mediastinal tumour is
encasing the aortic arch and
the proximal segments of
the brachiocephalic and
subclavian arteries

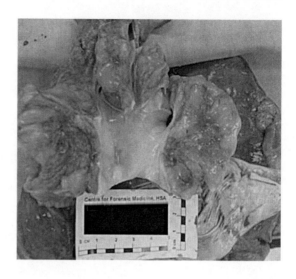

postresuscitative chest radiograph. The fleshy, hard lesion encased the ascending thoracic aorta, aortic arch, and the proximal segments of the brachiocephalic and subclavian arteries (Fig. 13.18), and also caused partial extrinsic airway compression.

Histologically, the tumour consisted of sheets of malignant, large lymphoid cells (CD1a−, CD3−, CD20+, CD30−, CD45+, CD68−) with pleomorphic, vesicular nuclei containing prominent nucleoli, as well as fairly abundant cytoplasm (Fig. 13.19A,B). Reed-Sternberg cells were absent. Immunohistochemistry for AE1/3, EMA and PLAP yielded negative results. There were areas of infarction as well as extensive perineural and vascular invasion. Malignant infiltration of the vascular adventitia and the superficial layers of the media were noted (Fig. 13.20). These features supported the diagnosis of a mediastinal diffuse large B-cell lymphoma, while largely excluding a thymoma or a germ cell tumour. Further examination also showed micrometastases to the tracheo-bronchial lymph nodes and the right adrenal gland (Fig. 13.21), but not to the bone marrow.

In all probability, the mechanical effects exerted by the advanced mediastinal tumour upon the airways and the thoracic cage, coupled with the pathophysiological effects of general anaesthesia on respiratory movement and airway patency, had led to the patient's sudden and unexpected demise in early pregnancy [7].

Case #8: Cerebral infarction complicating therapeutic embolisation of a facial cavernous hemangioma in an 8-year-old girl Approximately 2 h after undergoing elective angiographic embolisation of a large right facial hemangioma under general anaesthesia, an 8-year-old girl developed left-sided hemiparaesis. Computerised tomography revealed right fronto-parietal cerebral infarction, severe cerebral edema, and features of hypoxic-ischemic encephalopathy. Her

Fig. 13.19 A Case #7:
Malignant, large lymphoid
cells with pleomorphic
vesicular nuclei, prominent
nucleoli, abnormal mitoses
and abundant cytoplasm
(H&E ×400). **B** Case #7:
Intense positive staining for
CD20 (×200)

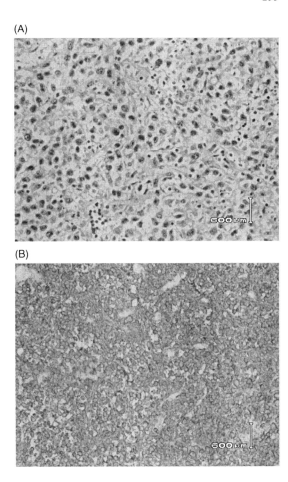

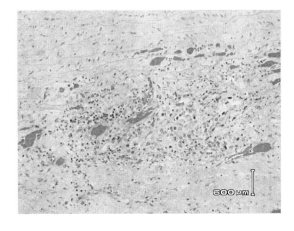

Fig. 13.20 Case #7: Malignant lymphoid cells infil-
trating the aortic
adventitia and the superficial layers of the media
(Masson-Trichrome ×200)

Fig. 13.21 Case #7: Right
adrenal metastatic
malignant lymphoma
(H&E ×4)

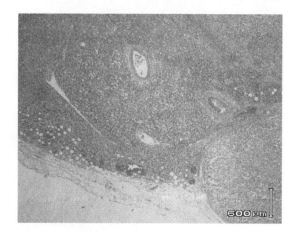

subsequent clinical course was dominated by neurogenic ventricular arrhythmia and pulmonary edema, recurrent episodes of cardiorespiratory arrest,
diabetes insipidus and progressive neurological deterioration culminating in
brain death two weeks later.

Microscopy of the facial soft tissues demonstrated presence of a cavernous
hemangioma (Fig. 13.22) with occasional foci of thrombosis and acute hemorrhage, but no evidence of malignancy. There were foreign body emboli, comprising strongly birefringent reticulated material (probably representing
polyvinyl-alcohol particles denatured by heat) which stained intensely black
with Verhoeff van-Gieson stain (Fig. 13.23).

Histologically, the brain showed an autolysed, pale-staining appearance,
accompanied by congestion and focal thrombosis of the cortical vessels. There
was cortical infarction (Fig. 13.24) mainly of both temporal lobes, with neuronal
liquefactive necrosis (mainly of the outer layers), accompanied by inflammatory

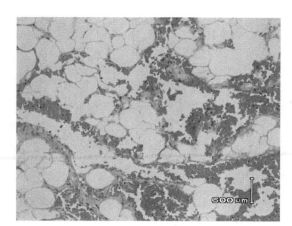

Fig. 13.22 Case #8: Dilated,
thin-walled blood vessels
interspersed with mature
adipose tissue (H&E ×100)

Fig. 13.23 **A** Case #8:
Foreign body emboli within
the cavernous hemangioma
(H&E ×100). **B** Case #8:
Marked birefringence
(polarised ×100). **C** Case #8:
Reticulated appearance
(Verhoeff van-Gieson ×200)

(A)

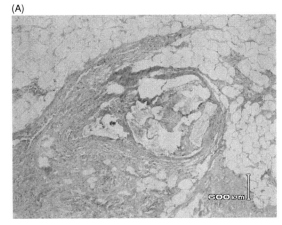

(B)

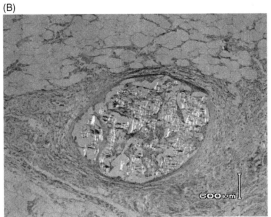

(C)

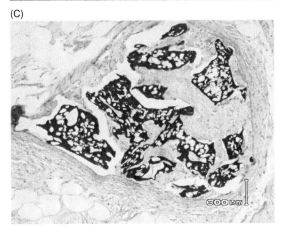

Fig. 13.24 Case #8: Cerebral
infarction (H&E ×100)

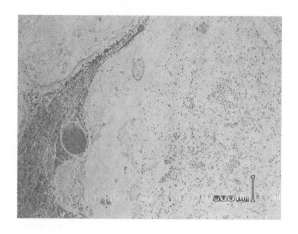

infiltrates of polymorph leukocytes and some foamy macrophages, together with early astrocytosis. Foreign body emboli, with features similar to those detected in the facial cavernous hemangioma (Fig. 13.25), were found in these areas, as well as in the occipital cortex and the basal ganglia. The cerebellar cortex showed diffuse liquefactive necrosis of the Purkinje cells, consistent with hypoxic-ischemic encephalopathy while the hippocampus was largely autolysed.

It appears that the angiographic embolisation of the facial hemangioma involved the selective and sequential catherisation of the right internal maxillary and facial arteries via the right external carotid artery, through a femoral approach. This was to enable a mixture of polyvinyl-alcohol particles (of sizes in the range of 150–250 μm) and gelfoam, suspended in radiocontrast medium, to be introduced into the main arterial feeders of the hemangioma, in order to achieve therapeutic occlusion of the relevant vessels. From a pathological perspective, it is entirely plausible that some of these particles might have entered the cerebral circulation through anastomoses between the right external and internal carotid arteries (e.g., the middle meningeal and ophthalmic arteries), and subsequently crossed over from the ipsilateral to the contralateral cerebral vasculature via the Arterial Circle of Willis, with fatal consequences.

Case #9: Accidental intraventricular administration of vincristine A 27-year-old female with acute lymphoblastic leukemia complicated by central nervous system (CNS) involvement was to receive an intensified course of chemotherapy, which included the administration of intrathecal methotrexate and intravenous vincristine, when the first course failed to bring about a remission.

A right frontal Ommaya reservoir which affords access to the cerebral ventricles was successfully implanted for this purpose. Unfortunately, a junior doctor who was assigned to administer these cytotoxic agents injected vincristine (2 mg) intrathecally, through the Ommaya reservoir. The mistake was realised the following day, whereupon a CNS washout was performed, but to

Fig. 13.25 Case #8: Foreign body emboli, virtually identical to those found within the cavernous hemangioma, in the cerebral microvasculature. **A** H&E ×200. **B** Polarised ×400. **C** Verhoeff van-Gieson ×200

(A)

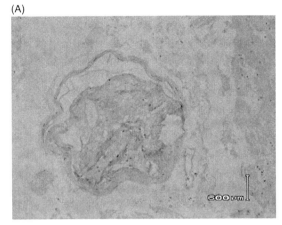

(B)

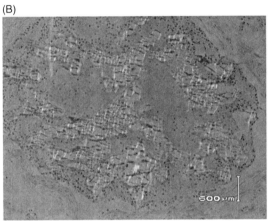

(C)

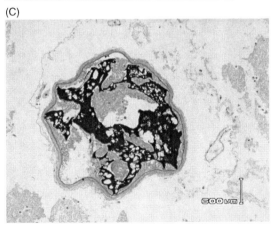

no avail. The patient developed progressive ascending paralysis, complicated by a persistent respiratory infection, eventually lapsing into coma to die approximately ten days after the lethal injection.

At autopsy, the brain was edematous, and showed diffuse discoloration of the cortical surface, with marked, generalised softening. The spinal cord was necrotic almost throughout its entire length, and particularly along the cervical, thoracic and upper lumbar segments, where necrotic brain tissue was present within the spinal subdural space (Fig. 13.26). The cerebellar tonsils were necrotic, too. Histologically, there was evidence of cerebral meningoencephalitis with extensive neuronal damage and astrocytosis (Fig. 13.27). The cerebellum showed leptomeningitis with focal loss of Purkinje cells. Sections of the brainstem showed a wide range of neuronal injury, ranging from ischemic-hypoxic changes to necrosis, accompanied by astrocytosis and focal perivascular hemorrhage, particularly in the pons and medulla. The spinal cord showed leptomeningitis with florid myelitis accompanied by widespread neuronal necrosis, particularly of the anterior horn cells (Fig. 13.28). Fragments of necrotic cerebellar tissue were present along the cervical and thoracic segments and around the nerve roots. There was no evidence of demyelination. There was also histological evidence of bronchopneumonia with heavy leukemic

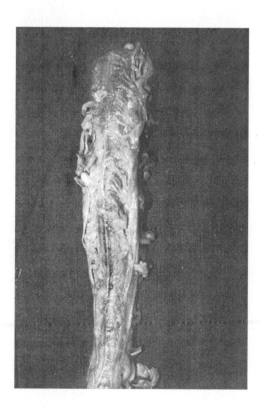

Fig. 13.26 Case #9: Necrotic cervical spinal cord with fragments of cerebellar tissue alongside it

Fig. 13.27 Case #9: Cerebral meningoencephalitis with perivascular lymphocytic cuffing (H&E ×200)

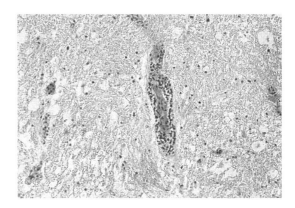

infiltrates within the myocardium, spleen, bone marrow, kidneys, and the portal tracts of the liver.

This case is but one of a good number of similar, if not identical, examples of an entirely avoidable medication error – that of administrating the right drug through the wrong route, as it were – which carries irreversibly tragic and lethal consequences [8].

13.2.5 As a Permanent Record of Lesions

It should be remembered that, even in instances where neither the cause of death nor any of the autopsy findings is in doubt, histological sampling of the major parenchymatous organs may yet provide permanent documentation of the presence or absence of any lesion deemed to be material to ascertaining the cause of death. This is particularly important for states and countries where cremation is the routine and preferred final procedure to put the deceased person to rest.

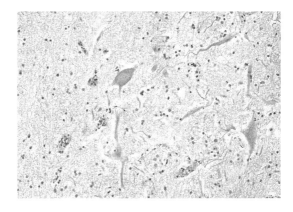

Fig. 13.28 Case #9: Neuronal necrosis and degeneration of the anterior horn cells of the spinal cord (H&E ×200)

13.2.6 As an Invaluable Resource for Teaching, Training, and Research

Last but not least, histological sections and material are an invaluable resource for teaching, training, and education. However, the extent to which this final advantage could be applied naturally varies from one jurisdiction to another.

13.3 Looking Ahead – The Future of Forensic and Autopsy Histopathology

Looking ahead, the role of immunohistochemistry and other molecular diagnostic techniques could be certainly expanded in forensic pathology practice. Although tissue quality is often the limiting factor in the application of these techniques, much could still be achieved in cases where autolysis is not advanced. The identification of the SARS coronavirus by in-situ hybridisation illustrated above is an excellent example.

There are currently many areas of research interest, as colleagues from many parts of the world continue to advance methods to refine post-mortem and forensic diagnosis. The following section is a brief, and by no means exhaustive or comprehensive, illustration of some of the research in this area.

13.3.1 Immunohistochemistry and Forensic Neuropathology

In recent years, the application of immunohistochemistry for ß-APP in the brain has spearheaded new understanding in the pathology of axonal injury, traumatic in origin or otherwise [9, 10]. Immunohistochemistry for ß-APP showed that traumatic axonal injury is much more common than previously recognised. It became clear also that axonal injury was a phenomenon that was not just restricted to trauma. For instance, ischaemia have also been shown to be associated with axonal injury.

13.3.2 Immunohistochemical Diagnosis in Cardiac Pathology

Sensitive and specific methods for diagnosing acute myocardial damage are particularly useful in forensic practice since cardiac disease is a very common cause of sudden death. Several applications of histochemistry have already been alluded to dating of myocardial infarcts above.

Recently, the significance of increased expression of complement C9 within myocardium damaged by ischaemia has been investigated. The authors reported increased but gradated differential expression of complement C9 in cases with histological evidence of acute myocardial infarctions, in cases with only electrocardiographic evidence of acute myocardial infarctions, and in cases with severe coronary artery disease but without evidence of acute myocardial ischaemia [11].

The detection of apoptosis within the myocardium by the TUNEL method has been investigated in cases of sudden cardiac death compared with controls. However, there was no significant difference in the proportion of apoptotic myocardial nuclei between the cases of myocardial infarction due to coronary artery disease and cases of sudden cardiac death without coronary artery disease. The authors suggested the application of the technique as a screening tool for the postmortem diagnosis of sudden death due to cardiac causes [12].

The immunohistochemical detection of cardiac troponin-C (cTnC) and cardiac troponin-T (cTnT) could serve as a tool for the detection of acute myocardial damage. The expression of cTnC was reported to be strongly positive, diffuse and more frequent than cTnT in cases of myocardial infarction [13].

Dettmeyer et al. [14] attempted to describe and differentiate dilated cardiomyopathy of an inflammatory aetiology from idiopathic/alcoholic dilated cardiomyopathy through the application of immunohistochemistry for markers of T-lymphocytes (LCA, CD3), macrophages (CD68) and tenascin. The criteria for inflammatory cardiomyopathy was suggested to be based on the visual quantification of >2 CD3 positive lymphocytes per high power field and >7 CD3 lymphocytes per square millimetre.

13.3.3 Immunohistochemical Diagnosis of Sepsis

The diagnosis of sepsis is important in forensic practice especially in sudden deaths and some cases of hospital deaths. The enhanced expressions of various cellular adhesion molecules, growth factors, and proteins in lungs of patients who had died with or from sepsis has been investigated [15]. E-selectin, which was not expressed in unstimulated endothelium of the pulmonary microvasculature, was found to be up-regulated in sepsis. ICAM-1 was up-regulated in endothelium and in leucocytes within the lungs, while lactoferrin and VLA-4 and were similarly up-regulated in pulmonary leucocytes. In contrast, vascular endothelial growth factor (VEGF), which is normally strongly expressed in normal alveolar and bronchial epithelium of healthy individuals, is down-regulated in sepsis-induced lung injury.

13.3.4 Wound Pathology

As previously alluded to, the histological ageing of wounds remains a problematic area. The ageing of wounds as well as establishing the vitality of wounds has been the focus of research for many years. Grellner et al. [16] reported that transforming growth factors (TGF)-alpha and beta1 were up-regulated in injured skin, reaching maximal intensity in 30–60 min after the injury. It was observed that both factors, especially TGF-beta1, remained detectable in elevated levels within wounded tissues after days to weeks. The authors suggested that the patterns of expression of the two factors could serve as a tool to aid the evaluation of wound age [16].

ICAM-1 was also found to be useful in correlation with the degree of skin wound inflammation as well as an early evidence of the vitality of the wound [17]. In addition, the degree of expression of VEGF in wound ageing has also been described but appeared to be useful only to indicate wounds aged seven days or more [18]. The value of the detection of p53, however, remained inconclusive in this field [19].

13.3.5 The Challenges Ahead

These adjunctive techniques mentioned above show great potential in forensic practice. Nevertheless, more research is required to reproduce and replicate some of the observations in order to refine them for application. In the future, perhaps more sophisticated molecular diagnostic techniques can also be applied to forensic diagnosis.

13.4 Conclusions

The authors believe that the practice of forensic pathology is entering a new era. While reliance on macroscopic observations and keen sense of acumen were the mainstay of the practice of yesteryears, the application of histological and molecular diagnostic techniques is finding new ground and being established as an essential part of the armamentarium in forensic pathology practice.

Acknowledgement The authors wish to thank Dr Angela Chong for contributing the photomicrographs reproduced in Figs. 13.1 and 13.2.

References

1. Saukko P, Knight B (2004) Knight's forensic pathology, 3rd edn. Arnold, London
2. Munro D, Merritt HH (1936) Surgical pathology of subdural haematoma. Based on a study of 105 cases. Arch Neurol Psych 35:64–78
3. Kintz P (2001) Deaths involving buprenorphine: a compendium of French cases. Forensic Sci Int 121:65–69
4. Lau G (2005) Iatrogenic injury: a forensic perspective. In: Tsokos M (ed) Forensic pathology reviews, vol 3. Humana, Totowa, NJ, pp 351–439
5. Lau G, Chan CL (2002) A case of massive hepatocellular necrosis: was it caused by Orlistat? A case report. Med Sci Law 42:309–312

6. Lau G, Lo D, Yao YJ, Leong HT, Chan CL, Chu SS (2004) "Slim 10" – slim chance. A fatal case of hepatic failure possibly induced by *N*-nitrosofenfluramine. Med Sci Law 44:252–263
7. Prakash UB, Abel MD, Hubmayr RD (1988). Mediastinal mass and tracheal obstruction during general anaesthesia. Mayo Clin Proc 63:1004–1011
8. Lau G (1996) Accidental intrathecal vincristine administration: an avoidable iatrogenic death. Med Sci Law 36:263–265
9. Geddes JF, Whitwell HL, Graham DI (2000) Traumatic axonal injury: practical issues for diagnosis in medicolegal cases. Neuropathol Appl Neurobiol 26:105–116
10. Reichard RR, Smith C, Graham DI (2005) The significance of beta-APP immunoreactivity in forensic practice. Neuropathol Appl Neurobiol 31:304–313
11. Piercecchi-Marti MD, Lepidi H, Leonetti G, Vire O, Cianfarani F, Pellissier JF (2001) Immunostaining by complement C9: a tool for early diagnosis of myocardial infarction and application in forensic medicine. J Forensic Sci 46:328–334
12. Edston E, Grontoft L, Johnsson J (2002) TUNEL: a useful screening method in sudden cardiac death. Int J Legal Med 116:22–26
13. Martinez DF, Rodriguez-Morlensin M, Perez-Carceles MD, Noguera J, Luna A, Osuna E (2005) Biochemical analysis and immunohistochemical determination of cardiac troponin for the post-mortem diagnosis of myocardial damage. Histol Histopathol 20:475–481
14. Dettmeyer R, Reith K, Madea B (2002) Alcoholic cardiomyopathy versus chronic myocarditis – immunohistological investigations with LCA, CD3, CD68 and tenascin. Forensic Sci Int 126:57–62
15. Tsokos M (2003) Immunohistochemical detection of sepsis-induced lung injury in human autopsy material. Legal Med (Tokyo) 5:73–86
16. Grellner W, Vieler S, Madea B (2005) Transforming growth factors (TGF-alpha and TGF-beta1) in the determination of vitality and wound age: immunohistochemical study on human skin wounds. Forensic Sci Int 153:174–180
17. Dressler J, Bachmann L, Muller E (1997) Enhanced expression of ICAM-1 (CD54) in human skin wounds: a diagnostic value in legal medicine. Inflamm Res 46:434–435
18. Hayashi T, Ishida Y, Kimura A, Takayasu T, Eisenmenger W, Kondo T (2004) Forensic application of VEGF expression to skin wound age determination. Int J Legal Med 118:320–325
19. Tarran S, Dziewulski P, Sztynda T, Langlois NE (2004) A study of p53 expression in thermal burns of human skin for determination of wound age. Med Sci Law 44:222–226

Part IX
Forensic Age Estimation

Chapter 14
Forensic Age Estimation of Live Adolescents and Young Adults

Andreas Schmeling, Walter Reisinger, Gunther Geserick and Andreas Olze

Contents

Abstract As a result of the global increase in migration movements in recent years, there is a growing demand for age estimates of live persons. The persons under examination are mostly foreigners without valid identification documents whose genuine age needs to be clarified for legal purposes. In many countries, the age thresholds relevant for criminal, civil, and asylum proceedings lie between 14 and 22 years of age. In line with recommendations issued by the *Study Group on Forensic Age Diagnostics*, for determining the age of live subjects a forensic age estimate should combine the results of a physical examination, an X-ray of the hand, and a dental examination which records dentition status and evaluates an orthopantomogram. To assess the age of persons who are assumed to be at least 18 years old, an additional roentgenographic or CT

A. Schmeling
Institute of Legal Medicine, University of Münster, Münster, Germany
e-mail: andreas.schmeling@ukmuenster.de

M. Tsokos (ed.), *Forensic Pathology Reviews, Volume 5*,
doi: 10.1007/978-1-59745-110-9_14, © Humana Press, Totowa, NJ 2008

examination of the clavicles is recommended. If there is no legal justification for X-ray examinations, the range of possible methods is limited to a physical and a dental examination. The present paper addresses the influence of ethnicity on the examined developmental systems. In so doing, the authors conclude that forensic age estimates should pay due heed to the proband's socio-economic status and ethnic origin. The effective doses from X-ray-examinations for forensic age estimations are given. There is no fear that the amount of radiation the examined individuals are exposed to during these X-ray examinations will have a detrimental effect on the person's health. At the end, research desiderata will be mentioned.

Keywords Forensic age estimation · Sexual maturation · Hand ossification Dentition · Clavicle ossification · Ethnicity · Radiation exposure

14.1 Introduction

In ancient times, age estimations of living adolescents were important. According to records in ancient Rome, adolescents were judged to be fit for service as soon as the second molars had erupted completely [1]. In England, a regulation from the year 1883 outlawed the employment of children less than 9 years of age in spinning mills and restricted the working hours of children between 9 and 13 years to 9 h a day [2]. At that time the minimum age of criminal responsibility was seven years [3]. It were mainly dentists who had to carry out age estimations. At a conference of the *Munich Medical Society* on April 1st, 1896, only one year after the discovery of X-rays, von Ranke came up with the idea that the age of children could also be examined by means of an X-ray of the hand [4]. In those days the Polish court pianist Raoul Koczalski, who is said to have given public concerts when he was only four years old and who had caused a sensation in Munich as a wunderkind, gave a performance in Munich. Von Ranke mistrusted the young court pianist and suspected that he was older than he had pretended. However, it is not known whether von Ranke verified his suspicion with an X-ray examination. A study of the ossification of the human hand published by Behrendsen [5] in 1897 was followed in 1909 by a publication of the American pediatrician Rotch [6], who believed that it is possible to estimate a child's readiness for school using the roentgenologic skeletal age assessment. There is a great time interval between these early publications and the systematic examinations about the time course of the ossification of the hand. The most famous are the publications of Greulich and Pyle [7], Schmid and Moll [8] as well as Tanner et al. [9, 10]. However, these atlases of radiographic anatomy were mainly used to diagnose disorders in skeletal maturity and not to estimate the chronological age of an individual.

The reason for the increasing importance of forensic age estimation of live individuals today is cross-border migration, which leads to an increasing rate of foreigners giving doubtful details about their age in numerous countries. The persons to whom forensic examination is to be applied are foreigners without valid identity documents who are suspected of making false statements about their age and whose genuine age needs to be ascertained in the course of criminal, civil, asylum, or old-age pension proceedings. In many countries, the age thresholds relevant for criminal, civil, and asylum proceedings lie between 14 and 22 years of age.

The *10th Lübeck Dialogue of German Forensic Physicians* in December 1999 provided the opportunity for a first transregional analysis of the current state of forensic age estimation of live subjects. At this conference, a proposal was made to set up a study group consisting of forensic physicians, dentists, radiologists and anthropologists with the aim of developing recommendations for carrying out forensic age estimates in order to standardize and optimize the still rather heterogeneous practices applied and to improve the quality of estimates. As a result, the international and interdisciplinary *Study Group on Forensic Age Diagnostics* was founded in Berlin in March 2000. This study group has drawn up guidelines for carrying out age estimates of live subjects for the purpose of criminal proceedings [11], and civil as well as asylum proceedings [12]. To assure the quality of age estimates, the study group organizes annual ring tests in which participants are sent the X-rays and results of physical examination of a set of subjects and asked to estimate their ages. Those participants who do so correctly are issued a certificate.

Age estimates carried out properly help enhance legal certainty by ensuring equal treatment of persons with or without valid identity documents. On the one hand, they help prevent persons from wrongfully benefiting from false claims to be younger than they really are. On the other hand, they supply exonerating evidence for persons who are erroneously suspected of making false statements about their age [13, 14].

14.2 Methods

In line with the recommendations of the *Study Group on Forensic Age Diagnostics*, age estimates carried out for the purpose of criminal proceedings should consist of a physical examination which also records anthropometric data, signs of sexual maturation, and potential age-relevant developmental disorders, an X-ray of the left hand; and a dental examination which records dentition status and evaluates an orthopantomogram. In addition, a roentgeno-graphic or computed tomographic (CT) examination of the clavicles is recommended to establish whether a person has attained 18 years of age [11]. If there is no legal justification for X-ray examinations, the range of possible methods is limited to a physical and a dental examination. With a view to increasing the accuracy of age estimates and improving the identification of age-relevant developmental disorders, a combination of all methods mentioned above should be used, and each examination should be carried out by an expert with forensic experience. All contributions to the overall age estimate should provide information on the methods or stage classifications as well as the reference studies used for diagnosing age, in addition to the age-relevant findings of each examination. They should also provide the statistical parameters of variation for each feature under examination, along with the diagnosis of the most probable age. The expert in charge of coordinating all contributions should compile the results in a final age diagnosis.

14.2.1 Physical Examination

The physical examination includes anthropometric measures such as body height, weight, and constitutional type, as well as visible signs of sexual maturity. In boys, these are penile and testicular development, pubic hair, axillary hair, beard growth and laryngeal prominence; in girls these are breast development, pubic hair, axillary hair, and shape of the hip.

Tanner's [15] staging for adolescence is commonly used to determine the status of genital development, breast development and pubic hair growth. Axillary hair growth, beard growth and laryngeal development may be assessed using the four-stage classification of Neyzi et al. [16]. The four-stage model of Flügel et al. [17] for determining sexual maturity is suitable for purposes of age estimation. On average, girls reach full sexual maturity at the age of 16 and boys at the age of 17.

Of the forensic methods recommended for age estimation, evaluating sexual maturity shows the largest range of variation and therefore should be used for age determination only in conjunction with an evaluation of skeletal maturity and tooth development. However, the physical examination is indispensable to rule out any visible signs of age-related illness and to cross-check whether skeletal age and tooth age correspond to overall physical development.

Most diseases delay development and are thus conducive to underestimation of age. Such underestimation of age would not disadvantage the person concerned in terms of criminal prosecution. By contrast, overestimating age due to a disease that accelerates development should be avoided at all costs. Such diseases occur very rarely and include, above all, endocrinal disorders, which may affect not only the attainment of height and sexual development, but also skeletal development [18]. Endocrinal diseases that may accelerate skeletal development include precocious puberty, adrenogenital syndrom, and hyperthyroidism [19].

The physical examination should look for symptoms of hormonal acceleration of development, such as gigantism, acromegaly, microplasia, virilization of girls, dissociated virilism of boys, goiter, or exophthalmos. If no abnormality is detected it may be assumed that the probability of such a disease occurring is well below one per thousand [20]. Another indication for a possible hormonal disease is a discrepancy between skeletal age and dental age, as dental development normally remains unaffected by endocrinal disorders [21, 22, 23].

14.2.2 Roentgenological Examination of the Hand

Roentgenological examination of the hand is the second pillar of forensic age diagnostics.

A basic prerequisite for roentgenological age estimation is a physical examination in order to establish whether the proband has a disease that may affect skeletal development, as noted above.

Criteria for evaluating hand radiographs include the form and size of bone elements and the degree of epiphyseal ossification. To this effect, either a given X-ray image is compared with standard images of the relevant age and sex (radiographic atlas) [7, 24], or the degree of maturity or bone age is determined for selected bones (single bone method) [9, 10, 25]. Various studies have demonstrated that although the single bone method requires more time, it does not necessarily yield more accurate results [26, 27, 28, 29]. Therefore, the two atlas methods developed by Greulich and Pyle [7] as well as by Thiemann and Nitz [24] seem to be appropriate for forensic age diagnostics.

The Greulich-Pyle atlas [7] is based on a reference population of the 1930s, whereas the Thiemann-Nitz atlas [24] uses a much more recent study conducted in 1977. With regard to the age interval relevant in forensic terms, Greulich and Pyle [7] identified a standard deviation ranging between 0.6 and 1.1 years for their method. Johnston [30] presented comparable results for the Greulich-Pyle method. The standard deviations identified for the Thiemann-Nitz method range between 0.2 and 1.2 years with regard to the relevant age interval [31]. The skeletal development of hand bones is complete at the age of 17 in girls and at the age of 18 years in boys.

Figure 14.1 shows a hand skeleton of a male subject with epiphyseal plates still open. Figure 14.2 shows a fully developed hand skeleton of a male subject.

14.2.3 Dental Examination

The main criteria for dental age estimation in the relevant age group are the following indicators of biological development: dentition status and tooth mineralization.

Tooth eruption refers to the gingival emergence of the apex of the tooth crown. It is diagnosed by inspecting the oral cavity of the person concerned and does not require an X-ray. Except for third molars, eruption of permanent teeth is complete around the age of 12, on average. Third molars usually erupt after age 17 (at least in Caucasian populations) [32]. After another two to four years, the occlusal plane is reached [33]. However, significant differences between individuals must be expected with regard to third molar eruption, so that examination results must be assessed carefully.

Tooth mineralization is evaluated using an orthopantomogram. Tooth mineralization begins with the development of the crown at the occlusal surface

Fig. 14.1 Hand skeleton of a
male subject with epiphyseal
cartilages still open.
Reported age: 13 years and
5 months. Estimated age
according to forensic age
estimation: approximately
16 years. True age: 16 years
and 6 months

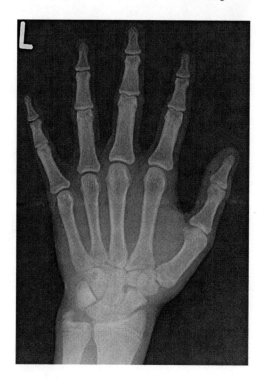

and progresses over the neck of the tooth down to the root. When the root is
fully developed, tooth growth is complete. Today, various classification systems
for assessing dental mineralization are available [34, 35, 36, 37, 38].

A study evaluating the different classification systems found that the one
developed by Demirjian et al. [34] is best suited to the purpose of forensic age
estimation, as it defines the stages on the basis of changes in form rather than
speculative estimates of length [39]. It defines four stages of crown mineralization (A–D) and four stages of root mineralization (E–H).

The degree of mineralization of second molars allows estimates of age
approximately until the age of 16 [40]. Various studies place the mean completion of tooth root formation between age 21 and 23 [40, 41, 42]. According to a
study by Olze et al. [42], the standard deviation of the stages E through H ranges
between 1.8 and 2.6 years. In impacted teeth, completion of root formation may
be delayed 3 years [36].

Figure 14.3 shows an orthopantomogram of a male subject with not yet
completed mineralization of the third molars. Figure 14.4 shows an orthopantomogram of a male subject with completed mineralization of the third molars.

After the third molar mineralization there are only epidemiologic features
such as the periodontal recession and the DMFT index for the dental age
estimation. Olze et al. [43] examined in a retrospective study, if the determination of the periodontal recession can provide an indication of whether a person

Fig. 14.2 Hand skeleton of a male subject, fully developed. Reported age: 17 years and 8 months. Estimated age according to forensic age estimation: at least 18 years. True age: 22 years and 8 months

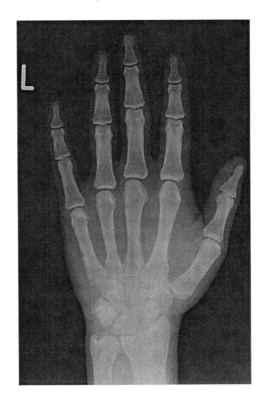

Fig. 14.3 Third molars of a male subject, mineralization not yet completed. Reported age: 13 years and 5 months. Estimated age according to forensic age estimation: approximately 16–17 years. True age: 16 years and 6 months

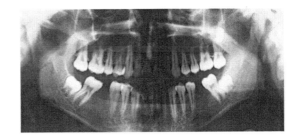

Fig. 14.4 Third molars of a male subject, mineralization completed. Reported age: 20 years and 10 months. Estimated age according to forensic age estimation: approximately 22 years or older. True age: 26 years and 9 months

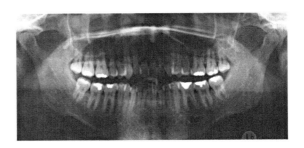

has attained the forensically relevant age of 21 years. For this purpose, 650 conventional orthopantomograms of German subjects aged 18–30 years were evaluated. The periodontal recession of the second premolars of all four quadrants was determined and four stages were defined. An increasing periodontal recession correlated well with an increasing age of the subjects. With incipient periodontal recession (stage 1) half of the examined individuals were at least 21 years old. Of the examined individuals with an advanced periodontal recession (stage 2), 75% were at least 21 years old. All of the male subjects with a severe periodontal recession (stage 3) were clearly older than 21 years; this stage, however, was hardly found in the examined age group. It was concluded that the periodontal recession seems to be suitable as an additional criterion for the forensic age diagnostics of young adults. However, the transferability of the presented reference data to individuals from other ethnic populations requires further examination in future studies. In another study [44] the suitability of different variations of the DMFT index for assessing if a person has attained 21 years of age was examined. On 650 conventional orthopantomograms of German subjects aged 18–30 years, the DMFT index of all permanent teeth as well as the DFT index of third molars projecting beyond the occlusal plane were determined. Due to the low age correlation and the considerable interindividual range, the examined DMFT index variations turned out to be unsuitable for the age estimation regarding the attainment of the 21st year.

14.2.4 Roentgenographic or Computed Tomographic Examination of the Clavicles

To answer the question of whether a person has reached the age of 18 it is particularly helpful to evaluate the ossification status of the medial epiphysis of the clavicle, because all other examined developmental systems have already completed their growth by then.

A number of studies are available examining the ossification of the medial epiphysis of the clavicle using either conventional X-rays or CT scans [45, 46, 47, 48, 49]. While traditional classification systems differentiate between four stages of clavicle ossification (stage 1: ossification centre not ossified; stage 2: ossification centre ossified, epiphyseal plate not ossified; stage 3: epiphyseal plate partly ossified; stage 4: epiphyseal plate fully ossified), Schmeling et al. [47] divided the stage of total epiphyseal fusion into two additional stages (stage 5: epiphyseal plate fully ossified, epiphyseal scar visible; stage 6: epiphyseal plate fully ossified, epiphyseal scar no longer visible).

If the fusion of epiphyses is complete and an epiphyseal scar is visible, it can be assumed, in the case of women, that the person is at least 20 years old, and, in the case of men, that the person is at least 21 years old. Total fusion of epiphyses with disappearance of the epiphyseal scar was first noted in both sexes at the age of 26 at the earliest [47].

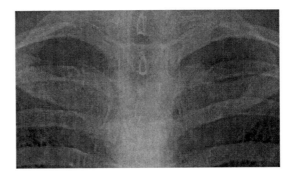

Fig. 14.5 Medial clavicular epiphyseal cartilage of a male subject, not fully ossified. Reported age: 15 years and 9 months. Estimated age: approximately 22 years. True age: 23 years

Figure 14.5 shows a not fully ossified medial clavicular epiphyseal cartilage of a male subject. Figure 14.6 shows a fully ossified medial clavicular epiphyseal cartilage of a male subject.

A CT-study by Schulz et al. [48] determined that the stages of ossification have partly been reached several years earlier than in the conventional X-ray study by Schmeling et al. [47]. The mostly large layer thicknesses of the analysed CTs were discussed as a possible cause.

In a study on the influence of the layer thickness on the ability to assess the stages of clavicular ossification, Mühler et al. [50] retrospectively analysed the CTs of 40 individuals which have been examined within the scope of age diagnostics. Scans with layer thicknesses of 1, 3, 5, and 7 mm have been reconstructed from the obtained data. Seven out of 80 clavicular epiphyseal plates showed differences depending on the layer thickness in the particular stages of ossification. In one case, a slice thickness of 1 mm led to a different diagnosis of the ossification stage than a slice thickness of 3 mm, in three cases the diagnoses differed between the slice thicknesses of 3 mm and of 5 mm, and in another three cases between 5 mm and 7 mm. The authors therefore concluded that for age estimation purposes the slice thickness should be 1 mm in order to ensure maximum accuracy and diagnostic reliability.

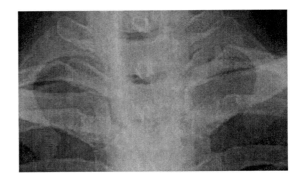

Fig. 14.6 Medial clavicular epiphyseal cartilage of a male subject, fully ossified. Reported age: 20 years and 11 months. Estimated age: at least 21 years, probably 25 years or older. True age: 26 years and 3 months

14.2.5 Overall Age Estimate

The results of the physical examination, the radiographic examination of the hand, the dental examination, and the radiographic examination of the clavicles, as the case may be, should be compiled by the expert in charge of coordinating all contributions in a final age diagnosis. The overall age estimate should include a discussion of the age-relevant variations resulting from application of the reference studies in an individual case, such as different ethnicity, different socioeconomic status and their potential effect on the developmental status, or diseases that may affect the development of the proband examined, including their effect on the estimated age. If possible, a quantitative assessment of any such effect should be given.

However, for age diagnoses obtained with a combination of methods, there is still no satisfactory way to determine scientifically the margin of error. While a number of reference studies collected data on individual features and some studies both on skeletal maturation and tooth mineralization [51, 52, 53, 54], there is still no reference study available analysing all required features for a single reference population. If independent features are examined as part of an age diagnosis that combines several methods, it may be assumed that the margin of error for the combined age diagnosis is smaller than that for each individual feature. However, it has not yet been possible to quantify this reduction. Combining methods makes it possible to identify statistical outliers, which should also reduce the scale of variation of the overall diagnosis to a certain non-quantifiable extent.

Indirect conclusions about the range of combined overall age diagnoses were possible after verifying age estimates carried out at the Institute of Legal Medicine in Berlin, Germany. To this effect, the court's case files of the persons originally examined for age estimation purposes at the institute were consulted to see whether the actual age of these persons was indeed established during the court proceedings. In the 43 cases where the age of the person concerned could be verified beyond doubt deviation between estimated and actual age ranged between plus or minus 12 months [55].

14.3 The Influence of Ethnicity on the Developmental Systems Examined

Since the subjects of forensic examination mostly belong to populations for which no reference studies are available that could be used for forensic purposes, the question arises whether there are significant developmental differences between various ethnic groups which would prohibit the application of relevant age standards to members of ethnic groups other than the reference population. In this respect, the term "ethnicity" shall be used only to identify the affinity of various populations in terms of origin.

Comprehensive studies of the relevant literature revealed that the major ethnic groups of interest to forensic age estimation achieve defined stages of ossification, dentition, and sexual maturity in the same natural sequence, so that it is generally possible to apply the relevant reference studies also to other ethnic groups [48, 49].

14.3.1 The Influence of Ethnicity on Skeletal Maturation

Numerous studies are available on skeletal maturation of all major ethnic groups (see overview in [56]). Because there are several potential factors of influence and their simultaneous action makes assessment of retardation a difficult exercise, all the more as the validity of some of those investigations seems to be limited due to small sample size, the exclusive consideration of non-relevant age groups, lack of information on health, ethnic identity and socioeconomic status and absence of confirmed data on proband age. Hence, for the problem at hand, greatest relevance may be claimed for studies on various ethnic groups of similar socioeconomic status and living in one and the same region or populations of one and the same socioeconomic status living in different regions. Such studies are available from the USA where research has been conducted on descendants of Caucasoids, Mongoloids, and Africans as well as from numerous ethnic groups of the former Soviet Union.

In a comparison with the Greulich-Pyle standards, Sutow [58] discussed racial differences as one of the causes of retarded skeletal maturation of Japanese children living in Japan. His findings were checked by Greulich [59] who referred to Japanese individuals living in the USA. He studied hand bone development in 898 children of Japanese descent aged between 5 and 18 years who where living in the San Francisco Bay area of California. While retarded skeletal maturation, in comparison with the Greulich-Pyle standards, was recorded by Sutow [58] for all age groups of Japanese living in their own country, such retardation was detected by Greulich only in boys aged between 5 and 7 years. Boys aged between 13 and 17 and girls between 10 and 17 years even exhibited comparative acceleration [59]. Greulich concluded that the significant retardation, in comparison with the Greulich-Pyle standards, recorded for children living in Japan was attributable to less favourable nutritional and environmental conditions rather than to racial differences [59]. Improved living standards in recent decades resulted in accelerated skeletal maturation even in Japanese living in Japan [60, 61] which, in the meantime has come to lie within the range of socioeconomically advanced European populations [62, 63].

Whereas some authors [64, 65] reported comparatively accelerated skeletal development in Africans in early childhood, ethnic origin obviously has no significant impact on the bone growth rate in later childhood and adolescence. Platt [66] studied skeletal maturation in 100 black inhabitants of

Florida, 143 blacks in Philadelphia and 100 whites in Philadelphia aged between 5 and 14 years. In none of these three groups was skeletal age, as determined by identical X-ray standards, significantly different from chronological age. Platt compared his results with studies on black residents of Africa. Mackay [67] recorded retardation by 1.5 to 2 years for East Africans, while Weiner and Thambipillai [68] recorded an average retardation of 16 months for West Africans. The assumption of an ethnic impact on skeletal maturation would justify expectation of a continuous series of phenomena ranging from severe retardation in blacks in Africa to moderate retardation in black Americans who had mixed with whites to absence of retardation in whites. Such continuous series do not exist, and Platt, consequently, postulated health and nutrition as the major factors influencing skeletal maturation. Skeletal maturation in 461 black and 380 white Americans in the Lake Erie region was studied by Loder et al. [69] between 1986 and 1990. Using the atlas method of Greulich and Pyle on the age group of 13–18 years, they recorded comparative acceleration of 0.45 years for white boys, 0.16 years for white girls, 0.38 years for black boys and 0.52 years for black girls. Johnston [30] studied the same age group of white Americans in Philadelphia by the same method and found acceleration values of 0.39 years for boys and 0.58 years for girls. Johnston's data for white Americans were almost identical with Loder's findings for black Americans, which seems to clearly underline that in the populations of the age group studied there were no ethnic differences with regard to skeletal maturation. Roche et al. [70, 71] investigated skeletal maturation in the context of race, geographic region, family income, and educational standards of parents in a representative cross-section of the US population aged between 6 and 17 years. They found no consistent black-white differences, no significant differences between regions, and no urban-rural differences.

Comprehensive studies were conducted on skeletal maturation in different ethnic groups of the former Soviet Union. Sixteen studies of 17 ethnic groups in different climatic and geographic zones of the former Soviet Union were evaluated by Pashkova and Burov [72]. Included were Russians, Ukrainians, Georgians, Armenians, Azerbaidjanis, Balkarians, Cabardines, Kazakhs, Tadchiks, Uzbeks, Ingushi, Chechenians, Udmurtians, Chukchen, Koryaks, Intelmenians and Evenkians. The range of variation at all stages of skeletal maturation was less than one year in all populations studied. However, the causes of those variations were attributed by the authors to relatively small samples, different methods and techniques used in the studies or undiagnosed diseases of probands but were not attributed to ethnic, regional or climatic differences.

Studies so far evaluated seem to suggest that there is a genetically determined potential of skeletal maturation which does not depend on ethnicity and may be exploited under optimum environmental conditions (e.g., high socioeconomic status), whereas less favourable environment may lead to retardation of skeletal maturation. Applying X-ray standards to individuals of a socioeconomic status lower than that of the reference population, usually leads to underestimating a person's age. In terms of criminal responsibility, this has no adverse effect on the person concerned.

14.3.2 The Influence of Ethnicity on the Eruption and Mineralization of Third Molars

Until recently, few comparative studies were available on the impact of ethnicity on mineralization of wisdom teeth. Gorgani et al. [73] studied 229 black Americans and 221 white Americans aged between 6 and 14 years. Crown mineralization of third molars in blacks was completed approximately one year earlier than in whites. Harris and McKee [74] studied 655 white and 335 black Americans aged between 3.5 and 13 years. While the blacks reached the early stages of third molar mineralization approximately one year earlier, minor differences were observed at later stages. This trend was confirmed by Mincer et al. [41]. They studied 823 Americans (80% whites, 19% blacks) aged between 14.1 and 24.9 years. The chronology of third molar mineralization did not reveal any significant differences.

In a recently published study, Olze et al. [75] investigated a total of 3652 conventional orthopantograms from 1430 German, 1597 Japanese and 584 black South African subjects, all aged between 12 and 26 with known dates of birth. All these assessments were carried out by the same observer. The authors found that if the predominant stage of mineralization in any given age group was considered, the Caucasoid sample occupied the middle position by age for each stage of mineralization investigated. For stages D-F (Staging according to Demirjian et al. [34]) the Mongoloid subjects were on average 1–2 years older, whereas for stages D–G the African subjects were about 1–2 years younger than Caucasoid subjects who had obtained the same level of mineralization. To enhance the accuracy of forensic age estimates based on wisdom tooth mineralization the authors recommend the use of population-specific standards.

With regard to the eruption of third molars, some studies have found significant differences between specific populations [57]. While in Caucasian populations third molars generally do not erupt before age 17 [32], Brown [76], Chagula [77], Otuyemi et al. [78], and Shourie [79] describe cases of eruption starting in African, Australian, and Indian populations already at age 13.

Comparative studies on the relation between age and third molar eruption are available for black and white Americans, Africans, and Asians. Garn et al. [80] studied the dentition of all permanent teeth in 953 black and 998 white Americans. In black Americans, the maxillary third molars developed 3.7 years earlier, and the mandibular third molars 5.6 years earlier, than in white Americans. Hassanali [81] compared the eruption times of third molars in 1343 Africans and 1092 Asians in Kenya. He found that in Africans third molars appeared two to three years earlier. Since age data for subjects of African origin are often not verified, further research is still needed.

14.3.3 The Influence of Ethnicity on Sexual Maturation

Data on sexual maturation is relatively scarce. Comparative studies on sexual maturation were conducted by Harlan et al. [82, 83], Channing-Pearce and Solomon [84], Wong et al. [85] and Huen et al. [86]. Between 1966 and 1970, Harlan et al. [82] analysed the sexual development of 6768 male Americans aged between 12 and 17 years. They found no significant differences between blacks and whites. In 1980, Harlan et al. [83] published a representative study examining the sexual maturation of a female American population of the same age group. This study observed relatively faster rates of maturation for blacks compared to whites. Channing-Pearce and Solomon [84] examined sexual development in a study involving 362 black and 355 white girls in Johannesburg, South Africa. Unlike Harlan et al. [83], they came to the conclusion that black girls on average reached full sexual maturity later than white girls. Wong et al. [85] examined sexual maturation in a 1993 study involving 3872 boys from southern China. They found that the time pattern of sexual maturation was comparable to that of Europeans, with the exception that Asians developed pubic hair later. Huen et al. [86] published a similar study including 3749 girls from southern China. They found that, according to the mean values for the individual stages of maturity, the examined girls were among the earliest to reach sexual maturity worldwide.

14.4 Radiation Exposure in X-ray Examinations

Since X-ray examinations are carried out for forensic age estimations without a medical indication, the question arises if the examined individuals have to fear detrimental effects due to the radiation exposure.

The effective dose from an X-ray examination of the hand is 0.1 microsievert (μSv) [87], from an orthopantomogram 26 μSv [88], from a conventional X-ray examination of the clavicles 220 μSv [87] and from a CT scan of the clavicles 600 μSv [89].

In order to assess the potential health risk of these X-ray examinations, the amounts of naturally-occuring and civilizing radiation exposure are compared to amounts of radiation exposure from radiological procedures. The effective dose from naturally-occuring radiation exposure in Germany is about 1.2 millisievert (mSv) on average per year. Apart from the direct cosmic radiation of 0.3 mSv and the direct terrestrial radiation of 0.4 mSv, the ingestion of naturally-occuring radioactive substances in the food contributes 0.3 mSv to the radiation exposure. For the inhalation of radon and its disintegration products 0.2 mSv must be added. This value increases by 0.9 mSv to a total of 2.1 mSv per year, due to the civilization-related stay in houses [90]. The highest contribution to civilizing radiation exposure yields medical procedures with about 2.0 mSv per inhabitant and year [90]. The radiation exposure from an intercontinental flight at an altitude of 12,000 m (7.45 miles) is 0.008 mSv per hour. It follows that the dose for a flight from Frankfurt to New York is 0.05 mSv [90]. A comparison of naturally-occuring and civilization radiation exposure with radiation exposure from X-ray examinations for forensic age diagnostics shows: in order to obtain the average naturally-occuring radiation exposure per day, 57 X-rays of the hand would be required. The radiation exposure from two orthopantomograms is equivalent to the radiation exposure from an inter-continental flight. Compared to the radiation exposure from an orthopanto-mogram the value from a conventional X-ray examination of the clavicles is 8.5 times higher and the value from the CT scan of the clavicles is 23 times higher. The radiation exposure from a CT scan of the clavicles is equivalent to the naturally-occuring radiation exposure of just under 3.5 months. On the basis of this comparison a relevant health risk as a result of X-ray examinations for forensic age estimations can be denied [91].

Concerning a possible health risk the biological effect of X-rays needs to be discussed as well. In this case a distinction between stochastic und non-stochastic radiation effects has to be made. Non-stochastic effects appear above 100 mSv and are therefore irrelevant to radiological diagnostics. DNA damage leading to mutations of the genotype and malignant diseases is one of the stochastic effects. To assess the risk of these stochastic effects in the low dose region the observed risk of high doses, e.g., of survivors of the nuclear bombs in Hiroshima and Nagasaki, is extrapolated to low doses on the assumption of a linear dose-effect-curve without a threshold dose. This procedure is a controversial issue. A group of radiation scientists even postulated biopositive effects, the so-called "radiation hormesis", in the low dose region, such as a stimulation of the cellular detoxication of chemically aggressive metabolic products, a stimulation of the DNA-repair and an improved immune defence. So far, these biopositive effects could only be detected at the cellular level [92]. By contrast, Rothkamm and Löbrich [93] recently found out in cellular studies that DNA-doublestrand-breaks after radiation exposure in the low dose region remained unrepaired, while DNA damages that were caused by high doses were repaired within a few days. To what extent the results can be transferred to the complete organism remains unclear.

On the assumption that there is a linear dose-effect relation without a threshold between the risk of radiation exposure and the delivered radiation dose and thus that even X-rays in the low-dose region can cause a malign disease, Jung [94] compared the mortality risk of X-ray examinations for age estimations with the mortality risk resulting from participation in traffic. He came to the conclusion that the mortality risk of an X-ray examination of the hand is comparable to participation in traffic for 1 h, the mortality risk of an orthopantomogram is comparable to participation in traffic for 2.5 h. Thus, the radiation risk of the X-ray examinations is as high as the risk the examined individual is exposed to on the way to the examination on the trial date. If the risk of an appointment for an age estimation seemed acceptable, this should also apply to the radiation risk of the X-ray examination [94].

As long as the discussion about the biological radiation effect in the low dose region is undecided, the so-called minimizing order remains valid without restrictions. It demands that any necessary examination is carried out with the minimum amount of radiation and without unnecessary exposure [95].

14.5 Prospects

While experience with age estimations shows that age estimations for forensic purposes with the accuracy required in criminal proceedings are possible with the range of methods used at present, further efforts in research seem to be desirable with regard to some questions.

One problem that has only been solved insufficiently is that statistically sound data must be provided on the range of age diagnostics for a combination of methods. There is no reference examination with all of the necessary features being determined synchronously. Reference studies for forensic purposes about the assessment of ossification of hands and clavicles are only available for ionizing imaging methods. In order to minimize the radiation exposure on the examined individual, it needs to be tested, whether comparable results can be gained with non-radiative methods such as magnetic resonance imaging or sonography. The mentioned research gaps are supposed to be filled by planned and partly started research projects of the *Study Group on Forensic Age Diagnostics*.

References

1. Müller N (1990) Zur Altersbestimmung beim Menschen unter besonderer Berücksichtigung der Weisheitszähne. Medical Thesis, Erlangen-Nürnberg, Germany
2. Loitz C (1992) Untersuchungen zur Entwicklung der Weisheitszähne als ein Kriterium der Altersbestimmung. Medical Thesis, Hamburg, Germany
3. Nortje CJ (1983) The permanent mandibular third molar. Its value in age determination. J Forensic Odontostomatol 1:27–31
4. Fendel H (1976) Die Methodik der radiologischen Skelettalterbestimmung. Radiologe 16:370–380
5. Behrendsen E (1897) Studien über die Ossifikation der menschlichen Hand vermittels des Roentgenschen Verfahrens. Dt Med Wochenschr 23:433–435
6. Rotch TM (1909) A study of the development of the bones in childhood by the Roentgen method with the view of establishing a developmental index for the grading of and the protection of early life. Trans Am Assoc Phys 124:603–630
7. Greulich WW, Pyle SI (1959) Radiographic atlas of skeletal development of the hand and wrist. Stanford University Press, Stanford, CA
8. Schmid F, Moll H (1960) Atlas der normalen und pathologischen Handskelettentwicklung. Springer, Berlin Heidelberg New York
9. Tanner JM, Whitehouse RH, Marshall WA, Healy MJR, Goldstein H (1975) Assessment of skeletal maturity and prediction of adult height (TW2 method). Academic Press, London, UK

10. Tanner JM, Healy MJR, Goldstein H, Cameron N (2001) Assessment of skeletal maturity and prediction of adult height (TW3 method). W.B. Saunders, London, UK

11. Schmeling A, Kaatsch H-J, Marré B, Reisinger W, Riepert T, Ritz-Timme S, Rösing FW, Rötzscher K, Geserick G (2001) Empfehlungen für die Altersdiagnostik bei Lebenden im Strafverfahren. Rechtsmedizin 11:1–3

12. Lockemann U, Fuhrmann A, Püschel K, Schmeling A, Geserick G (2004) Empfehlungen für die Altersdiagnostik bei Jugendlichen und jungen Erwachsenen außerhalb des Strafverfahrens. Rechtsmedizin 14:123–125

13. Schmeling A, Olze A, Reisinger W, Geserick G (2001) Age estimation of living people undergoing criminal proceedings. Lancet 358:89–90

14. Schmeling A, Reisinger W, Geserick G, Olze A (2005) The current state of forensic age estimation of live subjects for the purpose of criminal prosecution. Forensic Sci Med Pathol 1:239–246

15. Tanner JM (1962) Growth at adolescence. Blackwell Scientific Publications, Oxford, UK

16. Neyzi O, Alp H, Yalcindag A, Yakacikli S (1975) Sexual maturation in Turkish boys. Ann Hum Biol 2:251–259

17. Flügel B, Greil H, Sommer K (1986) Anthropologischer Atlas. Wötzel, Frankfurt/M, Germany

18. Heinrich UE (1986) Die Bedeutung der radiologischen Skelettalterbestimmung für die Klinik. Radiologe 26:212–215

19. Stöver B (1983) Röntgenologische Aussagekraft des Handradiogrammes. Röntgenpraxis 36:119–129

20. Schmeling A (2004) Forensische Altersdiagnostik bei Lebenden im Strafverfahren. Habilitationsschrift. Humboldt-Universität zu Berlin, Germany

21. Fleischer-Peters A (1976) Handskelettanalyse und ihre klinische Bedeutung. Fortschr Kieferorthop 37:375–385

22. Garn SM, Lewis AB, Blizzard RM (1965) Endocrine factors in dental development. J Dent Res 44:243–258

23. Prader A, Perabo F (1952) Körperwachstum, Knochen- und Zahnentwicklung bei den endokrinen Erkrankungen im Kindesalter. Helv Paediat Acta 7:517–529

24. Thiemann H-H, Nitz I (1991) Röntgenatlas der normalen Hand im Kindesalter. Thieme, Leipzig, Germany

25. Roche AF, Chumlea WC, Thissen D (1988) Assessing the skeletal maturity of the hand-wrist: Fels method. C.C. Thomas, Springfield, IL

26. Andersen E (1971) Comparison of Tanner-Whitehouse and Greulich-Pyle methods in a large scale Danish survey. Am J Phys Anthropol 35:373–376

27. Cole AJL, Webb L, Cole TJ (1988) Bone age estimation: a comparison of methods. Br J Radiol 61:683–686

28. King DG, Steventon DM, O'Sullivan MP, Cook AM, Hornsby VP, Jefferson IG (1994) Reproducibility of bone ages when performed by radiology registrars: an audit of Tanner and Whitehouse II versus Greulich and Pyle methods. Br J Radiol 67:848–851

29. Weber R (1978) Genauigkeit der Skelettalterbestimmungen und Größenprognosen nach den Methoden von Greulich & Pyle sowie Tanner & Whitehouse. Medical Thesis. Berlin, Germany

30. Johnston FE (1963) Skeletal age and its prediction in Philadelphia children. Hum Biol 35:192–202

31. Schmeling A, Baumann U, Schmidt S, Wernecke K-D, Reisinger W (2006) Reference data for the Thiemann-Nitz method of assessing skeletal age for the purpose of forensic age estimation. Int J Legal Med 120:1–4

32. Müller HR (1983) Eine Studie über die Inkonstanz des dritten Molaren (Fehlen, Anlage, Durchbruch). Medical Thesis. Dresden, Germany

33. Berkowitz BKB, Bass TP (1976) Eruption rates of human upper third molars. J Dent Res 55:460–464

34. Demirjian A, Goldstein H, Tanner JM (1973) A new system of dental age assessment. Hum Biol 45:221–227
35. Gleiser I, Hunt EE (1955) The permanent mandibular first molar: its calcification, eruption and decay. Am J Phys Anthropol 13:253–284
36. Köhler S, Schmelzle R, Loitz C, Püschel K (1994) Die Entwicklung des Weisheitszahnes als Kriterium der Lebensalterbestimmung. Ann Anat 176:339–345
37. Kullman L, Johanson G, Akesson L (1992) Root development of the lower third molar and its relation to chronological age. Swed Dent J 16:161–167
38. Moorrees CFA, Fanning EA, Hunt EE (1963) Age variation of formation stages for ten permanent teeth. J Dent Res 42:1490–1502
39. Olze A, Bilang D, Schmidt S, Wernecke K-D, Geserick G, Schmeling A (2005) Validation of common classification systems for assessing the mineralization of third molars. Int J Legal Med 119:22–26
40. Kahl B, Schwarze CW (1988) Aktualisierung der Dentitionstabelle von I Schour und M Massler von 1941. Fortschr Kieferorthop 49:432–443
41. Mincer HH, Harris EF, Berryman HE (1993) The A.B.F.O. study of third molar development and its use as an estimator of chronological age. J Forensic Sci 38:379–390
42. Olze A, Schmeling A, Rieger K, Kalb G, Geserick G (2003) Untersuchungen zum zeitlichen Verlauf der Weisheitszahnmineralisation bei einer deutschen Population. Rechtsmedizin 13:5–10
43. Olze A, Mahlow A, Schmidt S, Geserick G, Schmeling A (2004) Der parodontale Knochenabbau als Kriterium der forensischen Altersdiagnostik bei jungen Erwachsenen. Rechtsmedizin 14:448–453
44. Olze A, Mahlow A, Schmidt S, Geserick G, Schmeling A (2004) Radiologisch bestimmte Varianten des DMF-Index zur forensischen Altersschätzung bei jungen Erwachsenen. Arch Kriminol 214:103–111
45. Kreitner K-F, Schweden F, Schild HH, Riepert T, Nafe B (1997) Die computer-tomographisch bestimmte Ausreifung der medialen Klavikulaepiphyse-eine additive Methode zur Altersbestimmung im Adoleszentenalter und in der dritten Lebensdekade? Fortschr Röntgenstr 166:481–486
46. Kreitner K-F, Schweden FJ, Riepert T, Nafe B, Thelen M (1998) Bone age determination based on the study of the medial extremity of the clavicle. Eur Radiol 8:1116–1122
47. Schmeling A, Schulz R, Reisinger W, Mühler M, Wernecke K-D, Geserick G (2004) Studies on the time frame for ossification of medial clavicular epiphyseal cartilage in conventional radiography. Int J Legal Med 118:5–8
48. Schulz R, Mühler M, Mutze S, Schmidt S, Reisinger W, Schmeling A (2005) Studies on the time frame for ossification of the medial epiphysis of the clavicle revealed by CT scans. Int J Legal Med 119:142–145
49. Schulze D, Rother U, Fuhrmann A, Richel S, Faulmann G, Heiland M (2006) Correlation of age and ossification of the medial clavicular epiphysis using computed tomography. Forensic Sci Int 158:184–189
50. Mühler M, Schulz R, Schmidt S, Schmeling A, Reisinger W (2006) The influence of slice thickness on assessment of clavicle ossification in forensic age diagnostics. Int J Legal Med 120:15–17
51. Grön A-M (1962) Prediction of tooth emergence. J Dent Res 41:573–585
52. Lacey KA (1973) Relationship between bone age and dental development. Lancet 302:736–737
53. Lamons FF, Gray SW (1958) A study of the relationship between tooth eruption age, skeletal development age, and chronological age in sixty-one Atlanta children. Am J Orthod 44:687–691
54. Pfau RO, Sciulli PW (1994) A method for establishing the age of subadults. J Forensic Sci 39:165–176

55. Schmeling A, Olze A, Reisinger W, König M, Geserick G (2003) Statistical analysis and verification of forensic age estimation of living persons in the Institute of Legal Medicine of the University Hospital Charité. Legal Med 5:S367–S371
56. Schmeling A, Reisinger W, Loreck D, Vendura K, Markus W, Geserick G (2000) Effects of ethnicity on skeletal maturation – consequences for forensic age estimations. Int J Legal Med 113:253–258
57. Schmeling A, Olze A, Reisinger W, Geserick G (2001) Der Einfluß der Ethnie auf die bei strafrechtlichen Altersschätzungen untersuchten Merkmale. Rechtsmedizin 11:78–81
58. Sutow WW (1953) Skeletal maturation in healthy Japanese children, 6 to 19 years of age. Comparison with skeletal maturation in American children. Hiroshima J Med Sci 2:181–193
59. Greulich WW (1957) A comparison of the physical growth and development of American-born and native Japanese children. Am J Phys Anthropol 15:489–515
60. Kimura K (1977) Skeletal maturity of the hand and wrist in Japanese children by the TW2 method. Ann Hum Biol 4:353–356
61. Kimura K (1977) Skeletal maturity of the hand and wrist in Japanese children in Sapporo by the TW2 method. Ann Hum Biol 4:449–454
62. Beunen G, Lefevre J, Ostyn M, Renson R, Simons J, Van Gerven D (1990) Skeletal maturity in Belgian youths assessed by the Tanner-Whitehouse method (TW2). Ann Hum Biol 17:355–376
63. Wenzel A, Droschl H, Melsen B (1984) Skeletal maturity in Austrian children assessed by the GP and the TW-2 methods. Ann Hum Biol 11:173–177
64. Garn SM, Sandusky ST, Nagy JM, McCann MB (1972) Advanced skeletal development in low income Negro children. J Pediatr 80:965–969
65. Massé G, Hunt EE (1963) Skeletal maturation of the hand and wrist in West African children. Hum Biol 35:3–25
66. Platt RA (1956) The skeletal maturation of Negro school children. M. A. Thesis. University of Pennsylvania, PA
67. Mackay DH (1952) Skeletal maturation in the hand: a study of development in East African children. Trans R Soc Trop Med Hyg 46:135–150
68. Weiner JS, Thambipillai V (1952) Skeletal maturation of West-African negroes. Am J Phys Anthropol 10:407–418
69. Loder RT, Estle DT, Morrison K, Eggleston D, Fish DN, Grennfield ML (1993) Applicability of the Greulich and Pyle skeletal age standards to black and white children of today. Am J Dis Child 147:1329–1333
70. Roche AF, Roberts J, Hamill PVV (1975) Skeletal maturity of children 6–11 years: racial, geographic area and socioeconomic differentials, United States. Vital and health statistics-series 11. no 149. Government Printing Office, Washington, DC
71. Roche AF, Roberts J, Hamill PVV (1978) Skeletal maturity of youth 12–17 years. Racial, geographic area and socioeconomic differentials, United States. Vital and health statistics-series 11. no 167. Government Printing Office, Washington, DC
72. Pashkova VI, Burov SA (1980) Possibility of using standard indices of skeletal ossification for the forensic medical expertise of determining the age of children and adolescents living throughout the whole territory of the USSR [in Russian]. Sud Med Ekspert 23:22–25
73. Gorgani N, Sullivan RE, DuBois LA (1990) radiographic investigation of third molar development. J Dent Child 57:106–110
74. Harris EF, McKee JH (1990) Tooth mineralisation standards for Blacks and Whites from the Middle Southern United States. J Forensic Sci 35:859–872
75. Olze A, Schmeling A, Taniguchi M, Maeda H, Van Niekerk P, Wernecke K-D, Geserick G (2004) Forensic age estimation in living subjects: the ethnic factor in wisdom tooth mineralization. Int J Legal Med 118:170–173
76. Brown T (1978) Tooth emergence in Australian Aboriginies. Ann Hum Biol 5:41–54

77. Chagula WK (1960) The age of eruption of third permanent molars in male East Africans. Am J Phys Anthropol 18:77–82
78. Otuyemi OD, Ugboko VI, Ndukwe KC, Adekoya-Sofowora CA (1997) Eruption times of third molars in young rural Nigerians. Int Dent J 47:266–270
79. Shourie KL (1946) Eruption age of teeth in India. Ind J Med Res 34:105–118
80. Garn SM, Wertheimer F, Sandusky ST, Mc Cann MB (1972) Advanced tooth emergence in Negro individuals. J Dent Res 51:1506
81. Hassanali J (1985) The third permanent molar eruption in Kenyan Africans and Asians. Ann Hum Biol 12:517–523
82. Harlan WR, Grillo GP, Cornoni-Huntley J, Leaverton PE (1979) Secondary sex characteristics of boys 12 to 17 years of age – United States Health Examination Survey. J Pediatr 95:293–297
83. Harlan WR, Harlan EA, Grillo GP (1980) Secondary sex characteristics of girls 12 to 17 years of age – United States Health Examination Survey. J Pediatr 96:1074–1078
84. Channing-Pearce SM, Solomon L (1987) Pubertal development in black and white Johannesburg girls. S Afr Med J 71:22–24
85. Wong GW, Leung SS, Law WY, Yeung VT, Lau JT, Yeung WK (1996) Secular trend in the sexual maturation of southern Chinese boys. Acta Paediatr 85:620–621
86. Huen KF, Leung SS, Lau JT, Cheung AY, Leung NK, Chiu MC (1997) Secular trend in the sexual maturation of southern Chinese girls. Acta Paediatr 86:1121–1124
87. Okkalides D, Fotakis M (1994) Patient effective dose resulting from radiographic examinations. Br J Radiol 67:564–572
88. Frederiksen NL, Benson BW, Sokolowski TW (1994) Effective dose and risk assessment from film tomography used for dental implant diagnostics. Dentomaxillofac Radiol 23:123–127
89. Jurik AG, Jensen LC, Hansen J (1996) Radiation dose by spiral CT and conventional tomography of the sternoclavicular joints and the manubrium sterni. Skeletal Radiol 25:467–470
90. Bundesministerium für Umwelt, Naturschutz und Reaktorsicherheit (2002) Umweltradioaktivität und Strahlenbelastung im Jahr 2001. Bonn, Germany
91. Schmeling A, Reisinger W, Wormanns D, Geserick G (2000) Strahlenexposition bei Röntgenuntersuchungen zur forensischen Altersschätzung Lebender. Rechtsmedizin 10:135–137
92. Feinendegen LE (1994) Die mögliche Bedeutung günstiger Strahleneffekte in Zellen für den Gesamtorganismus. Röntgenpraxis 47:289–292
93. Rothkamm K, Löbrich M (2003) Evidence for a lack of DNA double-strand break repair in human cells exposed to very low X-ray doses. Proc Natl Acad Sci USA 100:5057–5062
94. Jung H (2000) Strahlenrisiken durch Röntgenuntersuchungen zur Altersschätzung im Strafverfahren. Fortschr Röntgenstr 172:553–556
95. Jung H (1995) Strahlenrisiko: Widersprüchliche Angaben verunsichern Öffentlichkeit und Patienten. Informationen. Deutsche Röntgengesellschaft 3/95:20–23

Index

Note: Page numbers followed by f for figures, t for tables.

Breinigsville, PA USA
10 June 2010
239521BV00005B/57/P